Magic, Faith, and Healing

Magic, Faith, and Healing
STUDIES IN PRIMITIVE PSYCHIATRY

Edited by ARI KIEV, M.D.

With a Foreword by JEROME D. FRANK, M.D.

JASON ARONSON INC.
Northvale, New Jersey
London

THE MASTER WORK SERIES

1996 softcover edition

Library of Congress Cataloging-in-Publication Data

Magic, faith, and healing : studies in primitive psychiatry /
    edited by Ari Kiev : with a foreword by Jerome D. Frank. — 1st Free
Press pbk. ed.
        p. cm.
    ISBN 1-56821-809-5 (pbk.)
    1. Psychiatry. 2. Medicine, Magic, mystic, and spagiric.
I. Kiev, Ari.
RC454.4.M32 1996
616.89—dc20   96-1266

Manufactured in the United States of America. Jason Aronson Inc. offers books and cassettes. For information and catalog write to Jason Aronson Inc., 230 Livingston Street, Northvale, New Jersey 07647.

To the Memory of My Mother

Mary Nover Kiev

A woman of valour who can find?
For her price is far above rubies . . .
Her children rise up, and call her blessed;
Her husband also, and he praiseth her:
"Many daughters have done valiantly
But thou excellest them all."

Proverbs 31

Jerome D. Frank, M.D.*

Foreword

THE INTERESTING accounts of illness and healing in nonindustrialized societies reported in this book may, at first glance, appear to have
little in common with psychiatric illness and healing in the industrialized
West. In perusing them, the reader may feel like a visitor at a zoo or a
passenger on a luxury cruise to exotic regions of the earth. He may be
entertained, even fascinated, by the outlandish healing rites of various
societies and impressed by the wealth of creative imagination they reveal,
but he does not immediately recognize that they have anything to do
with modern medical practice. And indeed conceptualizations of illness
and healing in nonindustrialized societies are superficially very different
from those in industrialized ones. Nor, at first glance, do the dramatic
and emotional activities of the shaman appear to have anything in common with the detached, quietly competent ministrations of the modern
physician.

In nonindustrialized cultures, illness is believed to have a variety of
causes, both natural and supernatural. These causes include noxious
environmental agents, the enmity of other persons, and the disfavor of the
gods, incurred perhaps by unwitting offenses against them. All illness,
therefore, arouses fear and self-doubt in the victim and disturbs his relations with his compatriots. Since illness may be evidence of the displeasure of supernatural forces and reduces the patient's contribution
to his society, it may also adversely affect the attitudes of others toward
him. Their concern may be tempered with fear and even rejection, which
feed back into the patient's own emotions, aggravating his condition.

The shaman, like the physician, tries to cure the patient by correcting
the causes of his illness. In line with his culture's concept of disease,
this cure may involve not only the administration of therapeutic agents

* Professor of Psychiatry, The Johns Hopkins University Medical College.

but provision of means for confession, atonement, restoration into the good graces of family and tribe, and intercession with the spirit world. The shaman's role may thus involve aspects of the roles of physician, magician, priest, moral arbiter, representative of the group's world-view, and agent of social control. His success may often depend more on his ability to mobilize the patient's hopes, restore his morale, and gain his reacceptance by his group than on his pharmacopoeia.

Industrialized societies hold quite a different concept of illness and healing. We fondly expect someday fully to comprehend the human being as a complex machine controlled by a computer in the skull. Disease will then be merely a derangement of the machine's functioning produced by noxious environmental agents in interaction with inborn or acquired vulnerabilities or errors of metabolism. Psychiatric illnesses are distinguished primarily by the fact that they manifest themselves in disturbances of thinking and behavior, leading to complications in the patient's interpersonal relationships. Ultimately, however, their etiology too will be found in derangement of brain function. Support for this position is afforded by the finding that the incidence of psychosis seems to be about the same in every culture. This finding suggests that cultural factors may not be causative but may merely determine the behavioral expressions of psychotic processes caused by chemico-physical abnormalities. It seems reasonable to expect, furthermore, that gains in knowledge of the biological bases of mental illness will lead to increasing effectiveness of pharmacological and neurophysiological remedies.

In this view, the physician is an expert scientist-technician whose job is to get the body into good running order again, and many psychiatrists dream of the day when they too can obtain triumphant cures with pills and injections.

The phenomenal triumphs of modern scientific medicine have been made possible by this emphasis on the physico-chemical aspects of health and disease, and greater triumphs are undoubtedly in store. Yet in one vital respect it will always remain insufficient. It does not take into account the powerful influence of meanings derived from the interplay of the individual with his family and his culture on his bodily states. Illness always implies certain meanings. It is never merely bodily pathology, but has implications for the patient's view of himself and for society's view of him. In industrial as well as in primitive societies, illness may create noxious emotions, raise moral issues, disturb the patient's image of himself, and estrange him from his compatriots. Barred from the front door, these intangibles sneak in at the back, and, unless the physician takes them into account, he will often fail. The widespread popularity of nonmedical and religious healers in twentieth-century America attests the fact that the physician must be more than a skilled technician if he is to help many of his patients.

The importance of cultural and spiritual factors in disease and healing is seen clearly in the chronically ill. The patient's loss of earning power, the constant reminder of the fragility of life and the inevitability of death conveyed by his disease, and the pity, scorn, or distaste of those about him are assaults on his self-esteem that often contribute more to his suffering and disability than the disease process itself. To rehabilitate him, the physician must not only treat his body but inspire his hopes, mobilize his environment on his behalf, and actively help him to resume a useful place in society. Sometimes this task includes helping the patient to achieve a philosophy of life compatible with his reduced expectations.

The complex interplay of illness, the physician, and society is also exemplified in suits for damages or workman's compensation following alleged injuries. The physician's estimate of the claimant's disability is supposed to be based solely on the latter's bodily condition, yet every physician knows that such motivational factors as discouragement or hope of financial gain may be much more significant. Furthermore, the ease with which physicians can be found to testify on both sides of such suits suggests that professional judgments involve implicit attitudes toward personal responsibility and self-reliance; the relation of the employee to the employer, of the private citizen to the state; and the like.

If the nonpsychiatric physician cannot often remain the impartial, objective scientist, the psychiatrist is even less able to do so. Not only is little known about the biological bases of mental disorders, but most such disorders also involve disturbances of the patient's self-image and social behavior. The diagnosis of mental illness is usually first made, not by a physician, but by persons in contact with the patient and is based on behavior that deviates from the accepted norms of the culture.

The social aspects of mental illness often require the psychiatrist, like the shaman, to function as a representative of the values of his society. Mention of damage suits is a reminder that the most difficult ones usually involve the testimony of psychiatrists, and they too can always be found to testify on both sides. Another example is afforded by the vexing question of criminal responsibility. One social function of psychiatrists is to make a judgment of the sanity of an accused person to determine whether he is able to stand trial for his acts. Unfortunately, the concept of insanity continues to elude precise definition. In actual practice the psychiatrist's judgment may be influenced by all kinds of considerations, implicit and explicit, that are remote from medicine. Judgment of the sanity or insanity of a defendant may be affected by cultural standards and by the psychiatrist's personal views on the nature of crime, guilt, expiation, and the interests of society.

Outside the courtroom but next door to it, as it were, society expects psychiatrists to "treat" certain socially unacceptable or morally reprehensible forms of behavior as if they were illnesses. Sexual deviations, for example, in some cultures may have a high social value or religious significance, while in others they are regarded merely as unfortunate or ludicrous quirks. Some Western societies, however, view sexual deviation as a cross between vice and illness. When he is asked to treat persons with these behavior patterns, the psychiatrist is really being asked to reform them.

Addicts and alcoholics dwell in the same no man's land between medicine and morals. At what point does heavy drinking cease to be a vice and become a symptom of the disease called "alcoholism"? Morphine and heroin, though addictive, are physiologically less harmful than alcohol in excess and, in societies that do not interdict their use, produce no antisocial behavior at all. Yet in the United States narcotics addiction is viewed as a more heinous vice than alcoholism, and in most communities an addict cannot get treatment unless he is branded as a criminal by being convicted as an addict. Furthermore, since opiates are obtainable only through illegal channels, they are forbiddingly expensive, so that most addicts are forced to steal. Behavior that is not even recognized as a problem in some cultures can thus become a severe medical and social problem in others.

These examples illustrate that, in industrial as in preindustrial societies, the definition of psychiatric illness is at least in part social, and successful treatment of psychiatric patients must take this point into account.

In industrialized cultures, the efficacy of medications and even of some surgical procedures may depend on their capacity to arouse the patient's hopes for cure, as do the shaman's charms and incantations. For example, patients with coronary artery disease have experienced spectacular relief of anginal pain and showed greatly improved ability to function following the tying of a blood vessel in the chest wall, which supposedly shunts more blood to the heart. Yet, a mock operation, mimicking the real one in all respects except the tying of the blood vessel, has proved equally effective. The ability of placebos—pharmacologically inert pills that serve as symbols of the physician's healing power—to relieve pain even in patients with organic disease is further evidence of the healing properties of emotions and attitudes aroused by the physician. In fact, since until recent years most medical remedies were either inert or harmful, the reputation of the medical profession actually rested largely on the power of the placebo. Since the effectiveness of placebos lies in their ability to counteract psychonoxious emotional states, it is not surprising that some of the beneficial results of psychotherapy can be duplicated simply by giving the patient a placebo. The psychiatrist therefore, must recognize, however reluctantly, that his treatment methods may rely on an important component of faith.

Furthermore, although his own thinking may be firmly anchored in the naturalistic world, not infrequently he must deal with supernatural or magical aspects of the world-views of his patients. Three patients recently treated in the psychiatric outpatient department of one teaching hospital, a veritable citadel of modern scientific medicine, come to mind. None was in any sense psychotic. One, born in Sicily, complained of intense nervousness and restlessness. He had flirted with someone's else's girl and sheepishly confessed that he believed his symptoms had been produced by the evil eye. He had gone to several fortune tellers whose reassurances had left him unconvinced. He is the spiritual brother of an Australian aborigine at whom the bone has been pointed. Another patient raised in the hills of West Virginia attributed her severe anxiety to a fortune teller's prophecy that her father was about to die. She stoutly affirmed the existence of vampires and was convinced that her grandmother was a witch. A third, a devout Catholic who had divorced her husband and married a Protestant, was more than half convinced that a miscarriage was God's punishment for having broken a religious taboo. For these patients, a priest or sorcerer might well have been a more suitable therapist than a scientifically trained psychiatrist.

These patients came from foreign or lower-class cultures and did not trouble to disguise their concern about possible supernatural causes of their distress. The better educated are more circumspect, but, as the current vogue among intellectuals for drugs that alter consciousness attests, some of them also try to solve their problems by seeking experiences that border on the supernatural. The introduction of these drugs into Western societies closes the circle between science and mysticism. Mind-altering agents are powerful tools for scientific investigation of brain processes in relation to conscious states, but some scientists and scholars take them in the hope of achieving experiences they do not hesitate to describe as "sacred." The parallel between an LSD party held in a setting designed to evoke religious emotions and a peyote ritual, for example, is uncomfortably close.

Most psychiatric patients seek to couch the moral or spiritual problems for which they seek psychiatric help in pseudoscientific terms, principally derived from psychoanalysis. Under the influence of the scientific world-view, the psychiatrist too views himself as morally neutral and believes that his therapeutic maneuvers are based on scientific principles. Yet much of his effectiveness depends not only on his capacity to inspire the patient's hopes but on his value system. The current popularity of existential forms of psychotherapy is in a sense no more than belated public recognition of what psychotherapists knew all along, although many were unwilling to admit it even to themselves. Although the psychotherapist may state his interpretations in neutral terms, many are nevertheless covert exhortations or criticisms based on implicit value judgments.

In all cultures, phenomena called "mental illnesses" disturb all levels of the person's functioning: bodily, psychological, and spiritual. They involve the sufferer's world-view, ethical values, self-image, and his relationships with his compatriots. These disorders result from or express the interaction of sociocultural stresses with vulnerabilities resulting from combinations of genetic, physico-chemical, and life-experience factors. The healer, whether psychiatrist or shaman, derives his healing powers from his status and role in the sufferer's society and functions, among other ways, as an evoker of healing forces, a mentor, a role model, and a mediator between the sufferer and his group. His task is to help the patient, whether he be a stockbroker, a research scientist, or an African tribesman, to mobilize his psychological and spiritual as well as his bodily resources.

These generalizations and others are amply supported by the rich and varied panorama of mental illness and healing in nonindustrialized cultures to be found in this book. Underneath its kaleidoscopic variety lie common features that serve to illuminate mental illness and its treatment in our own society. Lest the reader be dazzled by the passing show, the editor in his comprehensive introductory and closing chapters offers a firm and skillful guiding hand.

Preface to the 1996 Edition

LITTLE did I know, when I first invited contributions to this anthology, that it would become a standard textbook in anthropology courses throughout the world for some thirty years. But indeed this is what did happen. More than that, *Magic, Faith, and Healing* became a source of inspiration for at least three generations of scholars and a catalyst for the development of transcultural psychiatry. It spurred the federal government to fund studies of alternative medicine; and it helped create a climate of acceptance for insights from Ayurvedic medicine and Zen Buddhism and for the value of spirituality in therapeutic processes. It has also played a role in increasing the awareness of the needs and opportunities to assist in third-world development. There is, of course, still much to be learned, and it is my hope that this new issue of *Magic, Faith, and Healing* will have the same impact in the next thirty years as it has had in the last thirty.

ARI KIEV

Preface

SEVERAL years ago I had an opportunity to study the healing practices and beliefs relating to psychiatric disorders among the Vodun groups in Haiti. These people, although uneducated and impoverished— in fact living on a marginal subsistence level—have developed a therapeutically effective form of psychologial treatment centered around certain religious beliefs and rituals. Most striking was my finding that the relationship between healer and patient in this culture appeared to parallel in a number of ways the psychiatrist-patient relationship in Western society, despite the absence of scientific methods and knowledge of the discoveries of modern psychiatry. This finding suggested the possibility that certain general features of therapeutic relationships in various cultures—for example, the hope, expectation, and faith of the patient in the designated healer, coupled with the healer's use of meaningful symbols and group forces—might contribute more to therapeutic results than is ordinarily recognized in contemporary theories of psychodynamic psychiatry.

A subsequent search of the literature revealed few reports confirming these observations among other cultures, although many writers had reported on the psychotherapeutic features of primitive medicine *per se*. The search for further information led to contacts with various investigators who had gathered material relevant to this theme in the course of their studies. It was then decided to gather together in one volume a number of reports on psychological treatment in various primitive cultures and underdeveloped societies, with the aim of providing a necessary beginning for the study of this important area. It is the aim of this anthology to underline certain of the common as well as unique elements in the healing methods and beliefs of various groups throughout the world for the value such clarification will have in providing a clearer perspective on social and cultural factors in psychotherapeutic processes.

In addition to the various contributors who made this anthology possible, I am especially indebted to Dr. Jerome D. Frank, Dr. George Devereux, my parents Dr. and Mrs. I. Edward Kiev, and my wife Phyllis Eve Kiev, who read various portions of the manuscript and provided not only technical advice but encouragement to pursue the project. I am deeply grateful to Mrs. Martha Crossen and Miss Estelle Whelan for their superb editorial assistance during the final months of preparation. I am also grateful to Professor Sir Aubrey Lewis and the National Institute of Mental Health for providing me with the opportunity to prepare this anthology during the course of a Postdoctoral Research Fellowship at The Institute of Psychiatry—The Maudsley Hospital, London, England.

Dr. Alexander Leighton, Dr. Margaret Mead, Professor Meyer Fortes, Dr. William Caudill, Reverend E. F. O'Doherty, Professor R. T. Smith, Dr. James G. Roney, Jr., Professor G. W. B. Huntingford, Professor Raymond Firth, and Professor J. Clyde Mitchell were helpful in suggesting the names of many of the contributors. For their generous advice I am most appreciative.

ARI KIEV

Contributors

Catherine H. Berndt, Ph.D.   Visiting Tutor in Anthropology and Research Worker, University of Western Australia

L. Bryce Boyer, M.D.   Principal Investigator, Project for Field Research in Anthropo-Psychoanalytic Techniques, Department of Anthropology, University of New Mexico

John Dawson, Ph.D.   Research Lecturer in Psychology, University of Edinburgh, Scotland

J. Robin Fox, Ph.D.   Lecturer in Social Anthropology, London School of Economics and Political Science

Stephen Fuchs, Ph.D.   Member of Anthropos Institute, St. Augustin, Germany, and Visiting Professor of Anthropology and Indian Philosophy, San Carlos University, Philippines

Michael Gelfand, M.D.   Professor of Medicine, University College of Rhodesia and Nyasaland, and Physician, Harare Hospital, Salisbury, Southern Rhodesia

Jozef Ph. Hes, M.D.   Research Associate, Hebrew University, Jerusalem

Dale Johnson, Ph.D.   Clinical Assistant Professor of Psychology, Baylor University School of Medicine

Bert Kaplan, Ph.D.   Professor of Psychology, Rice University

Ari Kiev, M.D.   N.I.M.H. Postdoctoral Research Fellow, the Maudsley Hospital, London (1961-1962); Staff Psychiatrist, Wilford Hall USAF Hospital, Lackland Air Force Base (1962-1964); and Research Associate in Psychiatry, Columbia University College of Physicians and Surgeons, (September, 1964—)

Weston La Barre, Ph.D.   Professor of Anthropology, Duke University

T. Adeoye Lambo, M.D.   Professor of Psychiatry, University College of Ibadan, Nigeria

William Madsen, Ph.D.   Professor of Anthropology, Purdue University

Jane M. Murphy, Ph.D.   Assistant Professor of Anthropology, Department of Psychiatry, Cornell Medical College

Orhan M. Ozturk, M. D.   Instructor in Psychiatry, University of Ankara, Turkey

Raymond Prince, M.D.   Lecturer in Psychiatry, McGill University, Montreal, Canada

K. E. Schmidt, M.D.   Medical Superintendent, Sarawak Mental Hospital, Kuching, Sarawak

Victor W. Turner, Ph.D.   Visiting Professor of Anthropology, Cornell University

Michael G. Whisson, Ph.D.   Assistant Professor of Social Anthropology, University of British Columbia, Vancouver, Canada

xvii

Contents

Part Three

Part Four

Part One

The study of psychiatry and anthropology
uncovers many areas of interest common to
both disciplines, particularly the influence of
cultural factors on psychological treatment in
preindustrial societies. Cultural variations
in the form and meaning of
confession offer a prime example.

Ari Kiev

The Study of Folk Psychiatry

§ The Problem

MENTAL ILLNESS includes a wide number of abnormal states of mood, thought, and behavior, ranging from mild anxiety and tension to severe disorganizing psychosis, which arouse a multitude of emotions in onlookers and pose threats to the harmony of all social groups. Attempts to cope with the problems of the mentally ill have existed since ancient times, but only in the last two centuries have systematic and rational psychological treatments been employed; and only in the past fifty years has psychiatry developed into a recognized and scientific discipline.[1] This anthology is concerned with various forms of psychological treatment employed in a number of underdeveloped areas and in a number of primitive cultures. Its purpose is to add a further dimension to our knowledge of the basic processes of psychological treatment and to provide in one volume materials demonstrating both differences and similarities in psychotherapies throughout the world. These chapters emphasize the impact of cultural factors on the form and content of psychiatric theories and treatment, in order to demonstrate that culture, or a group's shared system of beliefs, practices, and behavioral patterns, contributes not only to personality formation and psychic conflict but to the development, perpetuation, and management of mental illness. While emphasizing sociopsychological factors, this approach recognizes the biological limits of human behavior; those limits account in part for the fundamental similarity of psychotherapies throughout the world.

Psychotherapeutic effects were no doubt produced in ancient times at the Asclepieion temples in Epidaurus and at such rites as the Dionysian mysteries, the worship of Mylitta, and the rites of Kali. Psychological benefits were provided by the Church in the Middle Ages, which offered sanctuaries, sacred retreats, the catharsis of the confessional, and the expiation of sins through purchase of indulgences. But not until the

3

eighteenth century was psychological treatment systematically studied.[2]

The study of hypnosis proved to be the starting point from which Freud created psychoanalysis in the twentieth century. The major features of the contemporary psychoanalytic model have been incorporated in many of the other systems of intensive psychotherapy developed over the past fifty years. Although often emphasizing different techniques and goals, these systems stressed intensive examination of the patient's history in an effort to correct distorted attitudes and behavior, unrealistic expectancies, and conflicting emotions.[3] While theoretical shifts in central motivational themes and therapeutic techniques have been further altered by the various offshoots of classical psychoanalysis exemplified by the work of Jung, Adler, and more recently Sullivan, Fromm, Horney, and Fromm-Reichmann, views of such fundamental issues as the role of the unconscious, the transference, and the abreaction of repressed affects have remained unchanged.[4]

In addition to providing a new model for psychological treatment, the early psychoanalysts devoted much attention to delineating the therapeutic factors in treatment. In the beginning, the encouragement of insight by the interpretation of repressed ideas was regarded as the crux of therapy, and effort was directed to uncovering the repressed pathogenic focus.[5] Later the resolution of transference distortions was emphasized. Still later the interplay of several factors—interpretation of the abreaction of affect, modification of the superego, and identification with the therapist—were emphasized. Some recent workers, following Alexander, have emphasized the "corrective emotional experience" of treatment; others the opportunity for the re-experiencing and retesting of interpersonal relationships.[6] Some workers have emphasized the value of consistent attention and permissive care in the treatment of schizophrenic patients, of providing them with the love they missed in childhood and helping them to re-evaluate distorted patterns of interpersonal attitudes.[7] Psychologists working in this area have in general emphasized the learning aspects of psychotherapeutic transactions in which the patient may learn to accept the therapist's positive feelings for him,[8] may unlearn behavioral patterns that interfere with subsequent learning,[9] and may be able finally to express previously inhibited fearful responses.[10]

In view of the amount of energy expended in the study and treatment of mental illness and the increasing knowledge in these areas, it is not unreasonable to expect that skilled psychiatrists using the most effective methods will obtain the most enduring results most frequently. Unfortunately that has not been the case. Recent studies have indicated that results with different treatments are markedly similar. Most statistical studies show that 65-70% of neurotic patients and 35% of schizophrenic patients improve after treatment regardless of the type of treatment received.[11] Long-term follow-up studies of treated patients have also demonstrated no differences among the various treatments.[12] These results, which have been repeated in various centers, suggest to some workers that specific therapies are of doubtful value and that psychotherapeutic theories and methods are unreliable. One critic has written:

> The therapeutic achievements of the psychogenetic movement do not necessarily depend upon real etiological knowledge of causal treatment. . . . It is quite possible that the therapeutic successes are essentially due to the same two basic mechanisms of confession and suggestion which are so little understood and which had been used with such success by the medicine man.[13]

In view of this orientation, which has characterized much of modern psychotherapy, particularly in America, it is not surprising that therapies used by primitive peoples have been neglected. Despite the fact that much work has pointed to its importance, primitive psychiatry has often been dismissed as consisting of brief suggestive techniques, study of which would add little to our knowledge of psychotherapy. It has been emphasized that treatment is too brief to be effective and that insight never results from such treatment. Some workers have, however, suggested that insight is not necessarily therapeutic, while others have suggested that insight, in the sense of ability to verbalize self-understanding, may be mistaken for genuine attitude change.[14] Some of the unproven assumptions about duration and frequency of treatment have also been called into question.[15] Furthermore, suggestion, reassurance, and direct influence may play a bigger role in rational psychotherapies than is ordinarily recognized. As Freud himself noted in 1904:

> An element dependent on the psychical disposition of the patient enters as an accompanying factor without any such intention on our part into the effect of every therapeutic process initiated by a physician; most frequently it is favorable to recovery but often it [suggestion] acts as an inhibition.[16]

Recent studies have indicated that suggestive factors operate even in psychoanalytic therapy (in which there is presumably the least active participation by the therapist), for the dreams of patients and their reports of improvement often conform predictably to the theoretical expectations of their psychoanalysts, and the patients often show shifts in values toward those of their therapists.[17] That therapists unwittingly influence the verbal behavior of patients by faint cues of approval or disapproval has also been demonstrated during interviews, and it is likely that they may influence patients' thoughts outside therapy sessions as well.[18] These and other studies suggest that the criticisms of primitive therapies are perhaps naive.

The complexity of psychotherapy is emphasized by the variety of studies focused on the components of the psychotherapeutic relationship. Some workers have found, for example, that psychiatrists' personality features are significantly related, not only to their choices of profession, but to the results of treatment and their particular treatment methods as well.[19] Others have found that cultural and socioeconomic factors influence the kinds of therapy doctors prescribe and patients accept.[20] Indeed the need for treatment is often affected by such nonmedical factors as local customs, ability to pay, availability of psychiatrists, and local definitions of mental illness. Whether or not individuals remain in treatment is also related to whether or not their values coincide with the goals of particular treatments and whether or not they are amenable to treatment *per se*—for some patients respond to "treatment" even when they are receiving only inert medicines.[21]

The difficulties attendant upon evaluating psychotherapy critically and objectively are thus very great. Different schools have adopted different criteria for improvement, emphasizing such elements as return to previous levels of adaptation, relief of symptoms, or reconstruction of personality. While it is theoretically desirable, in evaluating results, to consider not only the illness but also the therapist, the therapy, and the type of patient, it is rarely if ever possible to control these variables. Indeed, it is often difficult to know whether or not the patient has improved and if so whether or not his improvement is due to treatment or to other factors in his life.

Among the more provocative studies in recent years have been several that have examined various institutionalized forms of healing, persuasion, and influence with the idea that basic aspects of psychotherapy could be clarified by examining parallel systems of behavior. By shifting the orientation from the interpersonal level of analysis to one that takes into consideration the situational and cultural context, these studies have been most valuable in re-emphasizing the broader fabric in which psychotherapy occurs. The studies are of particular interest because of the attention they have focused on the cultural and social elements of psychotherapy, a particularly difficult step because of the twentieth century emphasis on intrapsychic features of mental illness and the two-person nature of treatment.

The methods used by communist interrogators for extorting information from prisoners have been of special interest to many.[22] In these
methods, physiological and psychological deprivation is used to increase
susceptibility to change, and an exhaustive review of past experiences is
skillfully manipulated by a sympathetic interrogator to arouse guilt for
presumed crimes against the state and to change the political beliefs of
prisoners. Fear, anxiety, and confusion are aroused by threats of punishment, and habits are disrupted by unpredictable treatment. In addition, the use of group pressures, isolation, overcrowding, and occasionally torture all contribute to the psychological conversion of the prisoner.
In the prolonged relationship between interrogator and prisoner and in
the permissive setting in which the prisoner is encouraged to confess,
thought reform differs from other methods of imprisonment and resembles psychotherapy. The prisoner is increasingly made to depend
and rely on the interrogator for emotional support, praise, and companion-
ship, which increases the likelihood of his accepting the beliefs of his
captors.

In *Battle For the Mind,* Sargant examined the parallel features of
such thought reform, religious conversion, and psychotherapy.[23] All these
activities were recognized as productive of excessive brain excitation and
emotional exhaustion, which facilitate emotional and ideological changes
by increasing receptivity to new ideas. Although these institutions focus
on very different beliefs and goals, they all induce alterations of basic
physiological processes through fundamentally similar procedures that
set the stage for the introduction of new ideas. On the basis of these com-
parisons, the efficacy of psychotherapy was attributed to the unchaining
of powerful physiological forces in patients by abreactive elements that
make them more amenable to the suggestive influence of the therapist
who, like the interrogator, is the agent of the group.

This comparative study thus emphasized one of the two major elements of psychotherapy—attitude change. These methods, as Frank has
noted, involve systematic means of arousing emotions in a context of hope
and potential support from the leader and the group. Such activities
characteristically require the participation of the sufferer, persuader, and
the group and involve methods designed to arouse a variety of emotions
including guilt, fear, and anxiety. As Sargant showed, these various techniques emphasize the importance of emotions in facilitating or producing
attitude change and the importance of the social situation in supporting
or challenging an individual's self-image and view of the world.

Likening psychotherapy to such forms of interpersonal influence and
persuasion as faith healing and thought reform, Frank has delineated their

common features.[24] The "influencer," acting as agent of a larger group, is committed to producing a desirable change in the sufferer, supplicant, or prisoner. He is able to do so by virtue of his superior status, by control of means of coercion, and by his ability to inspire the expectation of relief. He can, for example, impress the patient with his procedures through the use of familiar symbols and by his own knowledgeable and systematic approach to the procedures. His faith in his ability to help and in his methods increase the therapeutic value of the contact. Current methods of psychotherapy also share other features with other forms of persuasion and healing. They include initial distress of the patient, arousing of hope through dependence upon a socially sanctioned healer, a particular repetitive ritualistic relationship with the healer, a socially shared set of assumptions about illness and healing (the existence of which cannot be disproved by the sufferer's failure to respond), mobilization of guilt, heightening of self-esteem, detailed review of the patient's past life, changes in attitude, and social reinforcement of the new attitudes and behavior.

Examining methods of religious and magical healing, Frank noted that the core of their effectiveness seems to lie in their ability to elicit hope by capitalizing on the patient's dependence on others and an expectation of help aroused by the healer's personal attributes and his paraphernalia, which gain their power from culturally determined symbolic meaning. In addition:

> The ideology and ritual supply the patient with a conceptual framework for organizing his chaotic, mysterious, and vague distress and give him a plan of action, helping him to regain a sense of direction and mastery and to resolve his inner conflicts. . . . Methods of religious healing also have aspects that heighten the patient's sense of self-worth. Performance of the ritual is usually regarded as meritorious in itself. . . . In fact one factor in maintaining a cure may be the changed attitude of the group, which continually reinforces it. That is, if the patient relapsed, he would be letting the group down.[25]

Both the Sargant and Frank studies have highlighted the two core issues of this anthology: the universality of certain elements of the psychotherapeutic response and the relevance of specific cultural factors both to the content and to the technique of psychotherapy. This focus has been especially significant because the psychoanalytic model of psychotherapy underemphasizes emotional aspects of the therapeutic process, the nonspecific effects of therapy, the role of group forces, the powerful influence of the therapist, and the effects of culturally induced stresses. The induction of emotional abreaction underlined by Sargant and the use of persuasion and influence emphasized by Frank are dramatically demonstrated in primitive healing practices like those used by the Vodun priests and priestesses of Haiti.[26] On the basis of much observation and training, they have developed a theory of disease causation and special techniques for diagnosis and treatment. Their categories of both "natural" and "supernatural" psychiatric illnesses conform to clinically recognizable syndromes. They believe that natural illnesses that resemble depressive reactions are caused by frustration, a weak brain, or excessive intellectual effort—while supernatural illnesses that are schizophrenic in form are attributed to soul loss (through sorcery) or spirit possession (through violation of taboos). Divination by water-gazing, automatic handwriting, or card reading is used to distinguish supernatural from natural illnesses before treatment begins. Detailed histories are also obtained to ascertain whether or not the patient has offended either someone who has sought revenge through sorcery or a *loa* (deity) by violating a taboo.

Exorcism of a devil spirit includes washing the patient with pigeon blood, bloodletting, or spraying the patient with a foul liquid. Special ceremonies to appease the *loa* are held when illness follows transgressions. At these community ceremonies, the *hungan* (Vodun priest) performs various feats of magic and directs the complex healing rites while possessed by his *loa.** As in psychotherapy, the patient's favorable expectations are reinforced by the treatment setting and techniques and by the *hungan's* faith in his capacity to respond to the treatment. The *hungan's* initial pessimism, which introduces ambiguity into the situation, also increases the suggestibility and anxiety of the patient and promotes his desire to please the *hungan;* while the connection of treatment with dominant values, by enlisting the valuable support of the community, further reinforces the patient's faith in the *hungan* and his expectation of relief.

* Throughout this book no attempt is made to distinguish among the various types of individual concerned with the treatment of the sick or mentally ill. Some ethnologists have made such distinctions, most frequently between shamans and those who are not shamans. Loeb has defined "shaman" as an inspirational type of medicine man who is voluntarily possessed, who exorcises and prophesies, and through whom a spirit speaks. The prototype is the Siberian shaman. E. Loeb, "Shaman and Seer," *American Anthropologist,* 31 (1929), 61. The seer in contrast is a noninspirational type of medicine man. He does not become possessed but has a guardian spirit as does the common type of medicine man among American Indians. We shall make no such distinction, for we are primarily concerned with the function of healer *qua* healer rather than with the ethnology of shamanism. In some societies, specialization exists, and herbalists, singers, diviners, and medicine men all participate in treatment. No effort has been made to differentiate among these roles except when it is necessary to clarify who treats mental illness.

In Haiti, as in other primitive societies, the *hungan* utilizes certain popular notions of his own prestige and the influence of his person; these beliefs, coupled with his special techniques, permit him to avoid entering into intense emotional involvements with his patients. He receives institutional support for this "objective" and neutral behavior, which not only reinforces the patient's trust in the treatment but minimizes his fears of the *hungan's* motives. By adhering to a standardized social role, the *hungan* gains the power of the role regardless of his personal qualities or abilities.

In this setting, where germ theory, antibiotics, and steroids are unknown, the emotional, attitudinal, and interpersonal components of disease receive the chief emphasis. The Vodun groups have derived their medical practices from the conceptual framework of their society, and all its members share the same views of treatment. This unanimity no doubt increases the efficacy of Vodun treatment of functional psychiatric disorders. In addition, disease or illness is rarely regarded as a private affair. As in other subsistence economies, illness is a matter of group concern, for it often means loss to the community of able-bodied individuals or, in instances of violent psychotic episodes, threats to public safety. That treatment of mental illness is also regarded as a group responsibility in Western societies is attested by the fact that no other forms of illness have given rise to more theological concern and legislative effort.

Although primitive therapies are fundamentally magical, that is, nonrational attempts to deal with nonrational forces, they often contain elements of rational therapy.[27] The rubbing that often precedes sucking is a form of massage, and sucking itself is a form of bleeding. W. H. R. Rivers long ago noted the almost universal use of poultices, bloodletting, massage, vapor baths and counter irritants, which, though devoted to magico-religious purposes, often successfully relieve distress.[28] As Sigerist has pointed out, poultices are local applications of heat; bleeding relieves congestion in pneumonia and pleurisy; massage has been effective with lumbago or rheumatism; and sweat baths have physical therapeutic value. Furthermore, primitive pharmacopoeias, including infusions, decoctions, salves, ointments, inhalations, and enemas, have often served pharmacologically and physiologically sound ends throughout the world.

The influence of social and cultural factors is even more dramatically demonstrated in instances where they produce noxious effects, as in death from bone-pointing.[29] Victims of such magic become so resigned to death that they refuse food and help. Only the rapid administration of countercharms can save them from death caused by fear and despair.[30]

Among the Murngin of Australia, the community reinforces the victim's expectation of imminent death by withdrawing from him and arranging an elaborate mourning ritual designed to send his soul to the next world. Simmons and Wolff have commented on this phenomenon:

> Thus is man held captive by the culture of his time and place. Superimposed upon the purely physical processes of his life are the compelling social forces, pushing and pulling him toward illness or health. The influence which his sociocultural system exerts over his mental and emotional states alone may be sufficient to make up the difference for him between sickness and health or even between life and death. There is tremendous leverage in such a system for coping with life's emergencies. But when illy used or out of hand the power that saves can destroy.[31]

Analysis of *obeah*, the institutionalized witchcraft practices of the West Indies, reveals that such benefits as psychological catharsis and social control can arise from an illegal and ostensibly antisocial set of practices. According to Sereno, such benefits are possible because *obeah* is the result of channeling clients' aggressive drives.[32] Hiring such a purveyor of evil-doing as an *obeah* man has a salutary effect, in that it "is an effort to solve inner tensions through disbursement of money" and an attempt to "channelize hostile drives" by putting the actual manipulation of destructive elements into hired hands, thus shunning personal responsibility. Because personal hostilities can be handled in this way, individual violence is rare.

A review of development in Western psychiatry over the past two centuries and especially in more recent times suggests a predilection for studies that have not taken cultural and situational factors into consideration. The study of the *hungan* in Haiti, for example, beside its inherent interest and significance for ethnologists (because of its African associations), also serves to re-emphasize the structural elements of psychotherapy and the underlying mechanisms that indeed may be of greater significance than the specific content of native theories. These elemental features are highlighted by the cross-cultural study of primitive medicine, which also provides a more general perspective on the diversity and similarity of cultural materials.

§ Primitive Medicine

By emphasizing the significance of social and cultural factors in psychotherapy, this anthology focuses on the treatments for mental illness used in a number of cultures. This orientation is not original. Ever since the first travelers and missionaries reported on the "strange" ways and customs of the primitives, Western man has been fascinated by the medical beliefs and customs of primitive peoples.* From numerous studies, we have learned that primitive theories of illness have a universal pattern. Tylor suggested that concepts of disease causation through object intrusion had spread from one area by diffusion.[33] Clements supported this view, suggesting that the concept had spread to Asia and then America *via* the Bering strait during the Pleistocene era.[34] He found that there were only three or four basic explanations of disease causation in the world: loss of a vital substance from the body (soul loss); introduction of a foreign and harmful substance into the body (spirit intrusion, or possession); violation of taboos; and witchcraft.

In most societies these concepts are related logically to the medical techniques used. For example, where sorcery is suspected, countersorcery measures are used, or elaborate witchcraft hunts are performed until the culprit is found. Where harmful objects are believed to have entered the body, extraction of the supposed object by "sleight of hand" or ritualistic exorcism is attempted. From the crude magic of the aborigine to the sophisticated empiricism of the Plains Indians, medical systems have developed in all societies. To propitiate, exorcise, or coerce unwanted spirits possessing the sick, man has used prayer, sacrifice, fumigation, starvation, heat, frightening, bloodletting, catharsis, and scapegoats. To recover lost souls, confession, expiation, and purification of the sinner, as well as countersorcery and threats against the sorcerer, have been used.

To these causes of illness should be added a note on magic, most exhaustively studied by J. G. Frazer, for the techniques of magic are the vehicles for the various causes of illness.[35] Frazer recognized two forms of sympathetic magic—imitative and contagious—in which harm is done to the individual, who then suffers in sympathy. While imitative magic acts on a man's effigy, contagious magic acts on a part of his body—nail parings, a tooth, strands of hair—and is based on the notion that infection of a part affects the whole through magical contagion. The evil eye, a form of magic common to the Mediterranean, is based on the belief that whoever falls under the spell of the evil eye will suffer misfortune.

Who administers treatment depends on the extent of specialization

---

* By "primitive" (*naturels* or *Naturvolken*) we mean those societies isolated from the mainstream of Occidental or Oriental civilization, nonliterate, and organized on the basis of small local groups and kinship groups, with simple nonspecialized economies and technologies.

in a given society. In some priests and chieftains have been the medical specialists, while in others such functions were separated. In some societies, heredity determines the selection of medical specialists; other societies provide forms of training for the able and qualified; still others select individuals on the basis of certain temperamental or physical characteristics. Similarly, the aspect of the medical role that affords its possessor the "power to cure" also seems related to the technological complexity of his society.[36] Where there are little economic development and minimal division of labor, there is little medical specialization or organization. In simple food-gathering societies, medicine is dominated by magic, and the systematic organization of theories and practices is absent. Individuals only gain the power to heal by having special experiences with supernatural forces. Among the Australian Murngin, the healer gains this power in clandestine meetings with the spirits of the dead, and his magical rituals are exclusively owned and cannot be used by others.[37] A Cheyenne could study medical lore with an elder only after having had a unique dream experience; while the Shoshoni and southern Colorado Ute shamans obtained their powers from special dreams or visions.[38] The medicine men in these simpler cultures did not develop their own systems but relied on the beliefs of the group and their own supernatural capacities. Elaborate formulations were unnecessary for the continuation of their work, which yielded little extra reward in these barely subsisting societies.

In more complex fishing-hunting societies, where increased control of the environment (particularly food sources) made possible a division of labor, qualifications for the medical role are emphasized more. Religious and medical beliefs are more elaborate, strengthening the security and the authority of the medicine men. Eskimo shamans attain their influence by experiencing neurotic or hystero-epileptoid disorders, trance experiences, ordeals of physical isolation or adherence to special rituals and taboos.[39] Similarly, in the Andaman Islands the *oko-jumu* acquire power to communicate with the spirits that cause illness and the power to cause illness themselves through "jungle meetings" with the spirits, dream experiences, fainting episodes, or epileptic-type fits. They often bolster their reputations by circulating legends about their derived powers. Because of the influence they have attained, the *oko-jumu* receive a good share of the game caught by tribesmen. The northern Wyoming Arapaho medicine men derived much material gain from their work.[40] The enhanced social status of the medicine men in turn contributed to their personal power and the efficacy of their techniques. The Puyallup shamans of Puget Sound lived in bigger houses than their tribesmen.[41]

Much discussion has been directed to the nature of the behavior that precedes the assumption of the role of shaman or medicine man, most of it concerned with the special psychic experiences involved. Some writers consider it hysteria, others epilepsy, still others schizophrenia. Ackerknecht has suggested that, by accepting the career of shaman, an individual adjusts and becomes a useful member of society, the role serving essentially as a defense against a psychotic breakdown or the original illness.[42] Boyer has recently presented psychoanalytic and anthropological data on an Eastern Apache medicine man in support of the hypothesis that the usual shaman suffers from a hysterical personality disorder and possesses character traits of the impostor with strong oral and phallic fixations.[43] Whatever the psychodynamic and psychopathological issues, prerequisites differ in all societies and, in many instances, have become sufficiently stylized and ritualized so that even normal individuals behave in abnormal, albeit prescribed, ways before assuming the role of shaman.

Much as agricultural techniques alter the character of social units, they also lead to changes in the medicine man's methods of maintaining influence. In agricultural societies, there is increased competition for medical roles, more specialization, and emphasis on knowledge and heredity as qualifications. Illness is more often attributed to the sick individual's activities than to outside influences, which puts responsibility for the results of treatment on the patient. This sophistication is seen among the Nandi of Kenya, where the failure of a cure is attributed to the patient's neglect of specific instructions.[44] Specialization of medical roles is also prominent in agricultural societies. Among the Chiga of Western Uganda, poultices, herbs, and venesection are tried, first at home and then at the home of the neighborhood specialist.[45] The diviner, whose diagnostic and therapeutic techniques include purification and sacrifice, is consulted last. Among the Mano of Liberia, the midwife or an old woman is the first specialist to be consulted.[46] A priestess or the head of a girl's school may also be consulted. Next is a man of the medical guild, who may also be a priest of the boy's school. He has access to the ancestral spirits and knows magical remedies calculated to reach the evil influences causing the disease. Finally, a diviner is consulted to find out who may have cast a spell upon the sick. The guilty one can remove the spell by confession.

With growing reliance on empirical methods in many agricultural societies, cures are increasingly attributed to the medicines rather than to the supernatural powers of the practitioners. Among the Fox of Iowa, only intelligent children were taught the correct uses of herbs, and their prestige was maintained by broad knowledge of techniques.[47] In Tahiti,

only the able-bodied and sure-footed were candidates for medical training and were required to pass examinations after a training period.[48]
The Ashanti of West Africa required a three year novitiate with a master
for anyone who received a call to be a medicine man. In the first year,
the novice had to observe strict taboos—not tapping palm wine, not
setting fish traps, and refraining from sexual intercourse, for example.
If married, the candidate had to leave his wife for the training period.
During the second year, fetishes were worn, and ceremonial ablutions
were undertaken. In the final year, the candidate was taught water-
gazing, divining, and how to impregnate charms with various spirits. The
medical role was thus related to social organization and the dominant
beliefs and value system of a society. As economic differentiation becomes
possible, medicine men exert influences to obtain wealth and prestige
and use the social power of these advantages in their medical work.

Economics is also of some significance in terms of what seem to be
negative attitudes toward the sick. Some societies sacrifice the sick in
special circumstances like famine, drought, and forced migration. In New
Caledonia, the dying who are considered socially useless are left to themselves or killed.[49] Among the Zaparos of Ecuador, the sick are strangled
if family councils decide that they are useless.[50] Although preventive
motives (at time of epidemics, for example) sometimes play a part in
this attitude, economic motives predominate, as is demonstrated by different attitudes toward the sick among the young and among people of high
rank.

These studies of primitive medicine bear a special relationship to the
theme of this anthology. They paved the way for an appreciation of the
universality of medical theories and practices and of their significance,
not only as objects of esoteric interest, but as significant aspects of particular historical traditions and cultures. They have also made us aware
of the complexity of medical practice and the diversity of human responses
to the vagaries and stresses of illness.

§ Culture, Personality, and Psychopathology

While ethnographers like Codrington, Tylor, and Morgan in the nineteenth century and Frazer in the early twentieth century were primarily
concerned with describing and cataloguing such practices and beliefs as
we have been describing, twentieth-century anthropologists have sought
increasingly to relate their observations to more general theories of human
behavior. In these studies, the main heuristic device has been the con-

cept of culture, which in general has included those shared beliefs, attitudes, and ways of behaving from which have developed groups' world views and ways of life. It has referred not only to the patterning of social intercourse and the nature of economics, technology, and religion but also to the total pattern of interrelated activities and values. Gradually a view of primitive peoples has emerged that is quite at variance with the Rousseauian notion of the Noble Savage living peacefully amid natural splendor. We have learned that the beliefs and practices of various groups differ according to their respective cultures. An absolute norm of behavior is a mythical construct compounded of naïvete and ethnocentrism; unusual behavior is not necessarily abnormal in all contexts, and mental illness is not always expressed in abnormal behavior. Special experiences like glossolalia, spirit possession, trances, and visions have been recognized as acceptable forms of expression in certain cultures.[51]

Other scholars have examined the influence of culture on mental illness. In Java, Kraepelin noted that melancholia and mania were rare and that depressive reactions seldom contained elements of sinfulness.[52] Later Bleuler commented upon differences between English and Irish patients and between Bavarian and Saxon patients.[53] Others have described various "culture-bound" syndromes like *amok;* the Windigo psychosis of the Cree, Salteaux, and Ojibwa; *latah;* and Arctic hysteria.[54] More recently Tooth has described a special category of "delusional" states in West Africans, while Carothers has reported on "ill-defined" and "primitive" psychoses among the West Africans.[55] Other researchers have stressed the significance of cultural factors in the distribution of mental illness. Seligman noted in 1929 that confusional states were more common than systematized instabilities among the Papuans of New Guinea; and he could find no cases of manic depressive illness.[56] Berne noted that toxic confusional psychoses rather than the schizophrenias were the predominant illnesses among hospitalized Malays.[57] Carothers related Westernization to an increase in manifest paranoid behavior among patients in Kenya.[58] Spiro noted that there were no violent paranoid outbursts among the Ifaluk in the Carolines until after the Japanese occupation, and Slotkin emphasized paranoid schizophrenic phenomena among acculturated Menomini.[59] Opler found that lower-class Filipinos among the Hawaiian hospitalized had a high proportion of affective disorders and catatonic confusional states, while Carothers and Tooth found statistically low incidences of depression and suicidal states and relatively high incidences of confusional states among African natives.[60]

While some writers have offered theories to account for the differences in the forms and distribution of mental illness, others have argued that these various forms of illness, best exemplified by "culture-bound" syndromes like *amok* and *latah,* are merely variants of basic psychopathological states.[61] They claim that cultural factors are significant only in the determination of pathoplastic features of mental illness. This relationship has been best demonstrated in the study of delusions. Laubscher found that schizophrenic symptoms among Africans in Queensland included auditory and visual hallucinations with mythological content, delusions of being poisoned and bewitched, and delusions of grandeur (of becoming a chief or doctor); while the delusions of Europeans included influences operating from a distance through electricity, telepathy, and hypnotism.[62] Tooth found that the content of the delusions of the "bush" people in the North was associated with ramifications of the fetish system, while, among the more sophisticated people of the South and Accra, it included ideas of influence and control by electricity and wireless, along with Messianic delusions and delusions of grandeur.[63] Carothers noted persecutory delusions of bewitchment, ill-wishing, or condemnation to death among Africans. Stainbrook found that lower-class Bahian schizophrenics in Brazil suffer from anxieties and fears of retribution from African or Catholic deities, while middle-class delusions represent economic and class conceptions of power and such impersonal influences as electricity and physical waves.[64] Lambo found that among rural illiterate Yorubas, delusions are related to supernatural concepts and ancestral cults, while hypochondriacal delusions are prominent among literate Africans.[65] He explained the rarity of delusions of grandeur in terms of Yoruba culture, which "demands total allegiance to ancestral cults and nether world gods" and noted that "it is not always possible to delineate confidently where normal primitive beliefs cease and paranoid psychosis begins."[66]

In an intensive study of the delusions of ten West Indian schizophrenics in English mental hospitals, Kiev found a predominance of religious and magical themes that were strongly related to the beliefs of normal West Indian immigrants who set high value on a fundamentalist approach to the Bible, believed in the phenomenon of charismatic personalities, and were conversant with and receptive to notions of *obeah,* ghosts, and religious healing.[67] There were, however, distinct differences in the use of cultural materials by the normal and psychotic groups. The schizophrenics, rather than being humbled by their experiences, overpersonalized and distorted the significance of the Biblical message in what seemed to be unsuccessful restitutive efforts to explain their experiences. West Indian Pentecostalists claimed that such persons could be distinguished from those genuinely receiving the holy spirit because others could not "witness" (empathize with) a false spirit.

Unlike nonpsychotic individuals who participate in various religious cults and in the revivalist sects in which dissociative phenomena and possession are permitted and encouraged, the schizophrenic patients could not maintain sufficient control of autistic and regressive behavior to fit into the prescribed ritual patterns and made use of culturally accept-able notions in highly idiosyncratic ways—which accounted in part for the differences between their delusions and the belief systems. For individuals experiencing either early or late symptoms of schizophrenia, such religious beliefs and practices offer culturally acceptable explanations for strange happenings within and around them. Much as normal individuals may seek to express themselves in dissociative states, the psychotic individual may become convinced that what is happening to him is a religious experience.

In line with Benedict's suggestion that different societies tolerate and support different patterns of behavior, West Indian society seems to tolerate, to a greater extent than Western society, charismatic personality traits that find expression in such diverse institutions as *obeah* and Pentecostalism. It is generally believed that individuals can influence others through personal power or as agents of higher powers. Even those who deny belief in *obeah* are convinced that "belief kills, and belief cures" and cite instances of the powers of spiritualist healers and *obeah* sorcerers. Because this notion of personal influence is central to the beliefs of West Indians, individuals undergoing highly disturbing psy-chotic experiences need not resort to wholly idiosyncratic delusions as "security systems" or "defenses" against overwhelming disorganization. They may turn instead to readily available cultural explanations for other kinds of disinhibited behavior. In almost all the delusions of the patients studied, the content involved expression of special abilities to heal, to preach, and to help.

Although the delusions of patients are often rooted in culturally ac-ceptable beliefs, they are usually not identical with them and can be recognized as abnormal by most members of a particular culture. In some instances, the delusions are sufficiently overinclusive and the pa-tient's life so disorganized as to present no difficulty in diagnosis. In some instances, however, delusional content runs almost parallel with beliefs and presents a problem in diagnosis. In such instances, emphasis must be placed less on the strangeness of the ideas than on the relationship they bear to the inner insecurities and morbid experiences of the patient.

In the absence of other evidence of psychiatric symptoms, for example, a belief in *obeah*, ghosts, or the power to "kill and cure" cannot be taken as evidence of delusions. In equivocal cases, these beliefs must be considered in relationship to other facets of the patient's behavior. In addition, the doctor must look for exaggerations, misinterpretations, and distortions of culturally acceptable beliefs; recognition of such elements, of course, ultimately necessitates either familiarity with the culture or consultations with representative members.

It seems not unlikely then that mental illness is manifested in certain basic structural mechanisms and processes that recur together with certain regularity in the different clinical syndromes, providing a substratum on top of which the different cultures impose differences in content. There is little evidence to suggest that mental illnesses differ from culture to culture in any other way. With recognition of these basic structural limitations, there is still value in awareness of the native categories of illness and treatment, which, as Devereux has suggested, may occasionally fit the psychiatric realities of the tribe better than do modern categories in focusing on the sources of strain particular to a given culture.[68]

These twentieth-century studies of primitive cultures have been immeasurably influenced by psychoanalytic theory and the functionalist schools of anthropology. Functionalist theories associated with Radcliffe-Brown, Evans-Pritchard, and Malinowski held that cultures were social units kept stable by sets of complementary institutions.[69] Each institution contributed toward the maintenance of both the individual and the society and was functionally compatible with the other institutions. For example, religion and primitive medicine not only satisfied spiritual and physical needs and helped to integrate individuals into society but also contributed to the equilibrium of the society. Through the adherence to traditional customs and social relationships, institutionalized rituals and beliefs strengthened the meaning of the particular symbols expressed and reinforced the values of the group. Some studies have further suggested that other group rituals—like religious practices, sports, warfare, and drug-taking—contribute to reduction and rechanneling of energies and drives that might otherwise be pathologically repressed or misdirected and that they therefore had therapeutic effects. Mention should also be made of the large-scale responses to social change—for example, the Cargo Cults in the South Pacific and the Ghost Dance and Peyote religions of the Plains Indians—which appear to support old institutions with new supernatural sanctions and values and new forms of expression and to serve individual psychotherapeutic ends.[70]

Since the 1930s, another group of anthropologists has examined the

relationship between personality and culture. Studies in this direction
have led to the formulation of such concepts as Kardiner's basic personality type to explain the high incidence of certain personality characteristics in certain cultures.[71] The basic personality, consisting of the values
and attitudes shared by members of a given culture, was thought to be
the core of individual personality. With such a concept, the study of
psychopathology could proceed by examination of the culture rather
than of individual behavior. Along these lines, Benedict suggested that,
where cultural expectations conflict with personality patterns, mental
illness develops.[72] Evidence can be seen in situations where new demands
are placed on individuals brought up with different expectations of
themselves and life. Individuals raised as slaves on plantations, for instance, might reasonably find it difficult to adjust to freedman status;
soldiers returning from war might find it difficult to adjust to the tamer
life of peacetime. Similarly, an individual's role in life may conflict with
his idealistic nature, as, for example, when a religious individual, trained
to be honest and charitable, encounters the demands of business and the
market place. These strains can be seen particularly in times of social
change, even when technological advances increase opportunities for
people. Fromm, Ortega y Gasset, and others have written extensively on
the psychological stress attendant upon increased freedom, which often
upsets the comfortable *status quo* and disrupts old ways of dealing with
life.

Wolff elaborated this theme, considering the relationship between
changing sex roles in the twentieth century and changes in the incidence
of ulcers among men, emphasizing the interplay of cultural and social
factors in the production of physical illness.[73] He also reviewed a number
of studies that showed that perforations of ulcers in young women occurred frequently in the beginning of the nineteenth century but diminished at the beginning of the twentieth century. What was once principally a female disorder has become predominantly a male disorder. He
suggested that this shift can be understood in terms of an altered relationship between the sexes, reflected, for example, by a change of
woman's role in society and the family and a corresponding change in
attitude toward men following urbanization. Increasing emancipation of
women has lessened their dependence on men, while the increasing confusion of the male role has placed increased stress on men and afforded
them fewer opportunities to satisfy the dependency needs that previously could be satisfied under cover of their "dominant" role.

While culture-personality studies have been provocative and useful
in stimulating an interest in anthropological materials among psychiatrists,

they have often erred in misusing the concepts of psychiatry. While basic personality patterns have been meaningfully related to cultural experiences in particular societies, there has been an inclination to use psychopathological labels to describe what are characteristically normal behavior patterns for certain societies. The institutionalized patterns of suspicion, witchcraft, and grandiosity noted among the Kwakiutl were labeled paranoid, without due regard for the fact that the word did not have the same meaning in that context that it has in Western society. As Leighton has noted, the "use of clinical terms for conforming group oriented behavior involves a paradox."[74] This approach also led to psychodynamic formulations of social processes, despite the fact that psychodynamic concepts are derived from a different level of analysis and are inapplicable to examination of social forces.

Benedict's view that abnormality is relative to culture has been disputed by many, with some authors emphasizing the universal characteristics of psychopathology.[75] Few, however, have ignored her emphasis on the importance of cultural stress points in the development of maladjusted and disturbed personalities. Of special significance is the recognition that certain unusual mental states may be highly regarded in some societies, institutionalized in others, and greeted by ostracism in still others. Hysterical dissociative states were the necessary prerequisites for the priesthood in some societies; elsewhere, homosexuality was institutionalized, as in the *berdaches* of the Plains Indians and Mohave.[76] The mentally ill (believed to be possessed by frightening evil spirits) were often buried alive in Fiji and New Hebrides, while victims of witchcraft among the Bengala of the Belgian Congo were put to death to destroy the magic in them.[77]

In culture and personality studies, Benedict and later Mead[78] and others demonstrated to psychiatrists that group patterns of living are related to the patterning of the inner lives of group members. This relationship accounts for example, for the fact that, while the South Sea Arapesh were mild and gentle, their neighbors the Mudugamor were vigorous and aggressive and the Balinese withdrawn and isolated.[79] Underlining the importance of differential stress systems, Hallowell wrote:

> It seems likely then that as a result of differences in the social pressures imposed by varying cultural configurations, qualitative differences in cultural values bear some relation to the incidence and character of psychic stresses in different human societies quite additional to situational and organic factors.[80]

The best formulated theory and documented demonstration of this relationship between culture and the character of psychic stress have been made by Devereux in his study of a Plains Indian.[81] He has theorized that the structure of the basic personality is determined primarily by the experiences of the oedipal and postoedipal periods, the periods of life most significantly affected by the cultural ethos, and that a traumatic event can cause a severe neurosis only "if it affects the functionally most important segment of the personality."[82] This segment is the one in whose formation the tribal cultural pattern has played the greatest role between the oedipal and pubertal periods and in which are rooted the primary defense mechanisms.

This theory was supported by Devereux's observation of a Wolf Indian whose personality structure was determined primarily by the areal culture pattern of the Plains. "Although many of the external segments of his life history, behavior pattern and personality were affected also by his position as a marginal man in American society, the core of his personality was formed by the surviving Plains ethos and ideology which influenced him primarily between the oedipal and pubertal periods."[83] The ego of the Wolf was different from that of the average urban white patient, in that there was a more intense "cathecting of the nuclear 'body ego' which seems to determine a tendency toward systematization and a higher degree of libidinization of the musculo-skeletal system."[84] The order in which various defense mechanisms were used was determined by cultural factors tending to favor certain defenses over others. Dreaming and fantasy life were important Wolf defense mechanisms, and the reality-testing function of the patient's ego was severely taxed because of the very constricted and monotonous perceptual horizon of the Wolf child; but fantasy and dreaming were in conflict with the ethical codes and definitions of reality of the American social system.

A consideration of these factors was a critical part of the therapeutic relationship that Devereux formed with his patient. He recognized that the patient's racial background considerably constricted the range of social environments in which he would be permitted to function at his optimal level and decided that the reservation was the best *milieu* for the patient. There the absence of economic pressures and social discriminatory practices towards Indians would reinforce normal growth and happiness. Therapy was therefore aimed at rehabilitating the patient's "basic Wolf personality," which was compatible with the "means-end structure of his predictable social environment." The specific counseling objectives were to disengage the patient's basic personality and traditional reaction patterns from "underneath a rubble of ill-integrated, patchy and haphazardly acquired attitudes, which however useful they may be to the average white American are a source of constant disappointment to members of a depressed minority."[85] It was intended to restore the patient's Wolf Indian personality to its "normal" state.

The impact of social and cultural factors can be seen, not only on individual levels, however, but also on a larger scale, the study of which has long interested psychiatrists seeking to delineate relationships between mental illness and such phenomena as migration, mobility, and acculturation. Differentials among groups in rates of illness have been shown to vary with such factors as length of residence in a country, self-selection, the stresses of migration and adjustment, previous persecutory experiences, home ownership, and race—as well as with the impact of culture contact in non-Western areas.[86] In a recent comprehensive review of the subject, Murphy noted that, while there has been little doubt about the relationship between social factors and mental illness, only in the case of Westernization of non-Western peoples has there been unanimous agreement about the effect of social phenomena on the increase of mental illness.[87] One of the pioneering studies demonstrating this point was conducted by Carothers, who showed that the certification rate to mental hospitals for urban natives in East Africa was five times greater than that for natives living on reservations. Although the African rates were still lower than the whites, there was no question that they had risen, which could not simply be explained on the basis of improved medical facilities and diagnostic possibilities— a common explanation for changed rates.

The study of incidence and prevalence of mental illness in underdeveloped and primitive countries is very difficult. In many instances, modern facilities are lacking. When facilities are available, they are not always used by the natives, and when they are used it is often not for the same reasons as in the West. In these societies, there is often greater tolerance of mental illness and sometimes suspicion of Western hospitals as well. In addition, it is often difficult to distinguish etiological factors in diagnosis, particularly whether or not mental symptoms indicate underlying parasitic or infectious disease. Along these lines, Tooth noted that trypanosomiasis was the commonest cause of mental illness throughout large parts of West Africa, while Carothers noted that 3.4% of first admissions to mental hospitals in Kenya were due to malaria. Parasites, syphilis, and nutritional-deficiency diseases like pellagra and beri-beri must also be considered in diagnosing disease in primitive cultures.

Taking both individual and large-scale studies into account, Opler has noted that what is repressed, who are or who become cathected targets of projection or introjection, or what role models are available for sublimation—all of these conditions are matters which vary with the culture. In a comprehensive review of culture, psychiatry, and human values, he wrote: "The data on varying normative cultural behavior, and on differential psychopathology in these other cultural scenes demonstrate that the largest unresolvable 'differing stimulating conditions' affecting human conduct are cultural in essence."[88] This approach had been put forward as early as 1938 by Hallowell and based on his theory that responses learned from social interaction predominate over innately determined behavior patterns in humans; that such learned responses are related to definable bodies of traditional concepts, beliefs, and institutions, which transcend the lifetimes and experiences of the individuals whose lives they mold; and that, since the cultural traditions of mankind vary radically from people to people and age to age, it must be recognized that affective experiences are in part a function of cultural variables. Culture thus provides the primary frame of reference to which all learned behavior relates. It defines the situations that will arouse certain emotional responses, determines the degree to which responses are supported by customs or inhibitions, and defines the particular forms emotion and expression may take.[89]

It should be noted that, while classical psychoanalysis has been loath to acknowledge the significance of culture *qua* culture and, as Aubrey Lewis has noted, "makes the individual incorporate his environment rather than interact with it," various "neo-Freudians," especially Fromm and Horney, have stressed the significance of environment and cultural factors, reversing Freud's original contention.[90] Horney has emphasized the perpetuation of neurotic behavior through the peculiar demands of certain roles in American culture, while Fromm has redefined the meaning of "social character" even more elaborately along the lines of Kardiner's concept of basic personality structure. Fromm's *The Sane Society* is a classic exposition of the theme that the nature of society determines the character of the individual.[91] Fromm has suggested elsewhere that socially patterned defects can be detected as frequently in society and culture as in the patient and has argued that a sick society can produce only sick individuals and that attention should be focused on the system of values and attitudes prevalent in a given culture.

More practically, Frieda Fromm-Reichman has emphasized the use of cultural factors by patients in psychotherapy. She has noted that the patient's selection of subject matter for repression and dissociation is determined by the cultural standards accepted by the significant people in his immediate environment and in his group. Because of this cultural stress, the individual's behavior, styles of thought, and ways of reacting to life situations are influenced largely by the culture in which he lives and the ways in which his culture prescribes behavior for various situations.

These cultural anthropological studies, resting on a solid ethnographic foundation and fortified by functionalist and psychoanalytic postulates, have immeasurably enriched our knowledge of the meaning and signifi- cance of a great range of human behavior. They have been of especial value to psychiatry, emphasizing as they do the contribution of culture to personality strengths and weaknesses, to characteristic mental symp- toms, and to the frequency and distribution of psychiatric illness. As cultures produce characteristic tensions, they also provide mechanisms for the release of tensions. The study of these mechanisms is the main theme of this anthology.

§ Primitive Psychiatry

While many workers like Rivers, Clements, Harley, and Field have long been interested in primitive medicine, it is only in recent years that its psychotherapeutic elements have been examined.[92] Ackerknecht emphasized the presence of many psychotherapeutic features beside such objectively effective factors as baths, cauterizations, surgery, inocu- lation, and a vast pharmacopoeia to account for the success of primi- tive medicine.[93] Hallowell showed how psychic stresses arising from the violation of cultural proscriptions could be resolved by confession among the Salteaux Indians of Manitoba. In 1936, Morris Opler reported that a wide range of psychiatric illnesses, including tics, suicidal manias, and homicidal manias were treated by Apache shamans.[94] He noted that the shaman employed several devices to awaken the patient's expectation of relief but also avoided treating those skeptical of his ability. To spur credence, respect, and faith he would use *legerdemain*, boastfully recount his past successes, and spend much time learning about the patient in order to impress all with his omniscence. The treatment itself, a successful ceremonial "struggle" between the shaman, his "power," and the evil forces, could not fail to impress the patient.

The Leightons in their description of Navaho treatment methods emphasized group support and the invocation of traditional values.[95] When a pot of emetic was heated, the entire group would wash and drink from it along with the patient. When the Singer touched the patient with a brush of eagle and owl feathers, the others would be brushed as well. When hot pokers were applied to the patient's body, the others would receive the same treatment. It was only at the end that the patient was isolated from the others and had opportunity to reflect on the ceremony. Pfister, in an earlier analysis of the symbolic processes, the breakdown of the patient's unconscious resistances, and the detection of etiological factors by the shaman, demonstrated the close link between Navaho therapy and psychoanalysis. He maintained that the Indians penetrated to the unconscious motivation of the psychoneurotic disturbance under treatment and applied treatment individually. He wrote:

> There cannot be the slightest doubt that processes of this sort in which the distress, on the one hand, is recognized symbolically and, on the other is treated and overcome by a symbolic exposition of reality, have immense value and prophylactic and therapeutic significance in mental hygiene. . . . In these religious ceremonies the unconscious of the medicine man speaks to the unconscious of his patient and circumvents consciousness. He thus avoids resistance which would have been aroused had consciousness intervened.[96]

Other relevant studies of primitive psychotherapy include La Barre's study of the public confessions of Peyotist groups, Gillin's study of the healing of *espanto* or magical fright induced by fear of spirits in Guatemala, Field's study of treatment at religious shrines in Ghana, Kilton Stewart's study of therapy by shamanistic trance among the Negritos in the Philippines, and most recently an exhaustive study of Mohave ethnopsychiatry by Devereux.[97] From these and other studies, it has become clear that primitive psychotherapies encompass such complex and diverse techniques, the selection of which depends on various cultural factors.[98]

The value of these various primitive methods was recognized by Freud, who noted that they must be classed as psychotherapy; for to effect a cure a "condition of 'expectant' faith was induced in sick persons, the same condition which answers a similar purpose for us today."[99] Fenichel has provided a cogent analysis of the therapeutic value of such techniques.[100] He observed that a beneficial change in the conflict between undesirable impulses and associated anxiety or guilt (the basis of neurosis) could be effected by the prohibition of symptoms by an authority through suggestion or threats (symbolic castration). These methods may lead to a "substitute neurosis" in which the patient becomes afraid, introverted, rigid, and more dependent and to an increase of pressure on the repressed. Occasions are also provided for discharge, which may diminish the inner pressure and reinforce other repressions or may be accepted as a substitute for the spontaneous symptoms. According to Fenichel, baths, exercises, or physical measures may substitute for conversion symptoms; prescribed diets and ritual penances for compulsive symptoms; and prohibition for phobic symptoms. The efficacy of such methods then depends on whether the substitute fits the patient's personality, because "a hysteric cannot accept 'artificial compulsions' nor a compulsion neurotic 'artificial conversions.'" The substitute must also be pleasurable and sufficiently removed from the original instinctual meaning of the symptom to be acceptable. In addition, a "transference neurosis" develops in which repressed conflicts are represented in the emotional tie to the doctor, thus reducing the number of expressive channels needed. As Fenichel has written:

> The healing power of Lourdes or of a Catholic confession is still of a much higher order than that of the average psychotherapist for neurotics, who are persons who have failed in actively mastering their surroundings, are always more or less looking out for passive-dependent protection, for a "magic helper." The more a psychotherapist succeeds in giving the impression of having magic powers, of still being the representative of God as the priest-doctors once were, the more he meets the longing of his patients for magic help.[101]

While Fenichel's views have the merit of fitting a wide array of data into a single theory of human behavior, they lack proper attention to social and cultural factors. Little regard is paid to the culture-bound nature of symptoms and conflicts and to the specific cultural applicability of therapeutic maneuvers. Recently, however, Devereux has modified these psychoanalytic explanations. He has suggested that the shaman provides his patient with a whole set of "ethnopsychologically suitable" and congenial and culturally recognized defenses against his idiosyncratic conflicts. According to Devereux, the shaman, strictly speaking, provides not a "psychiatric cure" but a kind of "corrective emotional experience," which leads to a repatterning of defenses without real curative insight. This repatterning involves changing from idiosyncratic conflicts and defenses to culturally conventional conflicts and ritualized symptoms. Devereux also underlines the fact that such "remission without insight," while not a "cure" because the patient remains vulnerable, is nevertheless a "social remission" and therefore sufficiently valuable to the patient and the community to warrant recognition. This last point is of special importance because it demonstrates the relative merits of varying therapeutic ends, a view cogently emphasized by Frank, who has distinguished between the two distinct effects of psychotherapy: symptom relief and improved functioning. Symptom relief is rapid, independent of the type of therapy, and dependent mainly on the expectation of help. Improved functioning appears to be related to the type of therapy an individual receives—whether minimal, individual, or group—and is dependent not only on a learning process accelerated by the therapist but also on extratherapeutic social interactions. This view has the merit of recognizing the value inherent in a variety of techniques and in refocusing attention on those forms of treatment that may most profitably be utilized for the treatment of the vast numbers of patients in need of rapid treatment.

To substantiate the significance of cultural factors, Whiting and Child, in a recent study of about seventy-five primitive societies, found that magical medical beliefs are accepted more for their compatibility with personality variables than for their physiological utility.[102] Using the same approach and materials, Kiev also found that the use of various primitive therapies is related to personality variables.[103] Certain socialization experiences were found to lead to certain characteristic types of adult behavior, reflected in characteristic magical therapies. Many societies have practiced sacrifice to placate the dead or the evil spirits causing illness and to make restitution for the patient's arousal of the spirit. In these instances, it was hypothesized that the self-punitive nature of sacrifice, although empirically ineffective, had become instrumental in reducing the anxiety created by the threat of illness and related to earlier anxiety-laden socialization experiences, which were similarly resolved by self-directed aggression. In fact, it was found that sacrifice was most often used therapeutically in societies where aggressive behavior had been severely prohibited for children. A similar relationship between bloodletting treatment and the early inhibition of aggression in childhood was found to exist.

This connection between magical therapies and sociocultural factors was also clearly shown in Wallace's study of the changes in life-ways of the Iroquois, which were mirrored in their emotional needs and in their religious therapies.[104] In the 1600s, when the Iroquois were militarily powerful and politically independent, they placed great value on courage, indifference to pain or insult, truthfulness, generosity, and meticulousness in observing social responsibilities. The ideal Iroquois was expected to be not only autonomous and emotionally independent but also socially responsible, an expectation suggesting to Wallace that passivity—being given things; being taken care of; being irresponsible and infantile; and being assured of warmth, comfort, and love—would be the focus of repressed wishes in a great many individuals. He suggested that an individual's recognition in himself of such strivings would arouse anxiety; recognition of them in others, contempt, and fear. Iroquois

therapies were thus logical in concentrating on providing opportunities
ritually insulated from contact with life for the gratification of these
strivings. The cult of dreams, the False Face medicine rituals, and the
condolence rituals all allowed for the expression of repressed wishes.
During the False Face ceremonies, individuals wearing masks and im-
personating the gods, had opportunity to express attitudes and feelings
not ordinarily permitted to them. As Wallace has written:

> Membership in the society made it possible for the poised independent self
> controlled self sacrificing individual to express what he did not allow himself
> to feel: a longing to be passive, to beg, to be an irresponsible, demanding
> rowdy infant and to compete with the Creator himself and to express it all
> in the name of the public good.[105]

By the mid-1800s, the Iroquois had lost their territory and had been
politically and militarily emasculated by the white settlers. The male
prestige system, based as it was on hunting, warfare, and political roles,
no longer had meaning, for its ideals could no longer be realized. Failures
by their own standards and objects of contempt to the whites, the
Iroquois were less in need of opportunities to act out passive wishes
ritualistically than of control, order, and respectable images of themselves. These needs were provided by Handsome Lake, who inveighed
against self-indulgence, alcohol, dancing, card-playing, promiscuity,
witchcraft, and envy. Preaching the virtues of self-control and co-operation and the downfall of sinners, he instilled confidence and, according to
Wallace, increasingly organized the Iroquois perception of the world,
crystallized guilt associated with failure to achieve the ego ideal, and
provided for absolution by confession. In his conclusion, Wallace noted
that the psychotherapeutic needs of individuals tend to center on insti-
tionalized catharsis in a highly organized sociocultural system and on
control (the development of a coherent image of self and world and
the repression of incongruent motives and beliefs) in a poorly organized
system.

The papers in this anthology demonstrate that primitive psychotherapies are complex, culture-bound procedures. By extending our interest to non-Western cultures, we hope to delineate the contribution of
culture not only to the forms and content of primitive therapies but also
to the basic processes of psychological treatment. These studies evince
certain parallels with Western psychotherapy, showing how, as Frank
has noted, "a patterned interaction of a patient, a helper, and the group
in a framework of a self consistent assumptive world can promote healing."[106] Psychiatry has hardly begun to investigate the various forms

and organizations of treatment for the sick, which vary from culture to culture. These papers highlight further the fact that no one institutional model can meet the needs within all societies.

Since most human groups seem to have evolved definitions of and forms of treatment for mental illness, it seems probable that such illness is one of the oldest and most ancient modes of human behavior. Western nations have a growing obligation to introduce modern preventive and therapeutic techniques to nonliterate societies; in these circumstances, knowledge of the significance of local practices is important if disruptive effects are to be avoided. This anthology, then, by emphasizing the similarities underlying human groups, may further understanding and respect for differences among cultures.

Notes

1. Gregory Zilboorg and George Henry, *A History of Medical Psychology* (New York: W. W. Norton & Company, Inc., 1941).
2. Jules Masserman, *Principles of Dynamic Psychiatry* (Philadelphia: W. B. Saunders Co., 1946).
3. This observation is not true of modern Russian psychotherapy, in which persuasion and suggestion are still regarded as the primary element. See, for example, Ralph B. Winn, *Psychotherapy in the Soviet Union* (New York: Philosophical Library, Inc., 1961). Nor is it true of some so-called suppressive systems of psychotherapy.
4. Harry Stack Sullivan, *The Psychiatric Interview*, Helen S. Perry and Mary L. Gawel, eds. (New York: W. W. Norton & Company, Inc., 1954); Sullivan, *The Interpersonal Theory of Psychiatry*, Perry and Gawel, eds. (New York: W. W. Norton & Company, Inc., 1953); Erich Fromm, *Escape from Freedom* (New York: Holt, Rinehart & Winston, Inc., 1941); Karen Horney, *Our Inner Conflicts* (New York: W. W. Norton & Company, Inc., 1945); Horney, *The Neurotic Personality of Our Time* (New York: W. W. Norton & Company, Inc., 1937); Carl Jung, "The Psychogenesis of Mental Disease," *Collected Works*, R. F. C. Hull, trans. (London: Routledge & Kegan Paul, Ltd., 1960), Vol. 3; and Patrick Mullahy, *Oedipus, Myth and Complex: A Review of Psychoanalytic Theory* (New York: Grove Press, 1955).
5. Edward Glover, *The Technique of Psychoanalysis* (New York: International Universities Press, Inc., 1955).
6. Franz Alexander and Thomas French, *Psychoanalytic Therapy: Principles and Application* (New York: The Ronald Press Company, 1946); and Masserman, *The Practice of Dynamic Psychiatry* (Philadelphia: W. B. Saunders Co., 1955).
7. Sullivan, *Interpersonal Theory*; and Horney, *Neurotic Personality*.
8. Carl Rogers, *On Becoming a Person* (Boston: Houghton Mifflin Company, 1961).
9. O. Hobart Mowrer, *Learning Theory and Personality Dynamics* (New York: The Ronald Press Company, 1950).
10. John Dollard and Neil E. Miller, *Personality and Psychotherapy: An Analysis in Terms of Learning, Thinking and Culture* (New York: McGraw-Hill Book Co., Inc., 1950).
11. K. E. Appel, J. M. Myers, and A. E. Scheflin, "Prognosis in Psychiatry: Results of Psychiatric Treatment," *Archives of Neurology and Psychiatry*, 70 (1953), 459-68; H. J. Eysenck, "The Effects of Psychotherapy, an Evaluation," *Journal of Consulting*

Psychology, 16 (1952), 319–23; and E. E. Levitt, "The Results of Psychotherapy with Children," *Journal of Consulting Psychology,* 21 (1957), 189–96.

12. D. W. Hastings, "Follow-Up Results in Psychiatric Illness," *American Journal of Psychiatry,* 114 (1958), 1057–66.

13. Erwin H. Ackerknecht, *A Short History of Psychiatry* (New York: Hafner Publishing Co., Inc., 1959), p. 84.

14. Aubrey J. Lewis, "The Psychopathology of Insight," *British Journal of Medical Psychology,* 14 (1934), 332; and Jerome D. Frank, *Persuasion and Healing* (Baltimore: The Johns Hopkins Press, 1961).

15. Frank, *op. cit.*

16. Sigmund Freud, "On Psychotherapy," *Collected Papers* (New York: Basic Books, Inc., 1959), I, 249–263.

17. C. Fisher, "Studies on the Nature of Suggestion: Part I of Experimental Induction of Dreams by Direct Suggestion," *Journal of the American Psychoanalytic Association,* I (1953), 222–55.

18. Rogers, *Counseling and Psychotherapy* (Boston: Houghton Mifflin Company, 1942).

19. John C. Whitehorn and Barbara Betz, "Studies of the Doctor as a Crucial Factor for the Prognosis of Schizophrenic Patients," *International Journal of Social Psychiatry,* 6, (1960), 71–7; Betz and Whitehorn, "The Relationship of the Therapist to the Outcome of Therapy in Schizophrenia," *Psychiatric Research Reports,* 5, (1956), 89; Gerald L. Klerman, Myron R. Sharaf, Mathilda Holzman, and Daniel Levinson, "Sociopsychological Characteristics of Resident Psychiatrists and Their Use of Drug Therapy," *American Journal of Psychiatry,* 117 (1960), 111–7; and Karl Menninger, "Psychological Factors in the Choice of Medicine as a Profession," *Menninger Clinic Bulletin,* 21 (1957), 51–8, 99–106.

20. August B. Hollingshead and Fredrick C. Redlich, *Social Class and Mental Illness, A Community Study* (New York: John Wiley & Sons, Inc., 1958); and Jerome K. Myers and B. H. Roberts, *Family and Class Dynamics in Mental Illness* (New York: John Wiley & Sons, Inc., 1959).

21. Frank, L. H. Gliedman, S. D. Imber, E. H. Nash, and A. R. Stone, "Why Patients Leave Psychotherapy," *Archives of Neurology and Psychology,* 77 (1957), 283–99; and Gliedman, Imber, Stone, and Frank, "Reduction of Symptoms by Pharmacologically Inert Substances and by Short Term Psychotherapy," *Archives of Neurology and Psychiatry,* 79 (1958), 345–51.

22. H. G. Wolff and L. C. Hinkle, "Communist Interrogation and Indoctrination of 'Enemies of the State'" *Archives of Neurology and Psychiatry,* 76 (1956), 115–74; R. J. Lifton, "'Thought Reform' of Western Civilians in Chinese Communist Prisons," *Psychiatry,* 19 (1956), 173–95; and E. H. Schein, "The Chinese Indoctrination Program for Prisoners of War," *Psychiatry,* 19 (1956), 149–72.

23. William Sargant, *Battle for the Mind: A Physiology of Conversion and Brainwashing* (London: William Heinemann, Ltd., 1957).

24. Frank, *op. cit.*

25. *Ibid.,* p. 63.

26. Ari Kiev, "Spirit Possession in Haiti," *American Journal of Psychiatry,* 118 (1961), 133–8; and Kiev, "Folk Psychiatry in Haiti," *Journal of Nervous and Mental Disease,* 132 (1961), 260–5.

27. Henry Sigerist, *A History of Medicine,* Vol. I: *Primitive and Archaic Medicine* (London: Oxford University Press, 1951).

28. W. H. R. Rivers, *Medicine, Magic and Religion* (London: Macmillan & Co., Ltd., 1924).

29. W. L. Warner, *A Black Civilization: A Social Study of an Australian Tribe* (New York: Harper & Row, Publishers, 1941).

30. C. P. Richter, "On the Phenomenon of Sudden Death in Animals and Man,"

Psychosomatic Medicine, 19 (1957), 191-8; and W. B. Cannon, "'Voodoo' Death," *Psychosomatic Medicine,* 19 (1957), 182-90.

31. Leo W. Simmons and Wolff, *Social Science in Medicine* (New York: Russell Sage Foundation, 1954), p. 96.

32. Renzo Sereno, "Obeah: Magic and Social Structure in the Lesser Antilles," *Psychiatry,* 11 (1948), 15-31.

33. E. B. Tylor, *Primitive Culture* Part I: *The Origins of Culture* (New York: Harper & Row Publishers, 1958).

34. F. E. Clements, *Primitive Concepts of Disease,* (University of California Publications in American Archaeology and Ethnology, 32, [1932], No. 2).

35. James G. Frazer, *The Golden Bough: A Study in Magic and Religion* (New York: The Macmillan Company, 1922).

36. Kiev, "The Psychotherapeutic Aspects of Primitive Medicine," *Human Organization,* 21, (1962), 25-9.

37. Warner, *op. cit.*

38. Ackerknecht, "Primitive Medicine and Culture Pattern," *Bulletin of the History of Medicine,* 12 (1942), 545-74; Jack S. Harris, "The White Knife Shoshoni of Nevada," in Ralph D. Linton, ed., *Seven American Indian Tribes* (New York: Appleton-Century-Crofts, 1940); and Marvin K. Opler, "The Southern Ute of Colorado," in Linton, *op. cit.*

39. Paul Radin, *Primitive Religion: Its Nature and Origin* (New York Dover Publications, Inc., 1957).

40. Henry Elkin, "The Northern Arapaho of Wyoming," in Linton, *op. cit.*

41. Marian Smith, "The Puyallup of Washington," in Linton, *op. cit.*

42. Ackerknecht, "Problems of Primitive Medicine," *Bulletin of the History of Medicine,* 11 (1942), 503-21.

43. L. Bryce Boyer, "Remarks on the Personality of Shamans, with Special Reference to the Apaches of the Mescalero Indian Reservation," in Warner Muensterberger, ed., *The Psychoanalytic Study of Society,* Vol. 2 (New York: International Universities Press, Inc., 1962).

44. G. Huntingford, *The Nandi of Kenya* (London: Routledge & Kegan Paul, Ltd., 1953).

45. May M. Edel, *The Chiga of Western Uganda* (London: Oxford University Press, 1957).

46. George W. Harley, *Native African Medicine* (Cambridge, Mass: Harvard University Press, 1941).

47. Natalie Joffe, "The Fox of Iowa," in Linton, *op. cit.*

48. Radin, *op. cit.*

49. Sigerist, *op. cit.*

50. *Ibid.*

51. L. C. May, "A Survey of Glossolalia and Related Phenomena in Non-Christian Religions," *American Anthropologist,* 58 (1956), 75-96; T. K. Oesterreich, *Possession,* D. Ibberson, trans. (New York: Richard R. Smith, Inc., 1930); Jane Belo, *Trance in Bali* (New York: Columbia University Press, 1960); and Ruth Benedict, "The Concept of the Guardian Spirit in North America," *American Anthropological Association Memoirs,* 1923.

52. Emile Kraepelin, *Psychiatrie,* Vol. I (8th ed.; Leipzig: Barth, 1909).

53. Eugen Bleuler, *Dementia Praecox or the Group of Schizophrenias* (New York: International Universities Press, Inc., 1950).

54. H. G. Van Loon, "Protopathic Instinctive Phenomena in Normal and Pathologic Malay Life," *British Journal of Medical Psychology,* 8 (1929), 264-76; J. M. Cooper, "Mental Disease Situations in Certain Cultures," *Journal of Abnormal and Social Psychology,* 29 (1934), 10-7; A. I. Hallowell, "Culture and Mental Disorder," *Journal of Abnormal and Social Psychology,* 29 (1934), 1-9; Ruth Landes, "The Ab-

normal Among the Ojibwa Indians," *Journal of Abnormal and Social Psychology*, 33 (1938), 14-33; P. M. Yap, "The Latah Reaction," *Journal of Mental Science*, 98 515-64; and Yap, "Mental Diseases Peculiar to Certain Cultures: A Survey of Comparative Psychiatry," *Journal of Mental Science*, 97 (1951), 313-27.

55. G. C. Tooth, *Studies in Mental Illness in the Gold Coast* (London: Her Majesty's Stationery Office, 1950); and J. C. Carothers, *The African Mind in Health and Disease* (World Health Organization, Monograph Series No. 17, Geneva, 1953).

56. C. G. Seligman, "Sex, Temperament, Conflict and Psychosis in a Stone Age Population," *British Journal of Medical Psychology*, 9 (1929), 187-202.

57. Eric Berne, "Some Oriental Mental Hospitals," *American Journal of Psychiatry*, 106 (1950), 376-83.

58. Carothers, *op. cit.*

59. M. E. Spiro, "Ghosts, Ifaluk and Teleological Functionalism," *American Anthropologist*, 54 (1952), 497-503; and J. S. Slotkin, "Peyotism, 1521-1891," *American Anthropologist*, 57 (1955), 202-30.

60. Opler, *Culture, Psychiatry and Human Values* (Springfield: Charles C Thomas, Publisher, 1956).

61. H. J. Wegrocki, "A Critique of Cultural and Statistical Concepts of Abnormality," in C. Kluckhohn and H. Murray, eds., *Personality in Nature, Society and Culture* (New York: Alfred A. Knopf, Inc., 1948); and Yap, "Mental Diseases."

62. B. Laubscher, *Sex, Custom and Psychopathology* (London: Routledge & Kegan Paul, Ltd., 1937).

63. Tooth, *op. cit.*

64. E. Stainbrook, "Some Characteristics of the Psychopathology of Schizophrenic Behavior in a Bahian Society," *American Journal of Psychiatry*, 109 (1952), 330-5.

65. T. A. Lambo, "The Role of Cultural Factors in Paranoid Psychosis among Yomeba Tribe," *Journal of Mental Science*, 101 (1955), 239-66.

66. *Ibid.*

67. Ari Kiev, "Beliefs and Delusions Among West Indian Immigrants to London," *British Journal of Psychiatry*, 109 (1963), 356-63.

68. George Devereux, "Cultural Thought Models in Primitive and Modern Psychiatric Theories," *Psychiatry*, 21 (1958), 359-74.

69. A. R. Radcliffe-Brown, *Structure and Function in Primitive Society* (New York: The Free Press of Glencoe, 1952); E. E. Evans-Pritchard, *Witchcraft, Oracles and Magic Among the Azande* (London: Oxford University Press, 1937); and Bronislaw Malinowski, *Magic, Science and Religion and Other Essays* (New York: The Free Press of Glencoe, 1948).

70. Edward Norbeck, *Religion in Primitive Society* (New York: Harper & Row, Publishers, 1961); R. H. Lowrie, *Primitive Religion* (New York: Liveright Publishing Corporation, 1924); and Weston La Barre, *The Peyote Cult*, (Yale University Publications in Anthropology, No. 19 [New Haven: Yale University Press, 1938]).

71. Abram Kardiner, Linton, Cora DuBois, and J. West, *The Psychological Frontiers of Society* (New York: Columbia University Press, 1945).

72. Benedict, "Anthropology and the Abnormal," *Journal of Genetic Psychology*, 10 (1934), 59-82; Benedict, *Patterns of Culture* (Boston: Houghton Mifflin Company, 1934); and Benedict, "Continuities and Discontinuities in Cultural Conditioning," *Psychiatry*, 1 (1938), 161-7.

73. Wolff, *Stress and Disease* (Springfield: Charles C Thomas, Publisher, 1953).

74. Alexander Leighton and Jane Hughes, "Culture as Causative of Mental Disorder," *Causes of Mental Disorders: A Review of Epidemiological Knowledge Proceedings of a Round Table Held at Arden House, Harriman, N. Y., 1959* (New York: Milbank Memorial Fund, 1959), pp. 341-83.

75. Devereux, "Normal and Abnormal: The Key Problems of Psychiatric Anthropology," J. B. Casagande and T. Gladwin, eds., *Some Uses of Anthropology: Theoreti-*

cal and Applied (Washington, D. C.: Anthropological Society of Washington, 1956);
Yap, "Mental Diseases"; and Wegrocki, op. cit.

76. Linton, Culture and Mental Disorders (Springfield: Charles C Thomas, Pub-
lisher, 1956); and Devereux, Mohave Ethnopsychiatry and Suicide: The Psychiatric
Knowledge and the Psychic Disturbances of an Indian Tribe (Bureau of American
Ethnology Bulletin No. 175 [Washington, D. C.: The Smithsonian Institution, 1961]).

77. Sigerist, op. cit.

78. Margaret Mead, Coming of Age in Samoa (New York: William Morrow &
Co., Inc., 1928); and Mead, Growing Up in New Guinea (New York: William Morrow & Co., Inc., 1930).

79. John Honigmann, Culture and Personality (New York: Harper & Row, Publishers, 1954).

80. Hallowell, "Psychic Stresses and Culture Patterns," American Journal of
Psychiatry, 92 (1936), 1291-310.

81. Devereux, Reality and Dream, Psychotherapy of a Plains Indian (New York:
International Universities Press, Inc., 1951).

82. Ibid., p. 47.

83. Ibid., p. 48.

84. Ibid., p. 55.

85. Ibid., p. 108.

86. Benjamin Malzberg, Social and Biological Aspects of Mental Disease (Utica:
State Hospitals Press, 1940); Ornulv Odegard, "Emigration and Insanity: Study of
Mental Disease Among Norwegian Born Population of Minnesota," Acta Psychiatrica
et Neurologica Scandinavica, Supplement 4 (1932), 1-206; Malzberg and E. S. Lees,
Migration and Mental Disease: A Study of First Admissions to Hospitals for Mental
Disease, New York 1939-41 (New York: Social Science Research Council, 1956); J.
Bremer, "Social Psychiatric Investigation of Small Community in Northern Norway,"
Acta Psychiatrica et Neurologica Scandinavica, Supplement 62 (1951), 1-166; H. B.
M. Murphy, Flight and Resettlement (New York: UNESCO, 1955); and Paul Lemkau,
Christopher Tietze, and Marcia Cooper, "A Survey of Statistical Studies on the Prev-
alence and Incidence of Mental Disorders in Sample Populations," Public Health
Reports, 58 (December 31, 1943).

87. Murphy, "Social Change and Mental Health," Causes of Mental Disorders,
pp. 280-340.

88. Opler, Culture, p. 138.

89. Hallowell, "Fear and Anxiety as Cultural and Individual Variables in a
Primitive Society," The Journal of Social Psychology, 9 (1938), 25-47.

90. Lewis, "Points of Research Into the Interaction Between the Individual and
the Culture," J. M. Tanner, ed., Prospects in Psychiatric Research, The Proceedings
of the Oxford Conference of the Mental Health Research Fund, 1953.

91. Fromm, The Sane Society (New York: Holt, Rinehart & Winston, Inc., 1955).

92. Margaret J. Field, Religion and Medicine of the Ga People (London: Oxford
University Press, 1937).

93. Ackerknecht, "Natural Diseases and Rational Treatment in Primitive Medicine," Bulletin of the History of Medicine, 19 (1946), 467-97; Ackerknecht, "Psychopathology, Primitive Medicine, and Primitive Culture," Bulletin of the History of
Medicine, 14 (1943), 30-67; and Ackerknecht, "Primitive Autopsies and the History
of Anatomy," Bulletin of the History of Medicine, 13 (1943), 334-9.

94. Morris E. Opler, "Some Points of Comparison and Contrast Between the
Treatment of Functional Disorders by Apache Shamans and Modern Psychiatric Practice," American Journal of Psychiatry, 92 (1936), 1371-87.

95. Leighton and Dorothea Leighton, "Elements of Psychotherapy in Navaho
Religion," Psychiatry, 4 (1941), 515-23.

96. Oskar Pfister, "Instructive Psychoanalysis Among the Navahos," *Journal of Nervous and Mental Diseases*, 76 (1932), 251.

97. La Barre, "Primitive Psychotherapy in Native American Cultures: Peyotism and Confession," *The Journal of Abnormal and Social Psychology*, 42 (1947), 294-309; John Gillin, "Magical Fright," *Psychiatry*, 11 (1948), 387-400; Field, *Search for Security, An Ethnopsychiatric Study of Rural Ghana* (Evanston: Northwestern University Press, 1960); Kilton M. Stewart, *Pygmies and Dream Giants* (New York: W. W. Norton & Company, Inc., 1954); and Devereux, "Normal and Abnormal."

98. M. K. Opler, "Dream Analysis in Ute Indian Therapy," M. K. Opler, ed., *Culture and Mental Health* (New York: The Macmillan Company, 1959), pp. 97-118.

99. Freud, "On Psychotherapy," p. 250.

100. Otto Fenichel, "Brief Psychotherapy," Fenichel, *Collected Papers*, 2nd Series (London: Routledge & Kegan Paul, Ltd., 1955), pp. 243-59.

101. *Ibid.*, p. 253.

102. J. W. M. Whiting and Irvin L. Child, *Child Training and Personality: A Cross-Cultural Study* (New Haven: Yale University Press, 1953).

103. Kiev, "Primitive Therapy: A Cross-Cultural Study of the Relationship Between Child Training and Therapeutic Practices Related to Illness," Muensterberger and Sidney Axelrod, eds., *Psychoanalytic Study of Society*, I (New York: International Universities Press, 1961) 185-217.

104. Anthony E. C. Wallace, "The Institutionalization of Cathartic and Control Strategies in Iroquois Religious Psychotherapy," M. K. Opler, *Culture and Mental Health*, 63-96.

105. *Ibid.*, p. 80.

106. Frank, *op. cit.*, p. 36.

Weston La Barre

Confession as Cathartic Therapy
in American Indian Tribes

For A LONG TIME, psychiatrists have known the therapeutic value
in one person's simple, unfettered talking to another about his guilts and
worries. If the listener is not punitive—that is, if his own defensive anxiety
is not unduly aroused—then this "catharsis" is a kind of moral reality-
testing that tends to lessen anxiety in the person confessing. Such un-
burdening to a social other is often valuable enough, since it rescues the
sufferer from his aloneness. And if the listener is an older person, he may
appear (through unconscious transference) as a parent-figure, and the
value of the transaction may be correspondingly enhanced. Possibily even
private prayer, for some people, is a sufficient monologue with a projected Infinite Socius as William James called it, to procure this catharsis.
But for many, a still more potent way to liquidate guilt and anxiety
is to confess ritually to supernatural parent-surrogates or ancestors *via*
real human beings who are religiously sanctioned or otherwise socially
accredited for this function. Still another mode of catharsis is to confess
publicly to the whole society, in a culturally sanctioned context, one's
transgressions against the society's code. For example, in a certain sacrificial ceremony among the Karens of Burma, everyone must confess his
sins.[1] It is these last two methods—individual confession to a surrogate
for the supernatural and ritual public confession of sins—that I wish to
discuss here, in particular as they are found among American Indian
tribes.

The confession of sins among American Indians has been attributed
by some students to early missionary influence. Since such activity took
place extremely early among the Pueblo Indians and in Mexico and since
these regions were proselytized by Catholic priests, it is understandable

that both Parsons and Henry should have made this cautious and conservative imputation of the custom to them.[2] It is to a purely native hierarchy, however, that confession is made in the Pueblos as elsewhere; and for the Mexicans we have the specific statement of the contact-period authority, Bernadino de Sahagun, that "the Indians of New Spain considered it their obligation to go to confession at least once in their lifetime, and . . . they did this even long before they had any knowledge of the Christian faith."[3] Furthermore, the occurrence of the culture trait of confession in all American Indian culture areas, including regions remote from Catholic influence, makes it clear that ritual confession of sins is an aboriginal Indian custom.

For example, the thorough integration of the custom into the central pattern—warfare—of the Plains Indians is shown in the abundant references in the literature to public statements of sins, especially of sexual adventures, around the fire on a war party's first night out from camp. Explanations have been given for this custom, ranging all the way from the wish to avoid supernatural danger in war caused by unacknowledged transgressions to the need of a mechanism to control or liquidate in-group animosity in the face of a common enemy. It is true that this custom has also appeared to ethnographers to be anything from "boasting about sexual exploits" (to foment a kind of wartime Dutch courage) among some tribes to authentic sober confession (to avoid human or supernatural retribution) among others; but the same pattern is recognizable everywhere in the Americas—and the very fact of different phrasings and contexts in the tribes of one area attests the antiquity of a custom that has changed through cultural drift. The aboriginal authenticity of confession is shown not only in the early dates of many accounts but also in the fact that established *native* functionaries are involved—functionaries whose vested interests would lead them as conservatives to resist most strongly a new foreign influence like Christianity. For example, the Chol Maya

> were in the habit of confessing to their caciques [native chiefs] when sickness afflicted a member of the family, holding the belief that the sickness would end in death unless confession were made by son, father, or husband, etc. Should the whole community be suffering from plague or sickness, the confession of a serious sin would lead to the shooting of the sinner with bow and arrows.[4]

In the latter case, behavior tends toward the equally aboriginal pattern of finding a scapegoat. The specifically native status of the father confessor is fully evident in the priests found everywhere in South America,

from the mouth of the Orinoco to the Plata, and known variously as
carai (*cara-ìbe, cara-ìbe-bébé*), *pagé* ('Thevet says this word is equivalent
to "demi-god"), *piaye, pagy, boyé,* or *piache.* As Church writes:

> The influence of the Caraibes over the people was paramount. They were
> medicine-men, wise-men, astrologers, prophets, sorcerers, and devil-propiti-
> ators. . . . The sun, moon and stars obeyed their orders, they let loose the
> winds and the storms . . . the most ferocious beasts of the forests were sub-
> missive to them, they settled the boundaries of hunting-grounds, interpreted
> dreams and omens, were entrusted with all secrets, were father confessors
> in all private matters and . . . held life and death at their disposal.[5]

In each hand the *caraibe* held a sacred *maraca* or gourd rattle, which
contained the spirits that spoke to him; he was sumptuously dressed,
with large colored feather headdresses and bracelets, and he was accorded quasi-divine honors and deference.

Among the Aurohuaca Indians of the Colombian Sierra Nevada, all
sickness is believed to be punishment for sin. When summoned, a shaman
will refuse to treat a patient until he confesses his sins, for only then
can they be transferred into bits of shell or stone and exposed to the
radiant influence of the sun on the mountain tops.[6] The Inca of Peru,
after confession of guilt, bathed in a nearby river and repeated the formula, "O thou River, receive the sins I have this day confessed unto the
Sun, carry them down to the sea, and let them never more appear." The
uillac uma, "head that counsels," high priest of the empire and usually a
brother of the Inca, appointed the *ichuri,* who received confessions and
assigned penances. Wissler, indeed, lists as one of the chief characteristics
of Inca culture this "conventional confession of sins to a priest"; Karsten,
however, supposes that the Aymara of Bolivia had the practice of confession in their curing ceremonies before the Inca, their conquerors, ele-
vated it into an instrument of political control.[7] The Inca, it is true, have
borrowed much from the Aymara, and the modern Aymara on ceremonial
and festive occasions beg one another's pardon for any untoward behavior, believing that ill feeling destroys the effectiveness of the ritual;
but there is no reason to believe that the Inca did not also have the pre-
Columbian custom of confession.

Many of the ceremonies of the Ijca are introduced by confessions,
usually after some days of abstention from salt and alcohol. When the
confesser visits the *mama,* or priest, he carries with him a mnemonic device, made of corn shucks, and a knotted string of tree-wool, which are
to help him remember all the sins he needs to confess. The *mama* also

prompts the confesser, should he be disposed to leave out anything in the recital of his list.[8]

Confession was also a recognized native practice in Nicaragua:

> Andagoya says that it was made in the presence of a priest, but an assembly of chiefs of the Nicarao told Francisco de Bobadilla (Oviedo, lib. xlii, cap. iii) that "an old man is appointed for the purpose, in token of which he wears a gourd attached to his neck; and when he dies, we assemble in the council house, and appoint in his place the one who seems the most worthy; and thus the succession is kept up, and we regard the office as one of great dignity. And this old man may have no wife, and lives in his own house and not in any temple or oratory. . . . We tell him when we have broken any of our feast days, and have not kept them, or when we have spoken ill of our gods for not sending rain, and when we have said that they are not good; and the old men impose a penance upon us for the temple, and when we have confessed it, we depart, feeling much relieved and pleased at having told them, and as though we had not done wrong. . . . And the old men say to us: 'Go; and do not do this again.' We follow this custom because we know it to be good, and we believe that in this way we shall not fall into more evil, and will feel free from that which we have already committed."[9]

The testimony of the natives themselves indicates clearly that for them confession provides emotional catharsis. Also interesting is the choice of an old man for the function of confessor. Confession is not permitted until the age of puberty, and traditionally one confesses within a day of the fault, lest evil meantime befall. As with the modern psychiatrist, the old man is not permitted to disclose what is told to him.

In time of calamity, in several Guatemalan tribes, the people made a practice of confessing sins as a group. Similarly, in a personal crisis like childbirth, the midwife would order the woman in difficult labor to confess her sins.[10] Aguilar writes of the Maya of Yucatán:

> They also call old Indian shamans when a woman is in labor, and, with the words of their former idolatry, he will enchant her and hear her confession. They do the same with some other patients.[11]

In Yucatán, death and sickness were believed to be punishment for wrong-doing, and therefore a sick person confessed his sins to the priest or, in the priest's absence, to a parent or spouse. Friends and relatives would attend the sickbed and jog the memory of the sufferer, in case he omitted any; and sometimes, if the patient recovered, quarrels might

arise over confessed derelictions—from which it is clear that in some
regions public confession was not without its drawbacks.[12]

In Mexico, the confession of sins, particularly sexual ones, was a
prominent feature. The practice, reinterpreted in Catholic terms, was
even used by Spanish missionaries to root out peyotism, the ritual eating
of the dried top of the mescaline-containing cactus *Lophophora wil-
liamsii*, which they regarded as a peculiarly devilish rival to Christianity
in its use as a "sacrament." The confessional of Padre Nicholas de Leon
contains the following questions for the priest to ask the penitent:

> Dost thou suck the blood of others? Dost thou wander about at night, call-
> ing upon demons to help thee? Hast thou drunk peyotl, or given it to others
> to drink?[13]

Indeed, among the Chichimeca of Mexico, confession was part of the
peyote ritual itself.[14] Of this tribe, Sahagun writes that

> they gather on a level spot, where they dance and sing all during the day
> and night to their fullest pleasure, and this is on the first day because the
> following one all of them used to cry a great deal and they used to say that
> they were cleaning and washing their eyes and their faces with their tears.[15]

He adds further details of the Aztec confessional, whose patron was a
three-named tutelary goddess:

> [One] name of the goddess is Tlacqüani, which means eater of filthy things.
> This signifies that, according to their sayings, all such carnal men and
> women confessed their sins to these goddesses, no matter how uncouth and
> filthy they might have been, and they were forgiven. It is also said that this
> goddess or these goddesses had the power to produce lust; that they could
> provoke carnal intercourse and favored illicit love affairs, and that after such
> sins had been committed, they also held the power of pardoning and cleans-
> ing them of sin, forgiving them to the Sátrapas (priests).[16]

The Aztec confessional complex recalls a number of common laymen's
misconceptions concerning psychoanalysis. When the sinner is ready to
confess, he consults a priest, who chooses a favorable day for for him from
astrological tables, and brings a new mat and *copalli*-gum incense.

> After this he at once begins to tell his sins in the order that he has com-
> mitted them, with entire calmness and distinctness, like a person who recites
> a poem or legend, very slowly and well enunciated, or like one who goes on
> a very straight road without deviating to one side or the other.

According to the gravity of the offense, penances of fasting, piercing the tongue with a *maguey* thorn and lacerating it, or the like[17] are prescribed.

On the other hand,

> Confession of great sins, such as adultery, were only made by old men, and this for the simple reason to escape worldly punishment meted out for such sins; to escape from being condemned to death, which was either having their head crushed or ground to powder between two stones.

From this statement, it would appear that the aboriginal Mexican confessional breaks down at some points for the assuagement of the most grave anxieties of all.

The Huichol of southern Mexico confess their sexual sins at the time of the pilgrimage to the North to obtain *hikuli* or peyote for their religious rituals. Each woman prepares at home a string of palm leaf strips, with a knot for each lover, omitting none. She brings this string to the temple, and, standing before Grandfather Fire, mentions their names one by one, then throws the cord on the fire to be consumed. It is said that no hard feelings result from this confession, as otherwise the men would not find a single *hikuli* plant. The men similarly knot strings as they go along recalling their sins, and at a certain camp they "talk to all the five winds" and deliver their "roll call" to the leader to be burned by Grandfather Fire.[18] Since the quest for peyote is assimilated to the hunt in Huichol thought, the belief that confession is necessary recalls similar practices of confession on the ritual salt journeys of Mexico and on the war parties of the Southwest and Great Plains Indians.

The Athapascan tribes, perhaps universally, have the pattern of ritual confession also. In the Western Apache cult of Silas John Edwards,

> Confession is public and voluntary. It is not required of members of the cult coming to be cured, although such members may confess if they wish. There is no indication that new members are expected to confess, or that old ones must do so periodically . . . Although . . . no confession is required of a patient before submitting himself for a cure [the shaman] may ask him, "Have you done bad?"[19]

This description is in accordance with the most modern theory of psychosomatic medicine. The northern Athapascan groups also have the pre-Columbian confessional, although among the Tahltan of western Canada it is in a different context:

> Adolescent girls, secluded in a separate hut and subjected to many taboos,

underwent intensive training for from one to two years. Outdoors they covered their heads with robes so that no man could see their faces, and they often carried little sacks into which they confessed their wrongdoings and prayed for deliverance from further sin.[20]

The connection of ritual confession with the adolescent "puberty crisis" is one of psychodynamic significance in its relationship to the first menses. Among the related Carrier Indians, the crisis-context of the confessional is also evident:

> When . . . severely sick, they often think that they shall not recover, unless they divulge to a priest or magician every crime which they may have committed, which has hitherto been kept secret. In such cases they will make a full confession, and then they expect that their lives will be spared for a time longer. But should they keep back a single crime, they as firmly believe that they shall suffer instant death.[21]

Other Athapascans also make confession in similar circumstances. Among the Slave,

> If death seemed imminent, the patient confessed all his wrongdoings in the hope of delaying the fatal hour, a custom that prevailed perhaps among most of the northern tribes, since it has been reported also from the Dogrib and Yellowknife . . . In eastern and northern Canada many natives believe that public confession would blot out the offence.[22]

The Algonquian-speaking tribes also possessed the custom of confession. For example, among the Plains-Cree,

> the following peculiar sexual confession was sometimes held. A man would erect his tent over a spirit stone or a buffalo skull,[23] and, calling the men together would order them to recount their illicit sexual relations. This they were obliged to do, and truthfully, otherwise ill luck would overtake them.[24]

There is a suggestion that confession was an old pattern among the Shawnee too, for in a letter from Thomas Forsyth to General William Clark, the sixth "law" of Tecumseh's brother, the Shawnee Prophet Tensquatawa, is listed to the effect that

> All medicine bags and all kinds of dances and songs were to exist no more: the medicine bags were to be destroyed in presence of the whole of the people collected for the purpose, and at the destroying of such medicine, etc., every one was to make open confession to the Great Spirit in a loud

voice of all the bad deeds that he or she had committed during their lifetime, and beg forgiveness as the Great Spirit was too good to refuse.[25]

Among the Plains Ojibway,

It was formerly the custom to call a public confession of illicit sexual intercourse at intervals. Some man, given the right in a dream to call such an
assembly, gathered the people together in his lodge, where they owned up.
First the elders, then the youths, and then the women. A large painted spirit
rock was present, placed in the center of the floor, to render the occasion
one of solemnity. The stone heard their words, and disaster overtook all
liars. Men who did not tell the truth were certain to be slain on their next
war party [compare the warriors' confessional on the first night out on the
warpath among other tribes]. The participants sat in a circle in the tent about
the stone and were quizzed one after another by the dream-host.[26]

The Saulteaux, among other Algonquians, believed that sickness was the
result of sins, particularly sexual ones, to be cured only by confession; the
Blackfoot also had the public confessional rite.[27]

   The Blackfoot, among other tribes, also had what is perhaps the
reverse or positive side of confession in the ceremonial avowal of innocence. In the Blackfoot "All Smoking Ceremony," there is a rite involving
the cooking of buffalo tongues as the occasion for the avowal of female
virtue, sometimes in counterstatement to a braggart male's false "confessional" statement of sexual acts with her;[28] the buffalo-tongue "swearing rite" occurs in connection with the Sarsi sun dance, as well as with the
Blackfoot sun dance.[29] The Cheyenne[30] also practiced public ritual claims
on sexual matters. Among the Siouans, several Arikara ceremonies involved the avowal of sin or the assertion of sexual purity; in one of these
ceremonies,[31] a girl is given a rattle, which she holds up in challenge
to the men in the audience, who are bound to speak if any can dispute
her purity. The Arikara also have a

Test Dance, which was for the purpose of asserting the virtue of the females,
either married or unmarried. If slanderous tongues had falsely accused a
wife or daughter, the injured one went to her father or husband, asked him
to give a feast and made a dance. When everything was in readiness she
took an arrow, and, touching a painted buffalo skull, made a solemn oath
of chastity, and those who could not pass through the ordeal were for the
time abandoned to the lusts of whoever might desire them.[32]

In another Arikara ceremony, a girl touches a cedar bough at the top of a *tipi* if she is a virgin and gains "prizes" of cloth, vermilion paint, and beads; but if any know aught contrary to her avowal, the men challenge her, and she is publicly shamed.[33] Another Siouan group, the Dakota,[34] build a "virgin's lodge" if derogatory remarks have been circulated; at the feast that is arranged, the girl touches a knife blade, a stone, and the earth symbolically to evoke their revenge if she lies, and her accuser does likewise; but if the accusation is not substantiated, he leaves amid jeers. The Oglala[35] make an avowel of chastity at a special feast to confront a slanderer, with a similar ceremony for virgins male and female. These Algonquian and Siouan ceremonies in the Plains have the character of an ordeal or a law suit for slander; and, although these "swearing feasts" are in general the obverse of the "confession" rituals, the important point to note is that both ease the mind of the person publicly vindicated.

As for the custom of public confession itself, the Siouan-speaking peoples shared it with the Algonquian. A formal part of the Iowa peyote meeting is the command of the leader at midnight to confess:

"I want all of you to rise and confess your sins . . . if you repent." So the members get up, one after another and testify that they have given up drinking (peyote is believed to kill the taste for liquor), smoking, chewing, adultery, etc.[36]

The Crow, even before peyotism, had a similar confession; one recalls too the recitation of sexual exploits among the Crow when embarking on the warpath.[37] Confession is an integral part of Winnebago doctoring, and the sick person confesses and asks forgiveness of those praying for his recovery.[38] The "testimony" in Oto peyote meetings may be influenced by the practices of the Church of Latter Day Saints and the Russellites of Kansas, through the prophet Jonathan Koshiway, but Winnebago confession is amply documented:

At about twelve the peyote begins to affect some people. These generally rise and deliver self-accusatory speeches, after which they go around shaking hands with everyone, asking for forgiveness.[39]

Tribes of the Muskhogean language family of the southeastern United States may have had a similar practice. Adair, writing of an unspecified tribe, notes an annual atonement of sins, at which time all sins except murder are forgiven; and Bartram tells of a general amnesty at the annual "busk" of the Creek, when purgation by means of the "black drink" (*Ilex cassine*) is added, to give both spirit and physical purging.[40]

Still another linguistic group, the Iroquoians, had the pre-Columbian pattern of public confession. Before the "Maple Dance," the first in the spring, the people assembled for mutual confession of sins, as a religious duty in preparation for the council. In this "meeting for repentance," as it was literally called, one of the Keepers of the Faith took a white wampum string in his hand as he confessed his faults, then passed it around to old and young, men, women, and even children. The wampum was believed to record their words. Preparatory confession preceded all Iroquoian festivals, but three of them were particularly important.[41] Such universal confession on these solemn tribal occasions must have had considerable psychotherapeutic effect for the highly socialized Iroquois.

The aboriginality of confession in the New World is finally demonstrated by its presence among the Eskimo of Baffin Land and Hudson Bay. Nearly all Eskimo anxiety centers about transgression of taboos, a matter distasteful to Sedna, the mother goddess of the sea and provider of all food. Bad weather, poor hunting, and consequent starvation are always ascribed to the unconfessed sin of someone. Among the Eskimo, therefore, the wages of sin is starvation. If the guilty one confesses, then all is well: The weather improves, and seals allow themselves to be caught; but sometimes the *angakok* or shaman has to discover the malefactor in order to protect the community, and only prompt confession of some infraction of the rules can purchase immunity.[42] In all this belief and behavior, the Eskimo confuse superego-anxiety with ego-anxiety, moral guilt with natural fear; or, in other terms, unlike the Greeks, they have never made the necessary discrimination between *physis* and *nomos*, nature and custom.

The virtually pan-American distribution of the trait of confession, in one cultural context or another, leaves little doubt that it is a genuinely aboriginal psychotherapeutic technique. Indeed, we are probably dealing here with a custom already old in Asia, for the Paleo-Siberian Kamchadal of Kamchatka had a very similar conception of sin.[43] The great importance of public confession of sins in the liquidation of anxiety will be apparent to the psychiatrist. The focusing upon some concrete fetish or symbol of cultural authority—the "Father Peyote," buffalo skull, spirit stone, or wampum—is another valuable and dynamically significant aspect of the practice. The significance of a group ritual, as in the peyote cult (aided here by the awesome pharmacodynamic "authority" of the psychotropic drug mescaline), may serve to explain the survival through millennia of this kind of unwitting primitive psychotherapy and its persistence and spread in the modern religion of the Plains, the peyote cult.

Notes

1. Rev. Harry I. Marshall, "The Karen People of Burma: A Study in Anthropology and Ethnology," *Ohio State University Bulletin*, 26 (Columbus: 1922), No. 13, 236. More general works on confession include Raffaele Pettazzoni, "Confession of Sins among Primitive Peoples," *Congrès international des sciences anthropologiques, Compte rendu de la première session* (London: 1934), 294-5; and H. S. Darlington, "Confession of Sins," *Psychoanalytic Review*, 24 (1937), 150-64. See also Theodor Reik, *The Compulsion to Confess* (New York: 1959).
2. E. C. Parsons, *Pueblo Indian Religion*, II (Chicago: 1939), 1225; and Jules Henry, "The Cult of Silas John Edwards," *Mss.*, 1937.
3. Bernadino de Sahagun, *A History of Ancient Mexico*, F. R. Bandelier, trans., I (Nashville: 1932), p. 33.
4. J. Eric Thompson, "Sixteenth and Seventeenth Century Reports on the Chol Mayas," *American Anthropologist*, 40 (1938), 602.
5. G. E. Church, *Aborigines of South America* (London: 1912), pp. 31-2.
6. F. C. Nicholas, "The Aborigines of the Province of Santa Marta, Colombia," *American Anthropologist*, 3 (1901), 606-49. The belief that the sun sees all sins is widespread; compare Greek notions, the Osiris legend, the Finnish national epic (*Kalevala*, Runes xiv-xv), and Hindu beliefs. The sun is often symbolically the paternal eye, the eye of god.
7. Sir E. B. Tylor, in E. Westermarck, ed., *The Origin and Development of the Moral Ideas*, I, (London: 1924), 54; Sir Clements Markham, *The Incas of Peru* (London: 1910), p. 106; C. Wissler, *The American Indian* (2nd ed.; New York: 1922), p. 248; W. H. Prescott, *History of the Conquest of Peru* (New York: 1937), pp. 786-7; R. Karsten, *The Civilization of the South American Indians* (New York: 1926), p. 497; and Pettazzoni, *op. cit.*, p. 295-6.
8. G. Bolinder, *Die Indianer der tropischen Schneegebirge* (Stuttgart: 1925), pp. 139-40.
9. S. K. Lothrop, "Pottery of Costa Rica and Nicaragua," *Contributions from the Museum of the American Indian, Heye Foundation*, 8 (1926), Nos. 1, 2, p. 35. For similar Guatemalan practices, see H. H. Bancroft, *The Native Races of the Pacific States of North America*, 2 (5 vols.; New York: 1874-1876), 678; and A. E. Crawley, *The Mystic Rose* (London: 1902), p. 393.
10. Antonio de Herrera, *The General History of the Vast Continent and Islands of America, commonly call'd the West-Indies*, J. Stevens, trans., IV (6 vols.; London: 1725-1726), 148, 173, 190. See also T. Waitz, ed., *Anthropologie der Natürvolker*, IV (6 vols.; Leipzig: 1859-1872), 265. The significance of masochistic behavior in the solution of anxieties must not be overlooked in native America. As in Yucatán, the Nicarao "pierce their tongues from beneath . . . and some of them scarify the genital member" (Lothrop, *op. cit.*, p. 38). The Chorotegan (*ibid.*, pp. 82-3) "mutilate and scarify with small knives or flint their tongues, and ears, or genitals" and spill blood on corn that is later eaten as sacred food. In Yucatán, Indians "made sacrifices of their own blood, sometimes cutting their ears all around with rags which they had attached to them in sign of penitance; other times they made holes in their cheeks or the lower lip. Some cut pieces of flesh from certain parts of the body, or pierced the tongue slantingly, passing a wisp of straw through it with cruel suffering; others cut the upper part of the virile member, in such fashion as to leave it with two hanging ears" (Diego de Landa, "Relation des choses de Yucatán," in Waitz, *op. cit.*, p. 265). While genital and other mutilations are without doubt motivated, the Central American examples are done in penance. In the exorcism of life anxieties, compare the tying of buffalo skulls to skewers in the shoulder muscles of Plains sun dancers, who drag them around till the flesh is torn; or the tying of

such dancers in the same fashion to the center pole of the sun-dance lodge. The sacrifice in pain in these instances is intended to ensure success in war and hunting.

11. Pedro Sanchez de Aguilar, *Informe contra Idolorvm Cvltores del Obispado de Yucatan* (Madrid: 1639), in *Indian Notes and Monographs, Heye Foundation*, IX (1919-1920), 205. This Maya reference, like the Nicaraguan one, strongly indicates the aboriginality of the practice of confession in the very language of the descriptions made by the early Spanish explorers.

12. Diego de Landa, in Waitz, *op. cit.*, IV, 306-7; see also C. E. Brasseur de Bourbourg, *Histoire des Nations Civilisées*, II (4 vols.; Paris: 1857-1859), 114ff, 567; *ibid.*, III, 567-9.

13. Nicholas de Leon, *Camino del Cielo*, in Louis Lewin, *Phantastica, Narcotic and Stimulating Drugs* (New York: 1931), p. 96; also in W. E. Safford, "Narcotic Plants and Stimulants of the Ancient Americans," *Annual Report, Smithsonian Institution* (1917), p. 295. References to bloodsucking probably meant the sucking cures of Indian shamans, which the *padres* perhaps misunderstood but were anxious to combat; the second question evidently refers to something like the vision quest or to the animal familiars of shamans and others. In Fray Bartholomé's *Manual* of 1760 (p. 15) for the confessional of Indians in the area of San Antonio, Texas, the questions were asked, "Hast thou eaten human flesh? Hast thou eaten the peyote?" —neither of them an idle question among the cannibalistic peyotists of Texas.

14. On this question, see Weston La Barre, *The Peyote Cult* (Hamden: 1959) (reprinted from Yale University Publications in Anthropology, No. 19 [New Haven, 1938]), especially the chapter on "Psychological Aspects of Peyotism," pp. 93-104; see also La Barre, "Primitive Psychotherapy in Native American Cultures," *Journal of Abnormal and Social Psychology*, 42 (1947), 294-301, from which part of the present study is taken.

15. Sahagun, *Historia General de las Cosas de Nueva España*, C. M. de Bustamente, ed., IV (4 vols.; Mexico: 1829-1830), 3.

16. Sahagun, *History*, Bandelier trans., I, 29-33, from which are also taken the two subsequent quotations.

17. "Or he may say: 'You offended god by getting drunk, so you must appease the god of wine, called Totochi, and when you go to comply with your penance you are to go at night, naked with only a paper in front and one at the back to cover your privy parts; and when you are ready to return after your prayers are offered, you are to thow the papers that covered your front and back at the feet of the gods that are there" (*ibid.*, p. 32). The "paper" was probably aboriginal Mexican bark cloth.

18. Carl Lumholtz, *Unknown Mexico*, II (New York: 1902), 129. For the complex symbolism of Grandfather Fire among the Huichol, see La Barre, *Peyote Cult*, pp. 30-3. In the Plains peyote cult, it is the Father Peyote or fetish button resting on top of the crescent-shaped ground altar west of the sacred fire that is the focal center of the ritual and the palladium toward which all prayers are addressed. Father Peyote buttons are always handled with great reverence, are passed down as heirlooms together with stories of their powers, and if sold (as medicine bundles sometimes were) command extraordinarily high prices. Both in aboriginal Indian wars and in World Wars I and II, peyote buttons were carried on the persons of warriors and soldiers as protective fetishes. A Father Peyote figured in the shamanistic cure of a paranoid Oto (see La Barre, "Primitive Psychotherapy," p. 297). The psychodynamic significance of Grandfather Fire and Father Peyote as authority symbols will be apparent to psychiatrists.

19. Henry, *op. cit.*

20. Diamond Jenness, *The Indians of Canada* (Ottawa: 1932), pp. 373-4.

21. D.W. Harmon, quoted in Rev. Jedidiah Morse, *Report to the Secretary of War of the United States on Indian Affairs* (New Haven: S. Converse, 1822)

p. 345. The neighboring Algonquian tribes to the East have very similar ideas; see A. I. Hallowell, "Sin, Sex and Sickness in Saulteaux Belief," *British Journal of Medical Psychology*, 18 (1939), 191-7; Hallowell, "Fear and Anxiety as Cultural and Individual Variables in a Primitive Society," *Journal of Social Psychology*, 9 (1938), 25-47; and Hallowell, "Psychic Stresses and Culture Patterns," *American Journal of Psychiatry*, 92 (1936), 1291-1310.

22. Jenness, *op. cit.*, pp. 391 (citing Keith and Petitot), and 174 (citing Boas and Keith). In the Iroquois "White Dog" ceremony, after the confessions of communicants, their sins were cast into the scapegoat, which was then sacrificed.

23. Compare the fetishistic attitude toward the Father Peyote. The psychological function of the fetish is to give physical form and locus to some projected aspect of the person, at times of oneself, at times of another. Often as here the supernatural father, the fetish is also sometimes an amulet-projection of the phallic id; but the fetish can further be a projected superego or even an ego, whereby men disclaim responsibility for their own emotions, wishes, and acts. See the chapters on "Religion and Psychiatry," "Psychology of a Snake Cultist," and "Psychopathy and Culture," in La Barre, *They Shall Take Up Serpents: Psychology of the Southern Snake-Handling Cult* (Minneapolis: 1962) for a discussion of the multiple functions of the fetish.

24. A. Skinner, "Political Organizations, Cults, and Ceremonies of the Plains Ojibway and Plains Cree Indians," *Anthropological Papers, American Museum of Natural History*, 11 (1914), 540. The quotation continues: "Those who had unnatural intercourse with their spouses were obliged to confess it. Once . . . a girl refused to speak, and her father was sent for, who ordered her to make a clean breast of her sin, whereupon she confessed that she had transgressed with him."

25. T. Forsyth, in E. H. Blair, *The Indian Tribes of the Upper Mississippi Valley and Region of the Great Lakes*, II (Cleveland: 1912), 277. The letter is dated 1812.

26. Skinner, *op. cit.*, p. 506-7.

27. See Hallowell, "Sin, Sex and Sickness"; for the Blackfoot, see Skinner, "Societies of the Iowa, Kansa, and Ponca Indians," *Anthropological Papers, American Museum of Natural History*, 11 (1915), 726.

28. Wissler, "Societies and Dance Associations of the Blackfoot Indians," *Anthropological Papers, American Museum of Natural History*, 11 (1913), 445-7.

29. Leslie Spier, "The Sun Dance of the Plains Indians," *Anthropological Papers, American Museum of Natural History*, 14 (1921), 464.

30. G. Dorsey, "The Cheyenne," *Publications, Field Columbian Museum* (Anthropological Series 9 [1905]), Nos. 1-2, p. 158.

31. E. S. Curtis, *The North American Indian*, V (20 vols.; Cambridge, Mass.: 1907-1930), 79. It should be mentioned that in the Plains (as elsewhere in the Americas) there is a fetishistic attitude toward the shaman's rattle, a quality "emphasized in the sign language of the plains, where the sign for rattle is the basis of all signs indicating that which is sacred." F. W. Hodge, ed., *Handbook of American Indians North of Mexico* (Bulletin, Bureau of American Ethnology, No. 30, I [Washington, D. C.: 1907]), 355. The sacredness of this appurtenance of the shaman is extremely ancient in the New World and can perhaps be traced back to paleo-Siberian times.

32. W. P. Clark, *The Indian Sign Language* (Philadelphia: 1885), p. 45.

33. "Brackenridge's Journal," in R. G. Thwaites, ed., *Early Western Travels*, VI (32 vols.; Cleveland: 1904-1907), 131-2.

34. P. E. Beckwith, "Notes on Customs of the Dakotas," *Annual Report, Smithsonian Institution* (1886), Part I, p. 251.

35. Wissler, "Societies and Ceremonial Associations in the Oglala Division of the Teton-Dakota," *Anthropological Papers, American Museum of Natural History*,

49 CONFESSION AS CATHARTIC THERAPY

11 (1912), 1-110; see also Wissler, "Societies and Dance Associations," pp. 445, 447.

36. Skinner, "Societies of the Iowa," p. 726.

37. The woman chosen as tree-notcher in the Crow sun dance must be absolutely virtuous. The ceremonial leaders approach her with a buffalo tongue, and if she is not worthy of this honor she must openly confess, "My moccasin has a hole in it." She cannot then appear in the sun dance. R. H. Lowie, "The Sun Dance of the Crow Indians," *Anthropological Papers, American Museum of Natural History*, 16 (1915), 31. The Blackfoot women confess to the sun when they skin the tongues in the sun dance. Wissler, "Societies of the Iowa," pp. 236, 256.

38. Frances Densmore, "Winnebago Songs of the Peyote Ceremony," *Mss.* No. 3261, Bureau of American Ethnology, Smithsonian Institution (1932), p. 4; see also Densmore, *Mss.* No. 3205.

39. Paul Radin, "A Sketch of the Peyote Cult of the Winnebago," *Journal of Religious Psychology*, 7 (1914), 3; Radin, *Crashing Thunder* (New York: 1926), 177; Densmore, "Winnebago Songs"; and Mss. No. 3205.

40. J. Adair, *The History of the American Indians* (London: 1775), p. 150; W. Bartram, *Travels through North and South Carolina, Georgia, East and West Florida, the Cherokee Country, the Extensive Territories of the Muskogulges or Creek Confederacy, and the Country of the Chactaws* (Philadelphia: 1791), p. 507. The use of the black drink reminds us that, for the American Indian, cleansing from sin is often more literal and less symbolic than mere confession. The vomiting of peyote, which does indeed have a weedy, nauseating taste, is considered a punishment for one's sins, but it rids the body of uncleanness in the process. This symbolism is not an insignificant element to be brushed lightly aside: On one Arapaho fetish pouch collected by Kroeber, part of the beadwork depicts the "vomitings" deposited in a ring around the inside of the peyote *tipi;* the Osage (to the disdain of other tribes) go so far as to provide spittoons in their permanent, cement-floored churches. La Barre, "Primitive Psychotherapy," pp. 301-2. In a letter to the author, dated 1948, the late Dr. Edmund Bergler has kindly commented at length: "The astounding feature of verbalization of sins via an emetic casts doubts whether 'Father Peyote' does not camouflage 'Mother Peyote.' The child lives for a long time on the basis of alleged omnipotence, hence everything 'bad' comes from the outside, everything 'good' is taken for granted as provided by oneself. Sin means intrapsychically: 'Bad mother poisoned me.' Expelling the 'bad' via verbalization restores the original paradisiacal state of narcissistic bliss. The strange feature in Peyotism is the triad of hallucinatory exhilaration, vomiting, verbal confession. One could imagine that expelling bodily the 'poison of sin' supplements the expelling of the (swallowed) sin via words. In other words, Peyote vomiting is the pre-stage of confession, the bodily expression of the later confession. That trend of thoughts explains also the feeling of expiation after confession: sins are mutually forgiven because a community *of defensive alibis* is established: 'Mother, not I, is responsible.' . . . Peyotism adds an interesting feature to understanding of conscience. It represents a defensive alibi: via verbalization (psychic vomiting) the fantasy is maintained that all temptations comes from the outside. Thus the 'proof' is submitted that mother alone is the malefactor. The 'bad' milk is contrasted with the 'good' Peyote-'milk.' "

41. L. H. Morgan, *The League of the Ho-de-no-sau-nee, or Iroquois* (Rochester: 1851), pp. 170, 187-8. I believe that Morgan was mistaken in attributing Jesuit missionary origin to this confession.

42. F. Boas, "The Eskimo of Baffin Land and Hudson Bay," *Bulletin, American Museum of Natural History*, 15 (1901), 120-4; and Hodge, *op. cit.*, II: 406.

43. S. P. Krasheninnikoff, *The History of Kamschatka, and the Kurilski Islands, with the Countries Adjacent*, J. Grieve, trans. (London & Gloucester: 1764), p. 178.

Part Two

Traditional systems of psychotherapy rest
on widely accepted systems of belief
about the causes and cures of disease. Many
of these systems are highly differentiated
and incorporate such elements as
community participation and support
of the emotionally disturbed.

Jane M. Murphy

Psychotherapeutic Aspects of Shamanism on St. Lawrence Island, Alaska*

§ Introduction

THIS DISCUSSION of shamanism stems primarily from research experience in an Eskimo village on St. Lawrence Island, which is part of the State of Alaska. The St. Lawrence Islanders belong to a small group of arctic aborigines known as Siberian or Asiatic Eskimos who inhabit this island and a section of the coast of Siberia north of the Gulf of Anadyr. St. Lawrence, the largest island in the Bering Sea, is located near the Arctic Circle, 120 miles from Nome, Alaska, and forty miles from Indian Point, Siberia. Indian Point is the main village of Eskimos with which the St. Lawrence people were affiliated before communication was disrupted in the recent period of boundary control between the Soviet Union and the United States.

The island is situated at a transitional point between the Eskimo cultures of Alaska, the Canadian Arctic, and Greenland to the East and the Siberian cultures of the Chuckchee, Koryak, and Kamchadal to the West. Traditionally the St. Lawrence Islanders have displayed most of the characteristics typical of Eskimo cultures. The Eskimos generally are coastal and island people who depend primarily on arctic sea mammals for food and clothing, have well known patterns of dress and subsistence, and exhibit a characteristic theology centered on the shaman as a medico-religious practitioner. The cultural variations that set off the Si-

* The field work on which this paper is based was supported by the Cornell Social Science Research Center and Dr. and Mrs. Rex Murphy. The analysis was conducted as part of the Cornell Program in Social Psychiatry, directed by Alexander H. Leighton, with funds provided by the Ford Foundation. The Cornell Program is sponsored by the Department of Sociology in the College of Arts and Sciences, Cornell University, and the Department of Psychiatry of New York Hospital (Payne Whitney Clinic) and Cornell University Medical College.

berian Eskimos as a distinct group chiefly involve language and social structure. They speak a dialect of one of the two main branches of the Eskimo language—Yupik—which is spoken by the Siberian Eskimos and many groups in southwestern Alaska, in contrast to Inupik, which is the language group characteristic of the great majority of New World Eskimos. The St. Lawrence kinship system is organized on the principle of patrilineal clans, which is not the usual Eskimo custom.[1] Although they live in settlements that, during the years of recorded history, have gradually been amalgamated into two villages, they do not have the "community house" found in many other Eskimo groups. In several features, including the forms and practices of shamanism, they show marked affinity with the Siberian tribal groups, especially the Chuckchee.

The island was named in 1728 by Vitus Bering and was visited by a number of explorers of the North Pacific during the rest of the eighteenth century. It was relatively isolated from contact, however, until the period during the late nineteenth century when whale fishing flourished in these waters. In 1878-79 the islanders experienced a great famine, attributed by some to changed weather conditions that kept the winter ice and therefore the walrus away from the island. It is more generally believed, however, to have resulted from a prolonged debauch in which the Eskimos, drunk with liquor procured from whalers, did not lay in a supply of meat for the winter. Whatever the cause, the population was decimated, dropping from an estimated 1500 to 500, an attrition from which the island has never recovered. Following this famine, the St. Lawrence Eskimos instituted and have maintained a self-imposed restriction against the use of alcohol.

In 1894, the first permanent contact with the mainland was made when a combined school and mission was established by the Presbyterian Church. The school was built in the village of Sivokak, which was later renamed Gambell in memory of the first missionary. At the turn of the century, reindeer were introduced onto the island, and the second of the island's two villages, Savoonga, was formed at what had served for a few years as a herders' camp. At about the same time, a native-owned co-operative store was established, and goods from the white world began to be imported. In the early years of contact, the main sources of cash income were the sale of whale baleen and then of arctic fox pelts. But by 1940, the markets for both these commodities had essentially disappeared.

Although many changes had resulted from white contact—lumber houses, outboard motors, some education, and some religious conversion— until mid-century life continued to be directed primarily toward Eskimo goals. A reorientation of cultural patterns with pervasive influence from the modern world began to take shape after the Second World War, and, from that point on, the process of cultural change has proceeded at an extraordinarily accelerated rate. It has involved nearly continuous interaction with the personnel of armed-service installations on the island and for a time with the staff of a Civil Aeronautics Authority site near Gambell. Many islanders have lived temporarily on the mainland for work, further schooling, and especially hospitalization. Tuberculosis, the main cause of hospitalization among islanders, was exceedingly prevalent during the contact period until the late 1950s, when it was brought under control largely through a federal program of chemotherapy. There has also been some permanent migration to the Alaskan mainland, and a few St. Lawrence women have married white men and moved to places as far away as Pennsylvania and Arizona.

The research that resulted in these data about shamanism was conducted by two anthropologists and two psychiatrists.* During the summer of 1940, Alexander and Dorothea Leighton visited the island in order to study Eskimo personality development. During the year 1954-55, Charles Hughes and I lived in Gambell, in order to investigate social and cultural changes that were traceable in the period since 1940.[2] An additional purpose was to gain knowledge of the kinds and prevalence of physical and psychiatric illnesses on the island.[3] In all aspects of the field research, there was interest in the history, role, and techniques of the Eskimo medicine man or shaman.

The cultural history of St. Lawrence Island and the practice of shamanism are of psychiatric interest on three counts, only one of which will be considered here but all of which are to some extent intertwined:

1. St. Lawrence Island is in a geographical area where certain exotic forms of mental illness have been described. In the New World, the so-called "culture-specific" psychiatric syndromes characteristic of these peoples have been labeled "arctic hysteria" and *pibloktoq*.[4] The term "arctic hysteria" has also been applied to the "copying mania" (known by native terms like *amurakh*) that has been observed in the Siberian Arctic but does not appear to have crossed the Bering Strait into the New World.[5]

2. In varying forms and elaborations, seizures and possession also exist and have been given terminological recognition among these groups, some types being identified as psychiatric illnesses and others as part

* For this presentation, I have drawn on materials contained in my own unpublished field notes and in those of my colleagues. For the latter, grateful acknowledgment is made.

of the activity of shamanism. Possession as an aspect of shamanistic practice is found on both sides of the Bering Strait, but the wild paroxysms and peculiarly pathological tinge associated with shamanism in Siberia are the factors that have led some observers to equate the whole process of shamanizing with psychopathology and to question the psychic normality of virtually all shamanistic practitioners. The fact that the Siberian shamans described in early ethnographic works exhibited transvestism and other changes in sexually defined role—and sometimes homosexuality as well—in a manner not unlike that of the *berdache* among some American Indians, has also been taken as evidence of intrinsic emotional instability related to recruitment for and enactment of the shaman role. a sizable literature now exists on the topic of the normality or abnormality of shamans, but this issue is only tangentially relevant to the third point, which constitutes the theme of this chapter.[6]

3. Since the shaman role is culturally accredited for healing and curing, the established effectiveness of shamanistic treatment for certain kinds of illness has promoted interest in the therapeutic procedures entailed in shamanism. What follows is an effort to describe and analyze information about shamanism as practiced on St. Lawrence Island, in order to draw out the ways in which it is invested with therapeutic power.

§ St. Lawrence Island Shamanism

GENERAL DESCRIPTION

The term "shaman" as the name for a practitioner of healing rites is of Siberian origin. The terms "shamanistic" and "shamanizing," however, are commonly used to denote generic qualities of native medical practices, in Siberia and elsewhere, that involve certain types of magical and religious belief. Among the Eskimos of the New World, the medicine man is usually called *angahok*, with various dialectical distinctions employed in different groups. Among the St. Lawrence Islanders, he is known as *aliginalre*. In view of the similarities between the St. Lawrence Island brand of medical-psychiatric practice and that found among the Siberian tribes, the more familiar term "shaman" will be used here.

By 1955, most of the overt and dramatic manifestations of shamanism had disappeared from the life-ways of the St. Lawrence people. The years of white contact and the establishment of schools and missions have brought about a similarly marked decline in shamanistic activity in much of the Arctic. It may be that there are isolated pockets where it still flourishes openly, and various groups conceivably may have experienced or will experience shamanistic revival under circumstances of threatening cultural change, which, it has been observed, sometimes encourage revitalistic movements.[7] As far as St. Lawrence Island is concerned, by mid-century all but two of the total island population had become nominal Christians, and shamanism was considered the bulwark of the old ways that, outwardly at least, had been done away with. There were multiple evidences, however, that shamanism was still extremely viable at a less obvious level. Until the 1930s, there were reports that traveling ethnographers had actually witnessed shamanistic performances. In 1940 and 1955, it was not possible to attend a public, full-dress séance simply because they were nonexistent. Shamanism had taken cover in the face of the powerful odds of modern medicine and Christian evangelism.

Despite the recent submergence of shamanistic activity, the population of Gambell in the fifteen years between the two studies reported here included eighteen individuals who were said to have practiced or to be practicing some form of shamanism. A few of them had tried unsuccessfully to become shamans. Eight of these people were still alive in 1955. One of the two villagers who staunchly adhered to the Eskimo religion practiced what has been called familistic rather than professional shamanism. This distinction refers mainly to the fact that the professionals had more training and renown, were paid for their services, and accepted cases outside their own families. Two professional shamans in Gambell had joined the mission church but continued shamanistic practices on the side. One of them was a shaman of wide acclaim and reputation, and, during the 1954-55 investigation, it was reported that a few people visited or were visited by him in private sessions. The second was a younger man of lesser fame about whom there were rumors that he was "at it again"—also privately. The others had given up shamanism after accepting Western beliefs, and two of them were sufficiently attracted to a more modern way of life to have migrated to the mainland.

What can therefore be said about shamanism in its most recent form on St. Lawrence concerns continuing beliefs and practices that have been considerably attenuated and adulterated by the process of modernization. This statement applies to what was actually being done in 1955; general talk about shamanism provided a richer source of information. The earlier history of shamanism can thus be at least partially reconstructed from the recollections of days when more flamboyant performances were in vogue and from reports of early ethnographers and missionaries.

Both men and women have been shamans on St. Lawrence Island, as was commonly the case throughout the Arctic. A shaman usually entered the profession on the basis of a "call" reputed to be a subjective experience indicating that the candidate had been specially selected to fulfill the mission of healing. Initiation involved wandering alone on the tundra, going without sleep or food, and suffering a great deal of physical hardship and mental anguish. In a vision, the would-be shaman acquired a "spirit-familiar" with which he would later become possessed during the curing rites. In most cases, the spirit-familiar was a walrus or a polar bear or some other arctic animal.

On St. Lawrence Island, people are called "thin" if they seem to have telepathic perception—if they know uncanny things that other people do not know or are able to divine the future and find lost articles. Not every "thin man" is a shaman, but all shamans are "thin men." To "see things" brings prestige and is cultivated by many people. The mark of a shaman is his ability to put this power to use in curing. The difficulties of the initiation dissuade most people from the attempt, however.

It was reported by Eskimo informants on St. Lawrence Island that, during the time when candidates were trying to become shamans they would go "something like crazy for five days." The five-day period is said to be required by "Eskimo law" for shamanism. They do not eat or drink, yet they become so strong that even "ten men cannot hold them." One shaman told of staying outside during night storms, sleepless, crying to the spirits to help him obtain "the power to make the dead live." During these isolated wanderings, death and resurrection were enacted. The prospective shaman was supposed to break the bones of a bird five times and bring it back to life each time. It is said that people who became shamans felt very sick and perplexed during this time; they "go out of mind, but not crazy," and they felt all right again when they had "straightened up in their minds what was bothering them."*

Sometimes the shaman served an older mentor who trained him in the rudimentary techniques of primitive medicine and surgery and in ventriloquism and legerdemain, which also figure in the curing ceremony. Later, when he was called to heal a sick person or even to bring a dead person back to life, he performed a ritual attended by the patient's kin and many onlookers. His charismatic power and his frenzied mediumistic acts gave, by all reports, a heightened and distinctive aura to the performance. The séance was always carried out in a darkened room. It

* The phrases quoted from Eskimo informants here and throughout this section are taken primarily from the field notes of Jane M. Murphy and Charles C. Hughes. Page references are not given except for extended quotations.

began with singing and the beating of Eskimo drums. When an intense pitch of emotion and attention had been reached and while the audience continued to sing and drum loudly, maintaining seated positions in which no one touched his neighbor, the shaman would have a seizure. He would fall unconscious to the floor and would rise after a time, with changed visage and possessed by his spirit-familiar, to carry on the drama.

Although séances apparently varied considerably according to the special proficiencies of the shamans, histrionic possession by the spirit-familiar was an integral part of the curing ritual, as can be seen from the following description of a St. Lawrence shamaness, one who was reputed to be of only middling abilities and who would be classed as a familistic shamaness:

> When my brother was sick, my grandmother who was a shamaness tried her best to get him well. She did all her part, acting as though a dog, singing some songs at night, but he died. While she was singing, she fell down so hard on the floor, making a big noise. After about fifteen minutes later we heard the tapping of her fingers and her toes on the floor. Slowly she got up, already she had become like a dog. She looks awful. My grandfather told me that he used to hide his face with his drum just because she looks different, changed and awful like a dog, very scary. She used to crawl back and forth on the floor, making big noises. Even though my brother was afraid of her, he tried not to hide his face, he looked at her so that he would become well. Then my grandmother licked his mouth to try to pull up the cough and to blow it away. Then after half hour, she fell down so hard on the floor again (JMM, August 22, 1955, p. 21).

As an introduction to the curing rites or as part of the performance conducted during possession, the shaman would do a number of "tricks," as they are now called in the vocabulary of the bilingual St. Lawrence Islanders. The catalogue of magical tricks performed by St. Lawrence shamans is long and various. Bogoras, the famous ethnographer of the Chuckchee, reported that W. F. Doty, a missionary on St. Lawrence Island in 1898, had been present during a séance when the shaman was supposed to sink into the ground until only the hair of his head remained visible. In his diary, Doty described putting his hand on the shaman's head and feeling it sink lower. He attributed it, rightly or wrongly, to the shaman's ability to perform a turtle-like recession of the head into the body. Bogoras himself attended another St. Lawrence séance in which a shaman, with arms crossed on his bare chest, made a walrus skin adhere to his shoulders without the support of any visible straps or fasteners yet with sufficient tenacity to pull Bogoras, who was holding on to it, out of the room.[8]

One shaman, described as "very *aliginalre*" by Eskimo informants, was reputed to wrap a walrus skin rope around his neck and to direct two men standing on either side of him to pull it as hard as possible until it cut off his head. He would then wrap the head in a raincoat and have someone carry it down to the edge of the ice and throw it into the sea. When the errand was accomplished and the group reassembled, they would find that his head was fastened on again. A certain shamaness was said to gnaw her hands until they were bleeding and then, with her tongue, to lick them back into wholeness. Another reported trick was for a shaman to crush a stone between his hands, grinding it away until there was only a pile of sand at his feet, and then to pick up the sand and reform it into a stone. One shaman could make the parka of his patient rise from the ground and stand up with nobody in it and nothing for support.

It was recounted that, in a séance witnessed by the American physical anthropologist, Riley Moore, the shaman made "tin cans talk" during his seizure and threw his voice into other furnishings about the room.* One shaman had two spirit-familiars: They were said to carry on a conversation during the seizure; one of them spoke understandable Eskimo, the other "talked in tongues" or, as the informant put it, "didn't say the right words." Another trick during possession was for the shaman to produce sounds as though the spirits were walking around underneath the floor of the house—demonstrated by thumping and pounding until, as one informant recalled from her childhood, the house seemed to shake and rattle as though it were made of tissue paper and everything seemed to be up in the air, flying about the room. Still another shaman was noted for his fox spirit, which could be seen running around the rim of the drum while the shaman was in seizure.

It should be noted for the moment that some of the tricks were carried out preliminary to the main part of the curing rite, as if to set the stage, while some were performed during seizure. The "trick" aspect of the ritual provided considerable scope for the extemporaneous and individual talents of the shaman. Some shamans were more imaginative or better ventriloquists than others, while some were more dexterous at sleight of hand. Whatever the specific content of this part of the performance, the common purpose was the spectacular establishment of the preternatural powers of the chief actor in a drama before his audience.

The elements of shamanism described so far can be said to express the shaman's individual creativity and originality and to involve primarily

---

* Described by an Eskimo informant in the field notes of Alexander H. Leighton.

the interaction between the shaman and a group of onlookers. Many of the therapeutic measures standardized in shamanism involved a more direct relationship between the shaman and his patient and, at the same time, were more uniformly the outgrowths of indigenous concepts of the nature of disease. The shaman, in other words, activated cultural beliefs about the causes and cures of illness. It can safely be assumed that, without widespread subscription to these beliefs among the population at large, shamanism would be meaningless and impotent, and, in a group that had experienced a full revolution in modern scientific thinking, shamans would therefore be unable to function. The efficacy of shamanism in a group undergoing acculturation depends on compartmentalization of new and old beliefs and concomitant assignment of a province of truth to the old beliefs, to be separate from the new. It has been observed, for example, that a common way of making shamanistic beliefs about illness compatible with the ideas of Western medicine among the native population is to accept theories of germ transmission as explanations of "how" disease occurs but to adhere to shamanistic theories to explain "why" one person and not another is inflicted with disease.[9] In light of these considerations, some discussion of St. Lawrence ideas about the causes of illness is warranted.

ETIOLOGICAL ORIENTATIONS

For the organization of this discussion, it is useful to refer to the catalogue of indigenous etiologies employed by Clements[10] in a study designed to plot the distribution of various primitive theories of disease causation from a worldwide survey of ethnographic literature. He focused on five beliefs commonly found in non-Western groups. These beliefs are that disease is caused by soul-loss; breach of taboo; disease sorcery; object intrusion; and spirit intrusion. In the St. Lawrence Island study, analysis of the materials collected in investigations of the prevalance of physical and psychiatric illnesses indicated that this group of Eskimos made extensive use of the first four beliefs in explaining disease. The interpretation of data about spirit intrusion needs special explanation, which will be furnished later in this chapter. Each of these five categories is related to shamanism.

Soul Loss. The island is located in the same geographic area where Clements found a florescence of the idea that disease is caused by the loss of the patient's soul. This etiology was many times pointed out in the accounts of illness given by St. Lawrence informants. It is believed that a person's soul wanders abroad at night while he is asleep or that it departs from his body when he sneezes or is frightened suddenly. On any of these occasions, the soul may be captured by evil, predatory spirits that abound in the universe, and, until it is returned to the patient's body, disease holds sway.

This belief lies behind numerous preventive measures, as, for example, when the image of an open eye is painted on the eyelids of a child so that when he is asleep it will look as though he were awake and the malevolent spirits will be fooled and pass over him. It was also a supportive belief for the curative measures of shamanism. One of the most frequently employed techniques was for the shaman in possession to say that his spirit-familiar had departed from the premises of the curing rite and was searching the under worlds and the sky worlds for the lost soul of his patient. The son of one of St. Lawrence Island's famous shamans said that his father's spirit-familiar would undertake such an errand and could travel the eighty miles to and from Indian Point or Savoonga in less than five minutes—"just like electricity," he said—and would come back with information important to the search for the lost soul.

Many of the St. Lawrence folk tales deal with the experiences of shamans and their spirit-familiars in such pursuits. The same kind of adventure story-telling forms part of the shaman's performance during the séance. Needless to say, the narratives usually involve great feats of strength, endurance, perspicacity, and sometimes even a struggle between the evil spirit who wants to keep the patient's soul in thrall and the shaman's spirit who wants to release the soul and thus return the patient to health. The house-shaking thumps and rattles, which have been vividly described by St. Lawrence informants, were said to be the signal of the spirit's return from the nether world to the room where the rite was being enacted. Subsequently the shaman would make his report. Sometimes he would have to conduct more than one search during a séance or, presumably, during a series of séances before he could cure the patient. And sometimes, of course, he was forced to surrender in the face of death or continuing illness.

If the patient were repeatedly sick or did not respond to the soul-recovery ritual, the shaman might utilize still another therapy based on the soul-loss idea. This technique was used mainly for children and young people and involved a change-of-name ceremony, the purpose of which was to give the patient a new soul and to alter his appearance and disguise his previous identity so that the marauding spirits would not recognize him. In Eskimo ideology, the soul and the name are one phenomenon, and names are not sex-linked. The Eskimos believe in reincarnation through the successive generations of a family. When a person dies, he is believed to be reincarnated in the child upon whom his name is conferred. If the soul of a patient is constantly being attacked by evil spirits, however, the shaman may decide that a new name-soul will protect the patient from illness.

This kind of ritual was described as the shaman's "changing everything and making everything right." The customary prescription for a girl would be that she cut her hair like a boy's, start smoking a pipe, wear boy's clothing, and associate with male groups. For a boy, it would be to don girl's clothing and feminine demeanor. Such other kinds of disguise as blackening the teeth might also be advised. Despite the decline in shamanism, a number of villagers had experienced this kind of therapy in their early years and then had gradually resumed their normal sex roles. Presumably, if shamanistic belief were still orthodox and intact, some of these people would have maintained the sexual metamorphosis and might possibly therefore have been recruited to the ranks of the shamans who practiced transvestism and homosexuality. During the 1954-55 field trip, one ten-year-old girl was undergoing the change-of-name-and-sex therapy and for several years had dressed and behaved like a boy. She was the daughter of one of the remaining adherents to the Eskimo religion—and the practitioner of familistic shamanism mentioned earlier. Her deviance in dress was not very noticeable, however, in present-day circumstances—in which girls commonly wear blue jeans—and an outsider might easily have attributed it to "tomboyism" had it not been specifically pointed out.

Breach of Taboo. Another belief that had considerable currency among the St. Lawrence people was that disease is caused by a breach of taboo or the violation of Eskimo ethics and morals. In a variety of cultural groups, it is or has been believed that such acts as incest, sexual perversion, or masturbation are disease-provoking transgressions. Often these acts have been named specifically as the causes of insanity. In many such groups the "breach of taboo" concept of etiology is linked with a belief that the effects of such a transgression may be felt by people other than the offender—belief that the sins of the father are visited even to the seventh generation, for example—and that a whole family or community may be endangered by an individual's personal offense against societal regulations. As a counterpart to these beliefs, a shaman may bring the full force of his telepathic perception to bear on the problem of ferreting out the nature and content of the patient's iniquity or that of a relative. A usual accompaniment to this effort is an elaborate ritual of public confession, following which the shaman prescribes the appropriate acts of expiation that will bring about a cure.

Among the St. Lawrence people, the "breach of taboo" idea seemed to have a somewhat different quality in both its causal and curative manifestations, although it seemed firmly allied to the belief that the adverse results of sin could touch a wider group than the individual who committed it. This difference was apparent at least as these ideas were portrayed in the concrete examples by informants who were asked to discuss the actual illnesses of people living in the village. It should be mentioned here that most of the evidence presented in this chapter emerged from case-by-case analysis and that only on a few restricted topics were questions asked at the abstract level of what kinds of cause *could* lead to disease rather than what causes had led to this particular disease. Within this empirical context, it appeared that the main violations considered causal to illness involved maltreatment of animals and such offenses against the hunting code as not sharing meat equitably or claiming and pursuing to the kill a whale that had been sighted first by someone else.

The St. Lawrence Eskimos believe that, if the proper acts of respect and consideration for animals are not carried out, the animal spirits will be offended and will cause the animals to withdraw from the island so that they no longer offer themselves to humans as meat for subsistence. Thus the behavior defined as sinful enough to result in disease or death was that considered threatening to the survival of the group as a whole or an infringement of the laws about individual rights and social sharing relating to the administration of the most vital sources of food supply.

The definitions of "sin" and "transgression" always have a social context, but in terms of disease causation the St. Lawrence people emphasize the relatively public violations, which everyone is likely to know about and which affect the whole group, compared to the relatively private ones, which are confined to the individual or to sexual partnership and therefore require detection and confession.

Sexual deviance was not, however, ignored in their system of morals. Homosexuality, for example, was severely disapproved even though the transvestite shamans who sometimes practiced homosexuality were thought to be the most powerful. But it was not these relatively private kinds of sin that were considered to cause illness. It seems probable that the public nature of sins believed to be disease provoking is related to the fact that confessional seems to have been less important in St. Lawrence shamanism than were some other aspects. It was said, for example, that what the shaman did during séance was to find out what wrong had been committed and, through consultation with the spirit-familiars, to discover what atonement was necessary in order to rectify the situation and return the patient to a state of health. But, in comparison to some other Eskimo groups, the confessional *per se* does not appear to have been crucial. As a matter of fact, one could almost say that public transgressions affecting the whole group were so potent as causes of disease in the St. Lawrence ideology that they were resistant even to shamanistic cure. An outstanding example of this resistance was given in an account of a man who lost several relatives in succession, despite many efforts at shamanistic intervention—their illnesses being attributed in the last analysis to his abuse of the hunting law.

Disease Sorcery. The third concept in the Clements classification is disease sorcery. This concept, too, is a fully formulated belief in St. Lawrence thinking and has numerous concomitants in shamanistic practice. Where witchcraft is the suspected cause of disease, the techniques of the shaman and the sorcerer overlap to a large extent: The sorcerer's methods involve black magic directed at causing illness or voodoo death, while the shaman's efforts center on counteracting these forces by stronger and more effective magic.

The St. Lawrence term for sorcerer or witch is *auvinak*. As in other cultures, the sorcerer's art includes magical formulas and evil prayers, which are carried out in secret rituals. The specific content of witchcraft on St. Lawrence Island need not be spelled out here, for it involves the usual machinations with effigies and potions. A frequent custom was for the sorcerer to persuade a suggestible or possibly mentally defective person to obtain from his intended victim a piece of clothing, a strand of hair, or a nail paring. Then late at night, alone and away from the village, the sorcerer would boil the scraps of cloth and hair in an animal skull. If a person believed that he had been hexed or bewitched in this way, he would seek help from a shaman, who would try to intercept the malevolent magic. Part of the shaman's task in this kind of curing was to discover who was the witch and what form of black magic had been used, so that appropriate countermagic could be instituted.

The St. Lawrence people make a very clear distinction between the healing magic of the shaman and the black magic of the sorcerer, and apparently only a very powerful shaman would undertake cases that required countersorcery. It is said that shamans were reluctant to dabble in this kind of activity for fear that they "might get the habit of it." Nonetheless, preoccupation with witchcraft seemed to be rampant in the St. Lawrence population, and there were more accounts of people said to have died because they had been hexed than of people who had been saved from witchcraft by shamanistic therapy.

An obvious interpretation is that magical forces, in a group that subscribes to such beliefs, can be extremely potent forces for either good or evil ends, just as scientific acumen can be directed to both constructive and destructive goals. An awareness of the Janus-like quality of magic has led to measures of control in nonliterate groups, just as safeguards and ethics for the use of scientific knowledge have been developed in Western culture. For example, in a West African group where medicine men tend to band together in societies of specialists, it was found that, in order to qualify for membership, each individual had to swear a kind of Hippocratic Oath, promising never to use black magic and to employ his techniques only for healing. Such a ceremony was witnessed once by Alexander H. Leighton.[11]

In a highly individualistic pattern like that of the St. Lawrence shamans, where no medical society or priesthood exists, control of malpractice in the shamanistic arts is clearly informal—as indicated by the comment about shamans not wanting to have reputations for the "habit" of sorcery. Control may be not only less formal but also less effective in such a group. There was evidence in at least one of the St. Lawrence accounts that a fine line exists between the power to heal and the power to kill and that the balance tips one way or the other depending upon the individual practitioner. The following report gives some hints that the shaman was, in fact, dabbling in sorcery:

My father was very sick, and the shaman was going to help him to get well. He took five gravel rocks and told my father to eat them and that when his bowels move, he will throw away his sickness. It was dark in the room and then we heard the shaman's spirit come in, he was a great heavy fellow, it talks just like a man, and he was jumping around the room and the floors of our room were shaking. Then the spirit talked and he called the shaman foolish, and he said: "Don't fool your patient, you are not going to help him, you are just going to make him suffer more." I could hear that spirit slap the shaman. Then the spirit said to my father: "Those five stones will not make you well. They mean that your wife will get pregnant five times and each time one or two days after the child is born it will die. You will lose five children. The shaman is very foolish and he is telling you a lie that the stones will cure you. You shouldn't have believed him, now you have done wrong, you have just like thrown away those children." Then the spirit went away and we turned on the lights and the shaman sat there with his head down, and he said: "I'm not telling you a lie, that spirit, he is the one who is lying." But just in a little bit the spirit jumped again and said: "I'm listening to you. I'm here, and I'm not telling them a lie, you are." (JMM, August 12, 1955, p. 10)

The fact that the patient's wife *did* lose a number of children in succession no doubt lent credence to the accusation of sorcery, especially in the recollection of the event.

The shaman involved in this description was believed to be one of the most powerful and controversial practitioners on St. Lawrence Island during the period of investigation. In addition to accusations of evil practice, successful cures and unusually keen dramatic and magical abilities were attributed to him. The séance reported above is rather complex, and it demonstrates among other things that, in any given séance, the rites connected with more than one idea of disease causation may be employed. It is possible, for example, that the shaman was trying to establish that eating the five pebbles had been a "wrong" and to induce the patient, who was the father in this case, to *confess* this wrong and on the basis of the confessional to be cured. The pebbles can also be interpreted as "object intrusion," the next belief to be discussed.

Object Intrusion. The belief that disease can be caused by the intrusion of a foreign *object* into the patient's body was well developed in the St. Lawrence system although, like taboo breaking it, was not so important as soul loss. The meaning of the belief itself is self-evident. It involves the supposition that illness is created by a foreign element that must be extracted or expelled if health is to be restored. The shamanistic cures that stemmed from this belief varied in particular techniques, but in each the shaman was able to produce an object or objects that could be shown to the séance audience as proof that the disease had been cured.

Some shamans were known to suck at whatever part of the anatomy was in pain and then to spit out small stones that could be passed about as evidence. One St. Lawrence shaman was noted for another kind of "operation" involving object extraction. During the singing and drumming of the séance, he would appear to thrust his own drumstick into the stomach of the patient. When the stick was removed, there would be a writhing black thing—"something like a worm"—attached to the end of it. In the dimly lit room, the shaman would show the stick about and then eat the worm-like thing, demonstrating by this final act that the disease had been consumed by the spirit-familiar and was no longer noxious to the human patient. There were numerous

variations on this theme. In the example on page 66, the shaman told
his patient to eat five pebbles, saying that, when the stones had passed
through his system and been ejected in the stools, the patient would be
purged of his illness. In describing this incident, the informant, who
was an Eskimo woman of little education but who occasionally displayed
flashes of exquisite perception, said that this performance was "acting
out sickness."

Spirit Intrusion. The belief that a foreign *spirit* can be intruded into
the body of a human being has two aspects, which must be understood in the context of ideas about the causes and cures of illness. In
cultures where spirit intrusion is believed to cause disease, detecting
the spirit's identity is one of the diagnostic procedures of the curer,
and the therapeutic technique is ritual exorcism. Spirit intrusion in
this sense is usually invoked to account for insanity and episodic hysteria. The symbolic utterances of madness may be interpreted as the
voice of the supernatural being who resides in the insane person.
Similar phenomena have been reported among some of the central and
eastern Eskimo groups. A psychotic Aivilik Eskimo woman, for example,
was diagnosed as having stolen from someone else a fox, which was
causing her illness, and she later came to be believe that a fox was
living inside her. Her voice became hoarse from barking, and she clawed
a fester inside her mouth where she thought a fox hair was coming
out.[12]

The disease-causing aspect of spirit intrusion was not highly developed in the St. Lawrence system of beliefs. A comparable notion, however, was held by the St. Lawrence people. It was believed, as in
several other cultures, that the ghost of a recently deceased person might
hover about and attack a living relative with sickness, especially if
there were reason to blame that relative in any way for the death
through broken taboo. Such a ghost was thought to be particularly
efficacious in producing illness during the period of mourning. Gradually his power would wane, however, and it would be completely
vitiated when a new child was born into the family and named after
the deceased, thus indicating that reincarnation had taken place and
the wandering ghost brought into the human community again. There
are conceptual differences between ghost-attack and spirit intrusion,
although it seems clear that there is also an affinity in the two ideas.
If a shaman were called in to cure an illness based on a ghost attack,
his main contribution would be to diagnose the case in séance and to
prescribe or conduct acts of protection. It is of tangential interest at this
point to describe the clearest case in the St. Lawrence materials in

which this idea was employed. In 1955, after the sudden death of a man, the controversial shaman already mentioned, approached the daughter of the deceased and said that he could see the ghost of her father close beside her all the time. He suggested that she was likely to become sick unless she came to him for help. If through suggestibility the woman had developed an illness, the iatrogenic base would be clear. It is impossible to say how characteristic this kind of activity on the part of a shaman may have been. In view of the withering influence of shamanism by mid-century, it is conceivable that this particular shaman was attempting to maintain his practice through nefarious means. His effort in this case was ineffectual, and, although the daughter was visibly disconcerted by his pronouncement, her comment was, "That old shaman was only trying to frighten me; it is a good thing we have put away all those old stuffs."

The relative absence or at least the attenuated existence of the spirit-intrusion belief may well be the logical outcome of the emphasis placed on soul loss by these Eskimos. Concentration on the idea of driving out offending spirits seems incompatible with the emphasis among St. Lawrence shamans on restoring the soul to the patient after it has been captured by evil spirits. Whatever the reasons, shamanistic practice in this group does not focus on ritual exorcism, but, as previously indicated, spirit possession is a *sine qua non* of St. Lawrence shamanistic activity. The similarities between spirit intrusion and spirit possession have often led to confusion in interpreting data about primitive beliefs and practices. Some writers have viewed the possession syndrome as evidence of the shaman's intrinsic insanity.[13] It is useful to distinguish the two types of spirit residence in a human being. "Intrusion" covers those beliefs that indicate that spirits have caused illness and can be detected through diagnosis; "possession" covers phenomena that do not necessarily imply illness. From the St. Lawrence reports, it appears that the Eskimos themselves do not consider shamans insane— shamans were known, in the vernacular, to be "out of mind" during initiation and possession, but they *are not crazy.* Possession, to the St. Lawrence Eskimos, is the mark of curing abilities rather than of disease itself.

OBJECTIVE TREATMENTS

With the exception of the techniques of object extraction and the "sucking out cough" employed by the dog-inspirited shamaness, the shamanistic procedures flowing from the indigenous concepts of etiology just described have mainly involved psychological interaction between the shaman and his patient or between the shaman and the group of on-lookers. The St. Lawrence shamans also employed a number of objective therapies that entailed physical contact between the shaman and the patient. These therapies too hinged upon native views of the nature of illness. They included "blowing away," "sucking out," or "brushing aside" sickness. In the "blowing away" technique, the shaman would put his hand on the painful area of the patient's body, where sickness was thought to be attacking, and after reciting some incantations he would lift his hand and blow the sickness out of his palm. The "sucking" method described earlier—though not in the best hygienic tradition—was believed to permit the spirit-familiar inside the shaman to "magnetize" the sickness and draw it out of the patient's body into the spirit-protected body of the shaman. The "brushing" technique involved having the patient lie down, usually near an inanimate object like a log of wood or a saw but sometimes even beside a dog. With sweeping motions, the shaman would brush the sickness from the patient onto the object or dog. When the transfer had been accomplished, the object would be broken to pieces or the dog killed.

One instance was recounted in which a mother asked that her daughter's illness (reputedly pneumonia) be brushed onto herself. It was done, and the daughter recovered while the mother subsequently died—whether from having contracted the disease through infection or from autosuggestion and the psychological impact of the ritual will never, of course, be known. Nonetheless, this incident is somewhat similar to the ritual suicides that were formerly practiced on the island.[14] In these rituals, a parent might beg to have himself stabbed, shot, or hanged; and if he were sufficiently persistent, this execution would be carried out. Sometimes a parent would actually take his own life. A frequent motive was to save the life of a sick child by the self-sacrifice of the parent's life.

The concept that upholds these therapeutic measures is that disease has an objective reality, with a cause, a beginning, and a series of definable outcomes. Some of its characteristics may be uppermost in one phase of its course, while others are more prominent in other parts. There seems to be a fairly clear-cut belief that a disease is a defined entity that cannot be in two places at the same time; it is either in the body of the patient, or it is not. Its removal can be effected by the sucking, blowing, and brushing techniques. Allied with this concept is the idea of disease transmission, and, although it has little in common with germ theory in other regards, there is a straightforward recognition that disease can pass from one person to another or from a person to some kind of inanimate or supernatural agent.

In addition, disease is believed to flourish in certain habitats and to be rendered harmless in others, an idea that has considerable similarity with much of Western medicine. For example, a disease that might injure or impair a human being can be rendered ineffectual by blowing it into the air, where it becomes benign. Disease is also conceived as impotent if introduced into an immunized system—one protected by a spirit-familiar, for example. And finally, some kinds of disease are believed to run predetermined courses that can be terminated only by violent acts of destruction. If such a disease can be transmitted to some object considered more expendable than the patient, it can be destroyed by killing or breaking the surrogate disease-carrier. It is doubtful, of course, that the Eskimos would voluntarily generalize about their diagnostic concepts or their view of the nature of disease in exactly the words put forth in this analysis. Nevertheless, it is clear from their own descriptions of this system of belief and practice that they recognize the links between the therapies carried out by shamans and the body of thought that was crucial to the effectiveness of certain shamanistic procedures.

There was one other kind of therapy frequently employed by shamans, one that is more difficult to classify according to its psychological and physical import—lapping a wound with the tongue. It is not immediately evident whether it should be considered a magical or a medicinal technique. The St. Lawrence shamans were reputed to have cured "big cuts," smashed hands, gun-shot wounds, and frozen limbs by this means. Lapping can be viewed in the same frame of reference as can sucking and blowing, and perhaps these procedures were so intermingled that it would be impossible to disentangle their psychological from their physical significance. The saliva of many animals appears to assist healing. The descriptions of lapping cures suggest that they were modeled on the self-healing accomplished by dogs, a method that could be observed and copied by Eskimos. It is perhaps not too great a stretch of credulity to imagine also that, at one time, the arctic aborigines were freer of infectious organisms than they now are and perhaps also better equipped with certain types of native regenerative power than are city-dwellers. Whatever the explanation, lapping seems to have been a common shamanistic practice.

The kinds of damage to which lapping was apparently most frequently applied point up another characteristic of St. Lawrence beliefs about disease. Like virtually every known group, these Eskimos believed in natural causation and were in no way blind to the fact that injury follows accident, freezing comes from exposure, and natural death attends old age.

In addition to the techniques that primarily involve or are mixed with psychological elements—either in terms of beliefs about etiology, group support, the transcendant psychic power of the shaman, or the objectification of recovery—the shaman's repertory includes a number of even more strictly physical treatments than we have mentioned so far. The arctic pharmacopoeia is limited—probably in part because vegetable growth on permafrost is sparse and limited in variety—so that St. Lawrence shamanism is in that respect very different from the treatments of native herbal doctors in the tropics of Africa, for example. There were a few roots and leaves known to the St. Lawrence Islanders, however, as effective treatment for nosebleeding, for hastening the eruption of skin lesions in measles, or for clearing the sinus and throat—"like Vicks" as one informant put it. Urine was used extensively for cleansing and medicinal purposes, and ear wax was another "old-timer" prescription for sores and abscesses. Most of these substances were used as home remedies or by familistic shamans, although they also figure in reports of the practices of professional shamans.

Surgical amputation, trephining, lancing, and bloodletting were among the treatments practiced by professional shamans in the Bering Sea area. The arctic shaman's knowledge of anatomy stemmed from experience in dismembering animals after the hunt, which probably gave him a sense of familiarity in dissection and may also have provided insight into the placement of joints and muscles. Whatever the background, many shamans had reputations for admirable surgical and chiropractic skill.

Some of the early ethnographic reports give vivid testimonials to the unsanitary conditions in which shamans conducted their operations and registered amazement that any patient ever recovered. For example, a dirty lemming skin might be used to bandage wounds or to quench the flow of blood. Despite such invitations to infection, the shaman's power as a healer was attested in many reports of patients who recovered following these treatments. We can hardly judge the sanitary or unsanitary nature of his techniques since we know so little about the ecological balance between man and environment in such groups before contact was established with the outside world. It therefore remains a question how much credit belongs to the shaman and how much to "nature."

§ Analysis

On the basis of this description of the practices and beliefs related to St. Lawrence shamanism, it is now pertinent to analyze these ma-

terials in terms of the shaman's role in Eskimo society and the psychotherapeutic elements that the practice of shamanism entails.

THE ROLE OF THE SHAMAN IN ST. LAWRENCE ESKIMO SOCIETY

In a hunting and gathering culture like that of this Eskimo group,
most social tasks are divided between the men, who hunt, and the women,
who serve as gatherers and homemakers. The need for a healer is one
of the few prerequisites for maintaining a productive social group that
is not comprehended in the ascribed roles of sex and age or the basic
division of labor connected with subsistence. In the 1940 and 1955 investigations, relatively few people served as shamans: eighteen out of a
population of approximately 250 adults, to be exact. Such relative scarcity
may not, however, always have been the case. It has been conjectured,
for example, that professional shamanism developed out of family shamanism and that, in cultural history, female shamanism preceded male
shamanism.[15] If such an evolution of role did actually occur historically,
it probably took place in three stages: At one time, nearly all adult
women shamanized at least by the time they reached old age; then
most adult men, as well as women shamanized; and finally, in recent
history, the role has crystallized into a more exclusive professional
position involving considerable training and talent.

It is difficult to tell from the St. Lawrence data how accurately this
evolutionary paradigm applies or what difference it has made in terms
of both physical and psychological treatments employed. Reference has
already been made to evidence that shamanism was changing during
the period of the investigation—its decline in fifteen years is the foremost
demonstration. The vestiges of shamanism that remained, however,
were of both the professional and family type. Family shamanism involved the family as onlookers and demonstrated the same dramatic characteristics of possession and control by a spirit familiar as did professional
shamanism, although there seemed to be less emphasis on the preliminary
tricks performed. It is possible that family shamanism was a first line
of defense, the failure of which would lead to seeking the services of
a more renowned and expensive practitioner whose treatment would be
essentially the same in terms of the psychotherapeutic elements involved.
Also family shamanism may have been a more important aspect of social
functioning before the consolidation of isolated family settlements into
larger villages. Under conditions of isolation, it may well have been
necessary for each family to have one member who could undertake the
tasks of healing should disaster befall.

Whether or not the family-professional dichotomy means anything in
reference to the therapeutic aspects of shamanizing, it is apparent that

the St. Lawrence Islanders had a system of their own by which differences in shamans' proficiency were indicated. In English, the evidence lay in such phrases as "really shaman," "sort of shaman," "partly shaman," and "foolish shaman," the last term being used for anyone considered a "quack." The three or four people called "really shaman" were male practitioners. Whether or not this sex bias was a matter of the special history of these Eskimos and the smallness of the group cannot be determined. In the ethnographies of other Eskimo groups, a few shamanesses were reported to be similarly capable. The general orientation of the St. Lawrence group, however, was to foster male dominance and to expect men to fill the most eminent roles in the society. Being a man may therefore have played a part in establishing the accredited practitioner as a powerful individual in the eyes of the islanders.

In view of the fact that the role of shaman was an achieved role that only certain people could fill, it appears logical to conclude that certain kinds of individual deviance would incline people to it ("deviance" is used here to mean any characteristic that makes a person exceptional). The exceptional qualities of the people who became shamans may have further endowed the role with prestige and power and enhanced the group's view that shamans are special or omnipotent.

In an effort to understand what kinds of exceptional characteristic might fit people for the shaman role and thus invest the role itself with perceived power, the following list of qualifications has been drawn up from the St. Lawrence materials.

Age. Advanced age was undoubtedly a prestige factor for some shamans. Although age was not a necessary qualification, most of the shamans in the St. Lawrence population were adults or elders at the prime of their practice. In several St. Lawrence Island folk tales and in reports from the neighboring Chuckchee, a young person or even a child figures as a shaman.[16] Such was only the case, however, when the child was also an orphan, a factor that will be discussed later.

Sex. Both men and women shamanized, although it appears that men had a greater likelihood of being extraordinarily successful than did women. Sexual deviance, however, in the form of transvestism and homosexuality did characterize the role to some extent. An early report on the *Population of Anadyr District* by Gondatti and cited by Bogoras[17] indicated that at Indian Point the "transformed shamans have a great and baleful influence."* Gondatti tried to counteract this influence, and

---

* Bogoras used the term "transformation" to refer to all stages of the process of identifying with the opposite sex. Some of the more completely "transformed" male shamans for example, were reputed to lose the male desires altogether, to practice

Bogoras believed that he had been successful because, when Bogoras himself visited there, he saw only an invalid transvestite who had assumed female dress as a child to relieve himself of his chronic ailment.

Nevertheless, the tradition of transvestism and homosexuality either separately or as part of shamanizing has not been entirely extinguished on St. Lawrence Island. The St. Lawrence term for "soft man" or "womanly man" is *anasik*, and the counterpart for women is *uktasik*. In 1940, one informant recalled a "transformed" male visitor from Siberia who believed himself to be pregnant. He was so ashamed that he committed suicide by having himself abandoned on another island, and the story goes that the following year the corpses of an adult and a child were found where he had been left. In Gambell itself, the previous site of a *ningloo* house was pointed out as the abode of five men who lived together. They were all reputed to look like women and to dress in the female fashion. None of them hunted, and they were provided for by neighbors. All were said to be "good singers"—a comment that may have been an oblique reference to shamanism but not necessarily so. Another man was remembered as having had a feminine appearance and as never having had sexual intercourse with a woman, although he was considered a good hunter.

In the village population between 1940 and 1955, one man was said to be *anasik* and another "partly *anasik*," but neither one shamanized. It thus seems evident that, by mid-century, this aspect of the shaman's role had been suppressed, however effective it may once have been in underscoring the exceptional natures of those who became shamans. Nor can it be determined from the available materials that people who had pronounced *anasik* or *uktasik* tendencies in their personalities necessarily became shamans. In all probability, such characteristics were one factor in selective recruitment, but in other cases it was reported that, during the shaman initiation, the "call" from the spirit-familiar might include instructions that the candidate become sexually "transformed," exactly as a shaman might prescribe for a patient.

Orphan Status. Another element related to shamanism is the fact that orphans often went into shamanizing. That they did so was a prevalent idea in St. Lawrence lore even though it was not demonstrated in the life histories of actual shamans. Among the Angmagssalik Eskimos in Greenland, however, Rasmussen[19] noted that most of the shamans apprenticed

---

homosexuality in culturally recognized marriages with other men, and even to acquire the organs of women. Others similarly called "transformed" were known to be homosexual, to practice transvestism, to be allied to other men in marriage but to have female mistresses on the side, and even to produce children by them.[18]

to established practitioners were orphans and that an old shaman would spot such a child, encourage him to look for his dead mother in a vision, and then train him in shamanistic skills.

Physical Disability. Physical incapacity was another exceptional attribute. Of the shamans remembered in the St. Lawrence population, one had been blind and another had had palsy. It is likely that such people were sufficiently disabled so that they could not perform normal cultural roles and may have resorted to shamanizing, which, if they were successful, was likely to be lucrative and to offer prestige. A crippled man has difficulty hunting, and a barren woman cannot fulfill the biological role of motherhood. Both these defects might therefore promote the compensatory desire to become a shaman or shamaness.

Once the role was assumed, these defects may have been put to use and exploited to distinguish the shaman from the "common run" of people. The main trick of a blind shaman at Indian Point, for example, involved threading an ivory needle, for which sight was presumed to be a prerequisite.

Mental Disorder. A variety of psychiatric symptoms also seem, on occasion, to have had the effect of highlighting the shaman's difference from ordinary people. Like physical incapacity, psychiatric disability may have made it difficult for such a person to fulfill normal cultural roles and may therefore have served to encourage recruitment to shamanism. A Chuckchee shamaness of Bogoras's acquaintance had been violently insane for three years because of a spell cast by a rival. In fits of excitement, she lost the feeling in her wrists and sometimes in her whole body, and she would mutilate her hands by pounding them with stones. Her attacks on other people were sufficiently disturbing so that at times she had to be tied to a house-pole.[20] During lucid periods, she was apparently able to maintain her shamanistic practice.

Psychiatric disorder was not necessarily a prerequisite for shamanism. The group of shamans that came to attention in the St. Lawrence study appeared to reflect the population as a whole in distribution of psychiatric symptoms.[21] The well known shamans were, if anything, exceptionally healthy in this sense. As for those shamans who had suffered from psychiatric instability of one kind or another, it has been suggested that shamanizing is itself an avenue for "being healed from disease."[22] Whatever the psychiatric characteristics that may impel a person to choose this role, once he fulfills it, he has a well defined and unambiguous relationship to the rest of the society, which in all probability allows him to function without the degree of impairment that might follow if there were no such niche into which he could fit.

Intelligence. There is considerable evidence that a high level of intelligence is involved in the kind of shamanizing that reaches the stature of full accreditation. A number of observers, both natives and outsiders, have used the word "shrewd" in describing shamans.[23] This quality is best demonstrated in the St. Lawrence study by the ability of Gambell's most famous shaman to adapt to the changing times.

This old man had lived through the war years and the period of acculturation and had even been converted by Presbyterian missionaries without disturbing or shattering his ability to adjust. His shamanistic skill was still acute, although not so overt as before. He was held in both fear and respect by the villagers, despite the fact that he was not a leader in the mission or local government. He was one of the shamans who changed, not by giving up shamanism, but by adjusting shamanism to fit new circumstances—recognizing, for example, that Western medicine works for white man's diseases like tuberculosis while shamanistic medicine works for different illnesses.

He seemed to have come to terms with change, was concerned about educating his children, and was quite willing to give the modern world its due for airplanes, hospitals, and schools. In comparison to some of the other villagers, he appeared to have a stability that resisted wholesale enchantment with the "bright new world" and allowed him to assess the new as having both good and bad elements.

Even his shamanistic activities were not entirely outmoded by change, for his approach was to adapt his procedures rather than to discard them as old-fashioned. Before the Second World War, for example, his spirit-familiars were believed to be the usual walrus and polar bear. During the postwar years, when tension between the United States and Russia increased and propaganda accounts were heard against the communists, the old shaman added to his *ménage* of animal spirit-familiars the souls of four communists believed by the villagers to have died in shipwreck near the island. The expanded personnel of his spirit entourage was not viewed by local people as odd, stupid, or senile. The shaman was not suddenly thought "crazy" because he had communists working for him; he merely became more powerful and more to be feared. As a forecast of the village disposition based on a realistic assessment of the most effective means of preserving his position in a community fast losing faith in "walrus" and gaining tremendous respect and fear for "government," this addition to his armamentarium was both strategic and shrewd.

Emotional Control. Finally, for a shaman to become a successful healer he had often to display an exceptional ability in emotional control and in taking responsibility. Despite the pitch of frenzy reached in a séance and the seizure of possession, the performance as a whole is a highly stylized drama, the impact of which is largely related to its control by the key director—the shaman. In addition, the full-fledged shaman who is capable of dealing with the crises of illness and death and of offering psychological support to the groups of individuals taken into his spiritual custody displays qualities that can hardly be separated from those of leadership, responsibility, and power.

PSYCHOTHERAPEUTIC ELEMENTS IN SHAMANISM

A point has now been reached at which a broad summary can be made of the psychotherapeutic elements entailed in the shamanism practiced on St. Lawrence Island. Although these Eskimos recognize that some illnesses are predominantly physiological and some predominantly psychiatric, the therapeutic procedures of shamanism were uncompromisingly psychosomatic in approach. It did not seem, in other words, that physical treatments were exclusively employed for what were considered primarily physical disorders, not even in treating a frozen foot, for example. Nor was psychotherapy limited to psychiatric disorders. It seems wise, therefore, not to try to untangle one from the other but rather to view the process of shamanism as "whole man" therapy and to attempt to draw out the discrete facets of this orientation that make shamanism effective.

In order to do so, it is necessary to touch on "psychotherapy" as the term is employed in Western psychiatry and to outline its goals and the procedures by which these goals are accomplished. Since "psychotherapy" means different things to different people, definition is not altogether an easy task. Nevertheless there appears to be consensus that "psychotherapy" refers to verbal and nonverbal communications with patients, as distinct from therapies that utilize, for example, drugs, surgery, or shock.[24] Within these perimeters we can say that the term comprehends numerous kinds of activity believed to be therapeutic, among them suggestion, persuasion, hypnosis, catharsis, abreaction, identification, transference, psychodrama, group pressure, acting out, depth analysis involving the uncovering of unconscious materials through free association and dream interpretation, and education leading to the creation of insight.

In addition to these multiple approaches, psychotherapy can be directed toward several different goals. A useful outline is given by Kennedy in which he presents nine objectives of psychotherapy. The ordering, although not specifically explained, appears to be hierarchical, with the first goal considered more important than the second and so forth:

1. Relief of mental tension and its consequences.
2. Removal of functional disabilities.
3. More efficient use of mental potentialities.
4. Independence, especially to solve own problems.
5. Improved adaptation to circumstances.
6. Insight if this helps prevent relapse.
7. Increased capacity for responsibility.
8. Induction of a hopeful and positive attitude to problems.
9. Creation of a reserve to meet future stresses.[25]

Where does shamanism fit into this sketch of psychotherapy—what are its goals, and what techniques does it draw upon?

As indicated above, the distinction between physical therapies and psychological components like verbal and nonverbal communication with the patient does not hold in shamanism. It is also obvious from the description of Eskimo shamanism that its objectives are limited and that it focuses primarily on the removal of symptoms and relief from tension, anguish, and their consequences. Such other therapeutic goals as improved adaptation to circumstances, creation of hopeful and positive attitudes, and increased capacity for responsibility may be achieved as side effects and may even be conscious aims in the minds of some shamans. It is clear, however, that shamanism does not involve any standard procedures directed toward such accomplishments, and their achievement is probably more the result of a particular shaman's judgment and counseling abilities than of shamanism itself.

While shamanism appears to have remarkable strength to accomplish its limited aims, it is weak in encouraging independence[26] and producing insight. The effectiveness of shamanism in removing symptoms and giving release from anxiety rests upon the shaman's ability to demonstrate that he can repeatedly be depended upon for these ends. One might say that the encouragement of independence is, in fact, the opposite of what shamanism purports to do. With regard to insight, shamanism involves a body of thought about the causes of disease, but it does not involve a theory of personality. The insights produced through shamanistic activities have to do with cultural beliefs—discovering the patient's lost soul or his past transgressions, for example. Insight of this order is very different from what is meant, in Western psychiatry, by "insight" into the nature of the patient's personality functioning.

Turning, finally, to the psychotherapeutic techniques that make shamanism effective in accomplishing its main goals, we find that shamanism, like various other non-Western medico-religious treatments, utilizes several approaches.[27] It is not a therapy based solely on suggestion, for example, or exclusively on group involvement or controlled acting out. It is a combination of certain techniques familiar to Western psychotherapy. There are, however, numerous aspects of Western psychotherapy that it does not utilize—free association, dream interpretation, and character analysis, for instance.

The psychotherapeutic techniques of shamanism can be classified in the following manner:

Gaining Acceptance. Shamanism is related to a system of beliefs about the causes and cures of disease. The effectiveness of shamanistic therapy depends upon these beliefs' being widely held and emotionally accepted by the cultural group. In this regard, it is like various other forms of faith healing. Among the St. Lawrence people, the acceptance of this belief system was reinforced by folk tales, which were told for enjoyment, and by congruence with general religious views about the nature of the universe in both its human and spirit manifestations. During a curing rite, this whole system of beliefs was drawn into operation and given objective reality by the shaman.

Group Participation. The performance by the shaman takes place in a group context, and the drama of curing is given public recognition. The psychological interaction among shaman, patient, and audience is an aspect of the therapeutic force of the procedures. The patient is surrounded by familiar people in a ceremonial situation to which he has become accustomed through witnessing curing rites for others or participating in singing and drumming as recreation. In addition to the group's support of the patient and its desire for his well-being, the family's faith in the shaman and the curing rite is signaled in the payment of a fee at the close of the therapeutic séance. These aspects of shamanism bear some resemblance to techniques of acting out in psychodrama and of group pressure and involvement. They also set an atmosphere in which suggestion and persuasion can begin to operate.

Focusing Awe. A significant element in the shaman's ability to cure is his capacity to establish himself in the eyes of the audience as a person of extraordinary powers. This establishment may involve exploitation of any of the natural talents or unusual characteristics that probably inclined him to the role in the first place. Additionally, however, as an overture to the curing séance, he usually performs some act of magical perception or ability that reminds the group of his power. Through these means, the patient's and the group's expectations of a favorable outcome are enhanced through mechanisms somewhat similar to identification and transference.

Possession. Having revalidated his own position, the shaman becomes possessed by a spirit-familiar, which, in the group's system of beliefs, is more powerful than any human agent and able to determine human destiny. Possession is vividly demonstrated to the group by the shaman's seizure. It is as the agent of a spirit-familiar that the shaman engages the group's faith and brings into full play the cultural beliefs about the etiology of disease and its cure.

Diagnosis. A crucial aspect of the rite is diagnosis. While possessed by his spirit-familiar, the shaman is able to discover the particular causes of the patient's illness—such as soul-loss or breach of taboo— and then to prescribe the treatments, acts, and hygienic precautions that will promote health.

Treatment. In addition to the curing procedures that take place entirely on the psychic plane—retrieval of the patient's lost soul, for example—the shaman also conducts a number of objective treatments, some of which are medicinal, some surgical, some chiropractic, some (like bandaging) simply expedient, and some (like sucking out a foreign body) magical. Some of these treatments are undoubtedly therapeutic in themselves. In addition, the psychological effects of an objective demonstration that the disease has been dispelled or destroyed (the shaman's ingestion of the disease-causing worm, for example) should not be minimized in understanding the total process of shamanistic therapy. The objectification of recovery probably achieves its main force through suggestion.

Involving Patient. Not only does the shaman "do something" that is active and observable to indicate that the patient is passing from a state of disease to a state of health; he also prescribes that the patient carry out comparably objective acts, which are believed to stabilize further the cure or which demonstrate that a change has been achieved and recovery established. Although, in St. Lawrence shamanizing, confession is not the main route by which the patient is implicated in his own recovery, acts of atonement may be recommended. The commission of these acts has the psychological effect of enabling the patient to believe himself rid of the cause of his illness. Another important element of the ceremony in which the patient may be objectively involved is his assumption of a new name-soul, usually exhibited to his fellow beings by a change of sex identification in dress and demeanor. Through suggestion and the patient's personal involvement in the cure, these visible acts further promote in the patient a psychological realization that he is returning to a state of health.

In conclusion, it appears that, regardless of the significance of these discrete elements taken singly, shamanistic curing was an extraordinarily forceful combination of psychotherapeutic techniques, as long as the culture of the group in which it was practiced remained intact. Much of the particular content of the shamanistic procedures described here is directly related to cultural beliefs found on St. Lawrence Island, and, in these specific regards, shamanism will probably continue to wane with the waning of Eskimo avowal and acceptance of the underlying belief system. In terms of the processes and dynamics involved, however, these techniques have far wider generality and are fundamentally similar to the ways of handling psychic and somatic ills of man that have been found effective in modern as well as in primitive societies.

Notes

1. Charles C. Hughes, "An Eskimo Deviant from the 'Eskimo' Type of Social Organization," *American Anthropologist*, 60 (1958), No. 6, 1140-7.

2. Hughes, with the collaboration of Jane M. Murphy, *An Eskimo Village in the Modern World* (Ithaca: Cornell University Press, 1960).

3. Jane M. Murphy (formerly Hughes), "An Epidemiological Study of Psychopathology in an Eskimo Village" (Unpublished doctoral dissertation, Cornell University, 1960).

4. Zachary Gussow, "Pibloktoq (Hysteria) Among the Polar Eskimo: An Ethnopsychiatric Study," in Warner Muensterberger and Sidney Axelrad, eds., *Psychoanalysis and the Social Sciences*, VI (New York: International Universities Press, Inc., 1960).

5. Ralph Linton, *Culture and Mental Disorders* (Sprinfield: Charles C Thomas, Publisher, 1956).

6. A. L. Kroeber, "Psychosis or Social Sanction," *The Nature of Culture* (Chicago: University of Chicago Press, 1952), pp. 310-9; George Devereux, "Normal and Abnormal: The Key Problem of Psychiatric Anthropology," *Some Uses of Anthropology: Theoretical and Applied* (Washington, D. C.: The Anthropological Society of Washington, 1956); and B. J. F. Laubscher, *Sex, Custom and Psychopathology, A Study of South African Pagan Natives* (London: Routledge & Kegan Paul, Ltd., 1937).

7. Linton, "Nativistic Movements," *American Anthropologist*, 45 (1943), No. 2, 230-40.

8. Waldemar Bogoras, *The Chuckchee, The Jesup North Pacific Expedition*, VII, Franz Boas, ed. (2 Parts; New York: Memoir of the American Museum of Natural History, 1904-1909).

9. Edmund S. Carpenter, "Witch-fear Among the Aivilik Eskimos," *American Journal of Psychiatry*, 110 (1953), 194-9.

10. Forrest E. Clements, *Primitive Concepts of Disease* (University of California Publications in American Archaeology and Ethnology, 32 [1932]), No. 2, 185-252.

11. Alexander H. Leighton (Unpublished field journal of psychiatric observation in the Sudan and Nigeria, 1959).

12. Morton I. Teicher, "Three Cases of Psychosis Among the Eskimos," *Journal of Mental Science*, 100 (1954), 527-35.

13. Devereux, *op. cit.*

14. Leighton and Hughes, "Notes on Eskimo Patterns of Suicide," *Southwestern Journal of Anthropology*, 11 (1955), No. 4, 327-38.

15. M. A. Czaplicka, *Aboriginal Siberia, A Study in Social Anthropology* (Oxford: The Clarendon Press, 1914); and Erwin H. Ackerknecht, "Psychopathology, Primitive Medicine and Primitive Culture," *Bulletin of the History of Medicine*, 14 (1943), 30-67.

16. Bogoras, *op. cit.*

17. *Ibid.*, Part I, p. 455.

18. *Ibid.*, p. 451.

19. Knud Rasmussen, "Posthumous Notes on the Life and Doings of the East Greenlanders in Olden Times: The Angmagssalik Eskimos," H. Ostermann, ed., *Meddelelser om Grønland*, 101 (1938), No. 1.

20. Bogoras, *op. cit.*, Part I.

21. Murphy, *op. cit.*

22. Ackerknecht, *op. cit.*

23. M. E. Opler, "Some Points of Comparison and Contrast Between the Treatment of Functional Disorders by Apache Shamans and Modern Psychiatric Practice," *American Journal of Psychiatry*, 92 (May, 1936), 1371-87.

24. *A Psychiatric Glossary* (Washington, D. C.: American Psychiatric Association, 1957).

25. Quoted from Alexander Kennedy, "Chance and Design in Psychotherapy," *Journal of Mental Science*, 106 (1960), No. 422, 3.

26. Opler, *op. cit.*

27. Leighton and Dorothea C. Leighton, "Elements of Psychotherapy in Navaho Religion," *Psychiatry*, 4 (1941), No. 4, 515-23.

Raymond Prince

Indigenous Yoruba Psychiatry*

THIS STUDY is based primarily upon seventeen months' field work
with Yoruba healers in Nigeria between May, 1961, and September,
1962. My sample includes forty-six healers practicing in Abeokuta,
Ibadan, Ile-Ife, and Ijebu-Odi or in villages close to these towns. For
the first half of the study, I dealt with the healers themselves, gathering
data on their beliefs about mental illness and their therapeutic practices,
as well as more personal material. During the second half, I studied the
patient populations at sixteen treatment centers in the same areas, with
a view to assessing diagnosis and the efficacy of treatment.

There are really two kinds of institution dealing with mental illness
in Yoruba culture. The first involves treatment centers, healers, and
magical and herbal therapy, an approach not radically different from
that of the West. The second, the Orisa cult group, has no Western
parallel. It was only toward the end of my study that I realized the full
importance of these cults in the over-all treatment system.

All my interviewing was carried out through an interpreter who
was also a member of one of the main Yoruba healing cults. Interviews
were usually about two hours long, and each respondent (apart from
patients) was paid one pound at the end of the interview.

* This study was supported by the Human Ecology Fund, New York, to whom
I express my most sincere thanks. I must also acknowledge the many kindnesses
received from the Nigerian Institute of Social and Economic Research, particularly
from the director, Professor R. Barback. Mr. L. Obafemi, my resourceful interpreter;
Mr. Dosumu, secretary of the national organization of *babalawos;* and Chief
Durojaiye Aina, the head of the Abeokuta *babalawos* also deserve my special
gratitude. Plant identifications were made through the kind assistance of Mr.
D. P. Stanfield and Mr. R. W. J. Keay, both of the Federal Department of Forest
Research, Ibadan. Finally I acknowledge my indebtedness to Professor E. D.
Wittkower of the Section of Transcultural Psychiatric Studies, McGill University,
for his continuous advice, encouragement, and stimulation.

§ Culture and History

The Yoruba are a Negro group some six million strong occupying the Western Region of Nigeria, parts of the Northern Region, and Dahomey. They are best known to the world for their art; Yoruba wood carvings and espcially the "Ife Bronzes," a galaxy of portrait heads of unsurpassed artistry, have kindled the international imagination. The Yoruba have a highly complex social system: large cities; divine kingship with power controlled by a council of elders; a well developed system of trade with a network of markets and a monetary system; practice of both iron and brass metallurgies. On the other hand, fire and human muscle power are the sole sources of energy, and technological development is of a low order. Armstrong[1] has aptly characterized the Yoruba states (grouping them with the other great kingdom states of the Guinea coast—Ashanti, Benin, and Dahomey) as "very sophisticated adaptations to low energy economies." Before European contact in the nineteenth century, they did not employ the wheel, the lever, or the inclined plane, and writing was unknown.

Legends embody two conflicting accounts of Yoruba history. On the one hand, the holy city of Ile-Ife is said to be the cradle of life: Plants, animals, and men, both black and white, were created there—"The day dawned at Ife." On the other hand, there are stories and rituals associated with the installation of kings that suggest a migration from the Northeast, from Arabia or the Sudan. Willett's view seems best to resolve this contradiction:

> The Yoruba are racially very mixed, ranging from typically Sudanic negroes to pure Hamites, and it does seem likely that some of the peoples have come into the area from outside, very probably as a ruling group who eventually intermarried with the indigenes.[2]

It is possible that the legends of creation have come down from the ancient indigenous peoples, while the migration legends reflect the arrival of later immigrant groups. The Ife Bronzes (really brasses) support this view, for some of the heads are typically Negroid, others clearly Hamitic and Semitic.[3] Some indeed have an Oriental look, particularly about the eyes, which have epicanthic folds.

It was probably in Africa that man first emerged from his prehuman state. Central Africa is the home of man's nearest relative, the great ape; the fossil remains of scores of "near men," the so-called *Australopithecus africans,* have been discovered in East and South Africa.[4] Although the archaeology of West Africa has not been subjected to the same study as has that of the East and South (the rain forest of the West is not conducive to the preservation of fossil remains), Armstrong[5] suggests on linguistic and other grounds that West African groups are extremely ancient. The study of Yoruba folklore and ritual suggests a hoary antiquity; as the Yoruba say, "all these things come from the 'morning-time' of the world."

Clapperton and Landers were probably the first Europeans to penetrate Yoruba country when they traveled from Badagry to Old Oyo in 1826. In those early days of European influence, the Guinea coast was known as the "white man's grave"—Clapperton and Landers, like many of the missionaries and merchants who followed them, succumbed to malaria and dysentery. In the early 1840s, the first Christian missionaries settled in Abeokuta, and by 1860 Lagos had become a colony of Britain. Between 1914 and 1960, the whole of Nigeria was an official British protectorate and colony.

§ Indigenous Psychiatric Nomenclature

The Yoruba language contains a number of expressions for psychiatric disturbances. Many are used rather loosely by the healers, as well as by the general populace. Indeed the affixing of labels does not seem to assume much importance in the healers' minds. The following labels, however, seem to be used more or less consistently in the area studied.

THE PSYCHOSES

By far the commonest diagnostic label applied at native treatment centers was *Were.* It typically refers to a chronic psychotic who is careless in dress and vagrant, talks irrationally, and suffers auditory or visual hallucinations. The patient's harmlessness is generally stressed. Sometimes the term is applied to more acute psychoses. Many chronic and perhaps acute schizophrenics would be included in this category.

Asinwin is usually applied to an acute psychotic episode with sudden onset. Several informants emphasized that this kind of psychosis is the most dangerous, for the patient is more liable to commit suicide or homicide during this illness than during any other. The Western counterpart would be an acute schizophrenic episode, mania, catatonic excitement, or agitated delirium.

Dindinrin refers to a withdrawn, suspicious, and uncommunicative psychotic of a chronic schizophrenic type. Some healers say that *asinwin* might become *were* and that both *were* and *asinwin* might become *dindinrin* if they are not properly treated.

Danidani (*edani*) refers to either a severely regressed psychotic or a mental defective. None of the patients I observed at treatment centers was so labeled.

Were alaso (*were* that wears clothes) refers to a psychotic with a well preserved personality. "You may see him on the street and not realize he is mad. He is dressed properly and may speak sensibly at times, but he is still mad all the same."

Were agba denotes psychosis associated with old age.

Abisinwin is postpartum psychosis. "It generally starts about three days after delivery; I had one last year, and she strangled her child. It lasted three months. All such patients should have their children removed from them."

Were d'ile (*were* of the lineage) is, as it implies, hereditary psychosis.

THE PSYCHONEUROSES

Yoruba healers often do not make a clear distinction between physical disease and the psychoneuroses. This failure is understandable because many Yoruba neuroses present largely physical symptoms. The following diagnoses are commonly used and seem to refer to psychoneuroses, although they may include deficiencies and other organic ills in some cases.

Ori ode (hunter's head) is a designation that covers one of the commonest neuroses suffered by the Yoruba. The patient has somatic complaints of burning, crawling, or thumping in his head, which often spreads through the whole body. Visual symptoms like dimness of vision and "dazzling" of the eyes are common. Insomnia, dizziness, and trembling may occur. Several informants say that the patient may become psychotic if the *ori ode* becomes too intense. There are several native descriptions of the condition:

It is like an insect in the forehead; it starts in the nose and gets to the head; it knocks his brain and works through his whole body. His eyes will be no good; he can't see anything and his ears will be buzzing— it is a kind of mental trouble. . . .

Something will be striking in the brain as if to say a blacksmith is striking an anvil. He will be hearing a buzzing in the ears but no voices. There is burning in the head, and weakness. If it becomes too much, it may cover the eyes and the patient can't see, or sometimes the head is turned and the man runs mad . . .

Inarun, a condition "which comes from God," has as its common symptoms weakness, burning of the body or itching, skin rashes, dimness of vision, impotence or "black menstruation," deadness of the feet, paralysis of the legs, and occasionally organic psychosis: "Tired and weak, body scratching him, impotent, he feels hot on his body and might get paralyzed legs and may go mad; talking irrationally, he may look at an object for hours. He has memory loss and may cry a lot."

Aluro, egba, and *ategun* seem to cover both organic and hysterical paralyses, which were not clearly distinguished by my informants.

Gbohungbohun refers to hysterical aphonia.

Afota is a type of hysterical blindness.

Aiyiperi is a complex concept that includes hysterical convulsive disorders, posturings, and tics, as well as psychomotor seizures and probably tetanus. Some healers also include *warapa* (*grand mal* epilepsy) and *giri* (convulsions in children) under this designation.

Ipa were is madness associated with epilepsy.

In the cases I studied at the native treatment centers, there were fifty cases of *were,* thirteen cases of *dindinrin,* five cases of *asinwin,* four cases of *were alaso,* four cases of *were d'ile,* four cases of *ori ode,* two cases of *ipa were,* one case of *warapa,* one case of *inarun,* nine in a general category of other, and eight cases undiagnosed.

§ Concepts of Cause

Among the Yoruba, misfortunes including diseases are divided into three categories according to cause: natural, preternatural, and supernatural.

As most misfortunes have multiple causes, it is often necessary to take an herbal potion to deal with the physical aspect, to carry out a magical ritual to reverse the preternatural element, and to make a sacrifice to placate the supernatural agency. This principle of multiple causation enables the healer to carry out a series of different procedures, prolonged perhaps for several months, without losing face.

NATURAL DISEASES

A wide variety of illnesses is considered to be of natural origin. Such diseases, however, may be intensified by the activities of enemies or spirits. It is one of the witches' important practices to "spoil" the medicines of the healer so that the natural disease does not respond to the usual treatment.

Natural diseases are attributed to faulty diet, small insects or worms, black blood or watery blood, bad odors (as of feces or decaying flesh), hemp smoking and other toxins, or hereditary factors.

I do not wish to dwell upon these natural ills, which would take us too far into physical illness. Of the psychiatric disturbances, *were, asinwin, danidani,* and *dindinrin* are sometimes considered hereditary. *Inarun* and *aiyiperi* are regarded as natural illnesses and attributed to faulty diet and black blood. Psychoses due to the smoking of Indian hemp are frequent in the treatment centers. Illnesses attributed to natural causes accounted for 20% of the cases at the treatment centers.

PRETERNATURAL CAUSES

The preternatural causes of illness are believed to be malignant magical practices of sorcerers, curse, and witchcraft. These factors reflect hostilities and jealousies within the community. Many informants, in trying to account for the increase of mental illness since their fathers' time, emphasized that these factors were on the increase. They cited the growing tendency of women to leave their husbands for richer men and loss of respect for the elders as two important reasons for the increase in social tension, which finds release in sorcery and similar channels.

Sorcery. Sorcery is practiced by certain *babalawos*[6] or other elderly males. I have never met anyone who admitted to practicing sorcery, although one *babalawo* showed me a bad *Esu* (a rock, sacred to the powerful spirit *Esu,* commonly employed in sorcery); it was a small pock-marked stone protruding from the earth and covered with an inverted clay pot under some bushes. He insisted that it did not belong to him, although it was in his own compound!

The practice of sorcery often involves the use of human body parts—skulls, bones, limbs, organs, and so forth. It is difficult to know how frequent the practice is, but it is the unanimous opinion of the healers that it is extremely common. Indeed, one often sees in the local press accounts of murders committed to obtain body parts for "medicine" or descriptions of the discoveries of mutilated corpses that have presumably been used for the same purpose.

Yoruba sorcery follows patterns familiar from primitive cultures around the globe. Several elements are almost always found. As a means of "labeling" the victim and opening a passage through his defenses, the sorcerer uses either a substance that has been in contact with the victim—

his hair, excreta, or clothing, for example—or the victim's name (and often his mother's name so that there will be no error in identity). He often also carries out a ritual demonstrating, as it were, what will happen to the victim. Finally, the power is believed to be derived either from certain spirits who are summoned by invocations using their "real" names or from certain powerful medicinal substances—frequently human parts. I believe it is important to know the dead man's name, for the sorcerer summons his spirit to carry out the damage.

The following excerpts illustrate some specific patterns:

Ori ode may be caused by bad medicine. You take the hair of a man's head. You prepare medicine and put it with the hair and put them both in an ant hill. As the ants are circulating about the medicine, so the victim will feel it inside his head or you may put the medicine and the man's hair under an anvil, and every time the blacksmith strikes the anvil so he will feel it inside his head.

Some may use it in the thick bush. You hang it in a tree and when it is rotten it falls down. It is made of medicine and perhaps a black fowl, goat, and you may use a human leg in it. When it falls down, the man whose name you called is finished. Or you may use fire and immediately you put fire under it, the victim's body becomes hot, and if you let the thing fall into the fire and burn, the person will die.

If someone dupes anyone and he has no power to retaliate, he calls a native doctor to start *asasi;* Moslems do it too. When it is finished, the victim will be excited, talking irrationally, talking in his sleep, and may have dreams of *Egunguns* [a masquerade cult] chasing him. He will be hiding and saying the policeman is chasing him. When they use *asasi*, if it doesn't meet the person who it is sent against, the *asasi* will go to the crossroads and wait for the man there.

The following experience reported by a *babalawo* describes the experience of a victim:

It was in 1945, not long after I took another man's wife. It was five a.m., and I came out of the house to urinate. I saw a flash of light, I was stunned and felt as if to say someone got hold of me suddenly. I shook myself as if to release myself from the grip. I entered the house to call the woman to see if she was alright. I was afraid it might have damaged her. Then I took some medicine and gave some to the woman. Five days after, I heard the man was sick (the husband of the woman) because the *asasi* had gone back and met him. He died. If he had had preventive medicine he should not have died. If the person doesn't have preventive medicine he will either die, or if he is afraid, he will run mad.

Curse. Curse is one of the commonest causes of psychiatric disorder and has been described in detail elsewhere.[7] Curse is usually effected by the licking of certain medicine, followed by the emphatic utterance of certain commands in the presence of the victim. The results may be immediate or may not appear for several days, depending upon both the type of medicine used and the defenses of the victim. Cursing is usually done by males and is often associated with quarrels over women or land.

With *epe,* the man does what he is told to do. He may hang himself or run about the market showing his penis [or her vagina], or he may lay hold of a matchet and run about attacking people. He doesn't talk irrationally or see spirits; he does what he is told to do. *Epe* may take nine days to work. *Ase* works rapidly—perhaps within an hour. *Epe* is like a slow poison.

With *epe* the man runs into the bush, and he'll think he is going on a tarred road; he wanders about the bush thinking he is in town.

In Lagos there was a quarrel between two men. I don't know what it was about. They were quarreling loudly and abusing themselves. Then one shouted at the other, "as the corn goes to the farm nakedly, so too must you be walking nakedly!" I didn't see him using any medicine horn or anything, but he may have had something in his mouth. In a few minutes, the one who was cursed began to tear off his clothes, and all the people who had gathered around ran away. I had to run too.

Witchcraft. There was some difference of opinion on whether or not witches could be the *sole* cause of mental illness. Out of eleven healers who were questioned specifically on the matter, seven said that witches could cause mental illness, and four said they could not. Opinion was unanimous, however, about the witches' ability to spoil the power of medicine. Witches can also aggravate any disease.

I have described the nature and powers of the Yoruba witch at length elsewhere[8] and will not repeat that material here. At that time, however, I was not aware of the existence of a real witch cult and considered the beliefs I described to be a kind of cultural delusion. As far as my present information goes, there is certainly a real witch cult, composed mostly of elderly women with male leaders. It is very widespread, highly secret, and much feared by the people. Morton-Williams[9] was working in the town of Ilaro when the Atinga witch hunters from Ghana visited the town. He recorded several confessions made by the accused witches. The following confession offers what I believe to be an accurate account of how a woman may enter the cult:

My mother took no part in my witch society before she died. After she died, a woman came to me and said I should join an *egbe* [a friendly association]. I said that if it had a uniform, I would buy any cloth that they bought. She said it was not that kind of society. One day they called me to come and take soup with them. I ate it before I knew it was human flesh. This is how our society meets. We go in the night, leaving our bodies lying down, we go without them. The first time I went, I went in my own body to take the soup. Until I took the soup, they said I was the sort of person likely to give away their secrets.

Toward the end of my study, I met a prominent member of the Ibadan "chapter" of witches. She was an elderly woman, highly tatooed, and not unpleasant in manner. Before meeting her I had to send, through the healer who introduced me, a goat, a bottle of palm oil, and some eggs. Our dealings were always carried on in a darkened room, and I was cautioned to the greatest secrecy. Whenever I met her or when I was leaving, she always shook my hand and tickled my palm. I thought at first that I must be mistaken about the intention of this gesture, but later she made it quite clear that she wanted to have intercourse with me. That this desire was not merely her personal idiosyncrasy (or my personal charm!) is indicated by the remarks of one of the healers.

I always used to consult with the witches about my patients and get a sacrifice from the patients to give them. But now I do not, the reason is that the witch, no matter how old she is, always wants intercourse. I found that unpleasant.[10]

The following passages indicate some of the powers ascribed to the witches, powers that the witches themselves believe they have:

Witches can definitely cause mental illness. I know because I am one of them [this informant was one of the male leaders of a witch group]. All the medicines in the world can be stopped by them. They are the rulers of the earth. Witches have meetings in their real physical bodies and communicate with one another by a kind of "telephone" so that a third party would not know they are communicating.

Witches' powers lie in their eyes; they have no other power. They suck blood through the witch birds' eyes. The witches *okan* [heart-soul] changes into a bird inside her body and flies out of the mouth or anus. If that bird is killed, the witch cannot rise up again. This transformation occurs when the witch is asleep. When she is awake, however, she can see into the inside of the abdomen, she can see all the abdominal viscera.

Beside damaging medicines and causing or intensifying psychiatric disorders and some physical illnesses, witches are especially important for causing barrenness and impotence. Some healers collaborate with the witches personally, while others simply sacrifice to them as directed by various oracles.

Supposing a healer is going to a certain quarter of the town to treat a patient. If the witch there doesn't want you to treat the patient, the witch would stop you on the way and say that she didn't want you to go there again. Then the doctor would ask her if the patient had offended her, and then the doctor would beg her and ask what she would take to release the patient. The relatives of the patient must be prepared to pay a high price, maybe five pounds or some cloth that the witch wants, etc.

The witches have supernatural power over all the leaves and herbs the doctor uses. They may lay hands on the leaves and take the power. If they want to attack a person, they do it through the beak. It is the power given to them by God. At the university even and in each quarter of the town, there is a group and their leader. . . . If I have a patient who is not doing well, I go to them in person. They may ask for something from the patient. They may tell me to change the leaves I am using or they may say to use the same leaves but add some earth to it. Then the medicine works.

For the doctor that co-operates with them, they always send him to do some wicked things and cause trouble. They may send him to a person to demand what the patient can't afford. If they ask for ten things, the man can perhaps only afford five things, and, when they receive the five things, the witches will still not release the man, and then the patient and the relatives get suspicious of the doctor and think he is a liar and that he has kept the things for himself instead of giving them to the witches. They might ask, for example, for ten pounds and two bottles of gin.

I do not use the witches. I do not want to mix with them. I prefer to use *Osanyin* [medical *Orisa*]. I am against the witches because they are always dictating what animal and sacrifice should be bought and take part of your own salary away. I consult *Osanyin* [by divination], and if he directs that something should go to the witches I simply prepare it and put it out for them.

SUPERNATURAL FACTORS

The "Double" and the "Heavenly Contract." God created man in two parts, the being here on earth and a spiritual double (*Eleda* or *Ikeji*) in heaven. Before entering the world, a man makes a contract with his double, agreeing to stay away from heaven for a certain period, to do a certain kind of work, to have a certain number of wives and children—in fact all the details of his future life in the world are agreed upon with his double. After every decision, the gatekeeper of heaven rings his bell and pronounces "Amen." The details of the contract are then inscribed upon the soles of his feet and the palms of his hands. Before entering the world, the man embraces the tree of forgetfulness at heaven's gate.

Once in the world, the man cannot, of course, remember his contract, but should he fail to fulfill it he will not prosper and may even fall ill. If, on the other hand, the man abides by his agreement, the double, like a guardian spirit, ensures his good fortune and protects him from trouble and illness. Some believe that an offended double causes illness simply by withdrawing his protection; others, however, believe that he takes a more active role and dispatches spirits to damage his earthly counterpart.

The Ancestors. Yoruba ancestors are not so frightening as those of some other cultures. In interviews about the causes of psychiatric illness, they were never mentioned. They can, however, bring about "unrest of mind," lack of prosperity, and sometimes physical illness if they are not accorded proper burial and occasional sacrifices.

There is a very close relationship between a son and his deceased father, an element that emerged quite clearly in my conversations with the healers about their personal lives. All my healers were the sons of healers, often going back for four or five generations; most had studied medicine under their fathers for many years. All these healers communed with their fathers in dreams; the fathers would often advise them in the management of difficult cases. Several healers had, as young men, become Christians—often against the wishes of their fathers. Most of these men did not prosper as Christians or were not happy or had barren wives; through dreams or divination, it was revealed that the reason for their failures was that they were going against the wishes of their deceased fathers:

My father was a healer who used *Agbigba* [a form of divination]. As a boy, I felt no particular inclination to my father's work and became a Christian. Even though I was a Christian though, my father frequently asked me to help him, and I became very familiar with his work. Before my father's death, he handed over all his equipment to me and showed me how to use it. I packed it all in a box and hid it away.

I took training as a carpenter in the government and became a "master carpenter"; however, things did not go well for me. All the money I was earning I do not know what I did with it. I was highly respected everywhere but I never had any money. I had no wife and no clothes. I wouldn't stay in any one place for longer than two weeks, and then I had to move. I would get restless and have to move as though something were driving me. In my feelings I wasn't happy, and if I was playing with someone, it would change to a quarrel. My father's coworkers called me one day and said they were not pleased with my moving all about. They told me I should do my father's work. I consulted *Ifa* [divination], and *Ifa* told me I must do my father's work and would not prosper until I did. That was over twenty years ago. I did not like what the elders and what *Ifa* told me. I was very annoyed. That night I had a dream. I saw my father, and he took me to the box of instruments. He took everything out of the box and instructed me as to what each meant. When I awakened in the morning, I felt happy and decided to try it. I locked myself in a room with the box because I didn't want my Christian friends to see me. When trying it, I felt happy within myself, and, when I had developed some skill, I resigned my government job and devoted myself to my father's work completely.

When I have a difficult case, my father comes to me in my dream to help me. I would go to *Orisa Osanyin* [healing *Orisa*] with kola nuts and water and call upon him to enlighten me. Then he would teach me in my dream. I do this even today. Always what I am taught comes to pass. If I want to go somewhere, if it is not the place for me to go, I will dream and my father will advise me not to go there. As I sit here I do not sit alone, my father is here with me. After I took up my father's work, everything went smoothly for me. I gave up Christianity and had no time for it. I am fully pagan, and I am prepared to die at any time.

The Orisas. The *Orisas* are a host of minor deities who ensure health, prosperity, and fertility for their worshippers. Tradition says there are 401 of them, but there are probably many more. One or more *Orisa* are associated with each lineage, but an individual may be instructed by a diviner to devote himself to a different *Orisa*. In practice, as far as my observations go, people do not pay much attention to their *Orisas* except in times of misfortune or sickness. The *Orisas* are often deified cultural heroes fused with nature spirits (Sango, for example, was a legendary king of Oyo and also the god of thunder); some, however, like Esu, never had human embodiments. The *Orisas* have received attention from a number of authors; Farrow, Lucas, Bascom, Maupoil, and Idowu are probably the most important.[11] The *Orisa* cults (and similar institutions from Dahomey and other parts of West Africa) were transplanted through the slave trade to the New World, where they have flourished.

Psychosis or other psychiatric disturbances may result from neglect of one's family *Orisa*, especially Sopono (the god of smallpox); indeed, some informants believe that, if other *Orisas* are offended, instead of causing trouble themselves, they will send Sopono to punish the offender. Others say that the *Egunguns*[12] function as messengers for the other *Orisas* in this malignant way.

The following comments illustrate the role of the *Orisas* in causing psychiatric disorders:

Sopono is a spirit. It usually only affects a man who is supposed to worship him in his family. In his madness, he may be whistling and at times he may refuse to eat. If he is given medicine he will get worse, and when a *babalawo* [diviner] is consulted he will prove out that it is Sopono who is troubling him. When he meets Sopono it may be through whistling in the midday rather than that he should be worshiping him [it is taboo to whistle, particularly in the hot sun]. When he goes home, he will have high fever and come out in spots. If it is a man who is going to become crazy, his blood gets hot, and then it runs to his brain, and he will be mad. Sopono moves with the breeze; when the breeze blows on him, it will enter his body; it is like standing by a flame—it goes through his skin all over the body; If a man has spots from it, he will not run mad; it is only the internal kind that causes madness.

The man doesn't see Sopono, for he is invisible. He may hear him though. He will hear a voice, telling him someone is coming to injure him. He may hear it in the night and will get up and go out.

Sopono or other *Orisa*, if it is in the family and is neglected, will cause illness and madness. All *Orisas* when they want to cause madness send *Egunguns* to the man. The man sees *Egunguns* in his dreams. All the *Orisas* can get dressed up as an *Egungun*, one doesn't know who is under the garment of an *Egungun*. It is mostly Sopono who comes as an *Egungun*. The man seeing an *Egungun* chasing him in the dream will wake up frightened and become mad. Dreams of drowning in water mean that certain water *Orisas* are after the man, like Osun, Erinle, Yemoja, etc.

I had smallpox myself and saw spirits, thousands of them—some came out of the walls and were threatening me.

If Sopono is causing the trouble the man has a hot head, but his madness may be permanent though. In treatment you always sacrifice to Sopono. Sopono always pacifies the spirits that are causing it. You always sacrifice if you want a quick relief.

The main causes of the 101 cases investigated at the native treatment centers, according to the healers (the patients sometimes expressed other opinions), could be broken down into natural (20%), supernatural (18%), and preternatural (45%) causes. In the first category, the actual causes listed were heredity in eight cases, hemp smoking in four cases, bad blood in five cases, and other natural causes in three. Supernatural causes broke down into two categories—ten cases caused by Sopono and eight by other spirits. Among the preternatural cases, twenty-five people became ill through sorcery, twelve were cursed, and eight were victims of witchcraft. Of the remaining seventeen, four cases were assigned other causes, and in thirteen cases the causes were unknown.

§ The Therapeutic Network

There are two types of institution involved in the treatment of psychiatric patients: the treatment centers, which are in many ways like small private hospitals, and the *Orisa* cult groups, which form an intricate network linked together within the literature of the *Odus*. The *babalawo*, the distinctive Yoruba diviner, stands at the center of this network, commending the sufferer to the care of the appropriate *Orisa*.

THE TREATMENT CENTERS

In a secluded section of the town of Abeokuta stands a typical treatment center, that of Mr. F. His house is a one-story, L-shaped mud structure with a tin roof, set in a grove of palms. There are perhaps ten rooms, spacious, cool, and, apart from a few low stools, without furniture. The house is always a hive of activity, with his patients and his numerous wives and children cooking and eating, pounding *garri*, feeding babies, grinding medicines, and peeling kola nuts. Relatives of resident patients, friends, and outpatients are continually coming and going. Behind the house are two smaller buildings, one housing patients and the other a kind of "pharmacy" with three open fires and numerous pots for the preparation of medicines.

The hut for the patients is divided in two for male and female patients; in each section are two "seclusion" rooms with iron bars on the windows and chains hanging from the ceiling to put around the necks of disturbed patients. These rooms are also unfurnished; the mud floors are covered with grass mats. Behind the patients' hut there is a large grove of coconut palms. It is cool and pleasant there, but I have seldom seen it used by the patients, who seem to find the bustle of the big house more to their taste. The hut can accommodate eight to ten patients, and others may be given quarters in the main house. Psychotic patients (and the great majority of patients who "live in" are psychotic) are generally shackled for the first few days or weeks until they can be trusted not to abscond. The average length of stay in this center is from three to four months.

Growing around the patients' hut and also in a fenced-off garden nearby are many of the trees and herbs that are used in therapy *odundun*, *rinrin, ekan-ekun, ajeofole, agunmona, apikan, asofeyeje,* and many others.

The following extract from my notes illustrates something of the nature of the patient population at this center at the time of one visit:

August 2nd, 1961, 5 P.M.—F. was very busy and there were several people sitting outside who had been waiting to see him since the early afternoon. On my arrival F. was disputing with a patient's parents over the amount of money for food for their son. . . . There were ten patients "living in": One woman was living in the main house and was suffering from *ori ode* [psychoneurosis]. . . . Three women shackled in the patients' hut were suffering from psychoses due to *epe* [curse]; one of these was heavily sedated with *asofeyeje,* snoring loudly and stretched out on the floor. . . . He had also two new young boys with *warapa* [*grand mal* epilepsy]; he said that before they came they had two or three seizures a day, but now they had been free of seizures for several days. . . . There was one chronic elderly female there whom I had seen on several occasions before; she was sitting gloomily alone on a bench before the hut. Her illness is due to her failure to worship Obatala [one of the *Orisas*]; her relatives are Christian, and they refuse to pay for a sacrifice to Obatala and F. believes she will not recover until this is done. . . . There is also a psychotic girl from Ghana; F. says they do not know about *Rauwolfia* in Ghana. . . . Two partially recovered male patients were out on errands for F. and I did not see them . . .

Seven of the sixteen healers did not have separate buildings for their patients but used certain rooms within their own houses and did not have the spacious grounds enjoyed by Mr. F's patients.

THERAPY AT TREATMENT CENTERS

A psychotic patient is usually brought to the treatment center by a throng of relatives or by the healer, who, using his magical powers, may have captured the patient. If he is excited, he is bound or shackled. He may then be cooled down by a wash with snail's water, a clear, cool watery fluid found in the cone of the giant land snail. The patient may be stripped and his head shaved and rubbed with this fluid. He is then given a potion, usually containing *asofeyeje* root (*Rauwolfia*), and he goes to sleep. Some healers give a purgative-emetic mixture to "weaken" the patient before giving the sedative or tranquilizing agent.

Generally speaking, each healer has his own standard approach to treating patients, and it is only when he sees that the patient is not responding that he changes his medicine. He sometimes decides on the cause in this way; that is, he gives the patient *epe* (curse) medicine, and, if that does not cause improvement, he decides that it is Sopono's work and applies *ero Sopono*. Alternatively, he uses divination or consults with the witches if the patient is not doing well.

Some healers routinely carry out blood sacrifices at admission. Such a sacrifice may be a sheep, goat, or fowl and is aimed at appeasing the witches or spirits involved. In cases where *epe* (curse) or *asasi* (sorcery) is the cause of the trouble, a detoxifying procedure is carried out—medicine is introduced into the blood through razor cuts in the scalp, a procedure that will be enlarged upon later.

Treatment with tranquilizing and other herbal medicines (generously laced with magic) usually continues for three or four months. Doses are given daily or every two days.

As the patient improves, the shackles are removed, and he is given the run of the treatment center and the healer's house. He may work on the healer's farm or hire out as casual labor to other farmers. He may be allowed to go to market or run errands for the healer. Most healers require that a relative of the patient stay at the treatment center, especially during the early period. Relatives provide nursing care and feed the patient.

When the patient is ready to return home, a discharge ceremony, aimed at preventing a recurrence of his psychosis, is held for him. This ritual includes a blood sacrifice and is often performed beside a river. Some of the ceremonies are quite elaborate and expensive; they symbolize final cleansing of the illness and sometimes "death and rebirth" into a new life.

Charges for treatment vary from twenty to seventy pounds—at least, that is what the healers claim; how much they do actually receive is hard to say. One of their favorite topics of conversation, however, is the perfidy of relatives who do not pay their fees. They also emphasize that, if they are properly paid, they can do a much more rapid and complete healing job. These healers certainly do not suffer from "therapeutic nihilism," and almost all were most emphatic about their ability to cure all illness—"If there is money!"

Word Magic. The power of the word in a magical sense is a very prominent element in Yoruba thought. The importance of the curse has already been described, and the same kind of thinking emerges in the healers' magical subduing and control of obstreperous patients. Sometimes horns of medicine like those used in curse are used for subduing purposes also. One healer showed me his pair of horns, both filled with a solid black medicine that protruded from the top of the horn; one was a cow's horn and showed evidence of constant use, for the black medicine was worn away in the shape of his mouth; the other was a twisted antelope horn, and thrust into the medicine were a cobra fang and a pin, made he said of copper and lead. To use it, he pulls out the pin and rubs it over the tip of his tongue; then whatever he says will come to pass. I have reason to believe that the former horn is the one he uses for patients, and that the latter is for *epe* (curse), but the healer vehemently denied it. He insisted that he uses the horns every morning to give him the power to control his patients; similarly, if he has to go out and capture a patient, he licks them before going.

Akaraba is another device for subduing the patients. The one I saw consisted of a pig's skull partially covered by a cloth. A long cord was attached and wound around the skull. The healer said that a really potent *akaraba* is made from the skull of a person whose name is known. In the presence of the excited patient, an incantation is recited invoking the spirit of the dead man and instructing him to "bind up" the patient. The healer shouts, "Catch him! Catch him!' and at the same time winds the cord around the skull.

Another device used by healers for the same purpose is called *betu betu*. It is a small pellet of medicine wrapped round with black and white thread and held in the healer's mouth while he commands the patient.

Ritual. The following ritual is common in treating psychosis due to *epe* (curse) or *asasi* (sorcery). It is used during the early stages of treatment after the patient has been calmed. (It is not employed in cases caused by Sopono—"It would make the sickness worse.")

The patient's head is shaved. Shea butter, palm oil, pap, and banana* are kneaded together and then generously plastered on the scalp; next, juices of certain leafy plants (*odundun, rinrin, tete abalaiye***) are squeezed into a pail of water to make a cooling shampoo. This shampoo is used to wash off the oily plaster. Finally, a series of shallow razor cuts is made over the scalp in the form of a cross (from brow to occiput and from ear to ear). Into these cuts is rubbed a medicine composed of cer-

---

* Shea butter is a semisolid oil made from the nuts of *Butyrospermum Parkii*. It comes in grayish or cream-colored loaves of somewhat the consistency of cheese. Palm oil is a red oil expressed from the nuts of *Elaeis guineensis*. Pap is a common maize food the color and consistency of *blanc mange*. All are commonly used in sacrifices or medicines.

** *Odundun* (*Kalanehoe erenata*) is a small herb with fleshy leaves, believed to be one of the first created plants. Dalziel, in 1937, noted its use in the Gold Coast as a sedative for asthma and palpitations, but whether or not it is active physiologically I have not been able to discover. *Rinrin* (*Peperomia pellucida*) is a common weed regarded as the first created herb. *Tete abalaiye* was unidentified at the time of writing. I consider these plants to have purely placebo effects because of the small doses used and the lack of physiological response to their use. In any case, they are deeply embedded in the medical lore of the Yoruba and figure prominently in some of the medicinal verses of the *Ifa Odus*.

tain roots, the filings of a human tooth, and a small quantity of fluid collected from a putrifying human corpse. The oily mixture soothes the patient's agitation, while the shampoo cools his overheated brain. The medicine enters the patient's blood through the cuts, "fights" with the toxic agents caused by the *epe* or *asasi,* and expels them in the feces and urine. This technique of cutting to introduce substances into the blood is very widely used. The cuts are made near the seat of the trouble, that is, in the case described above, in the head; in cases of visual hallucinations or the nightmares of children, they are made under the eyes; for auditory hallucinations, they may be made in front of the ears.

Discharge Ceremonies. As in the West, Yoruba psychiatric patients suffer frequent relapses. Many of the patients studied at the treatment centers had previously received treatment in one or more other centers (including Aro, Lantoro, and Yaba Hospitals, the Western-style psychiatric hospitals in the Region). The healers usually attributed these relapses to inadequate previous treatment because of relatives who were not able to pay the required money. This high rate of relapse is reflected in the healers' preoccupation with discharge ceremonies. These ceremonies take highly diverse forms, depending upon the healer and upon the cause of the illness. The common feature is the sacrifice of an animal or bird accompanied by incantations to assure that the illness will never return.

I observed the following ceremony at Ife. It was performed for a young woman who had just recovered from a psychotic episode. It took place in a secluded part of a river about five miles from the town. On the river bank, the patient put off her clothes and dressed in a new white wrapper. The healer, his assistant, carrying three white doves, and the patient waded into midstream where the waist-high water flowed swiftly. The patient's head was shaved. The healer placed a piece of soap on the breast of one of the doves. Using it as a living sponge, he dipped it into the water and lathered the patient's head and body. The body of the drowned dove was thrown downstream. The second dove was decapitated, and its blood was spattered over the patient's head and smeared over the upper part of her body. Again she was washed and the dove flung downstream. A cross of razor cuts was made over her scalp, and into the cuts was rubbed a mixture of blessed camwood, chalk, and the blood of doves (which had been prepared previously). The patient was divested of her white wrapper, which floated away downstream. Ashore, her body and head were again generously rubbed with camwood and chalk, the last dove was decapitated, and the blood again spattered over her body. She then stood on the body of the dead bird, incantations were recited, the bird's body was flung into the river, and the ceremony was complete.

After her return to the doctor's house, another dove was sacrificed and its blood sprinkled over the threshold. Palm oil was poured up the steps, over the threshold, and into the house. The patient could then enter.

Several incantations were recited during the ceremony. A rough translation of one of them follows:

> *Eji Ogbe*
>
> He who awakens and makes a bargain with God.
> He who awakens and is God's peer.
>
> Health is the bondsman of my father
> and I crossed the river to seek him
>
> Let this woman have health today
> Doves dwell in tranquillity
> All men are at peace with water
>   Of it we take to bathe
>   Of it we take to drink
> Let *asinwin* pass from this woman today
> Let *were* pass from this woman today
> Let *dindinrin* pass from this woman today
> Let *danidani* pass from this woman today
> Let all the evil on her head follow the water away
>   If it is the work of an *alfa**
>   Or a *babalawo's* curse
>   Perhaps a hunter or farmer paid money for this evil·
>   Or a sorcerer or a witch or any other cause of evil upon her.
> As she drinks and bathes in water,
> Let water bear all things evil away.
> Let only peace and contentment follow her home.
> Water always flows forward—it never comes back,
> Water always flows forward—it never comes back.

The symbolism of the ceremony is partially apparent. Doves are symbols of peace, their blood mingled with that of the patient brings tranquillity. The evil, which is partly present in the patient's blood and partly a kind of coating over her head and body, is borne away on the bodies of the doves and the white cloth (anyone picking up the doves or the cloth will contract the illness). Some elements suggest death and rebirth—wrapping in white cloth, the use of the camwood and chalk, the

* An *alfa* is a Moslem diviner.

spattering with blood are all features of Yoruba burial ritual. At any rate, the ceremony is clearly a "rite de passage"[13] from the sick mode to the healthy mode.

A Case History. On January 31, 1962, Mr. F., *babalowo* and native healer of Ife, was called upon at his house by the kin of one Taiwo who had "run mad" in his village about ten miles distant. They were afraid that Taiwo would kill someone, for he was a hunter and had a gun that he had fired off twice in the village. He was abusing everyone and had demolished his own house. He had not slept for ten days and had been mad for five. They gave F. three pounds and implored him to come and take charge of the man.

F. and his brother went to the village. Most of the villagers had fled. Taiwo was sitting in his partly demolished hut sharpening his machete. He said that people had told him that he was to become a councilor or a minister but that all the money he had been sent had been stolen by his fellow villagers. He had decided to kill them all. F. urged him to come with him, promising that he would help him to arrest the villagers. Taiwo refused. F. touched him with his medicated ring and began reciting incantations. With this magical help, the illness was partially "quenched," and F. seized the man, bound him hand and foot, bundled him into a taxi, and took him to his own house in Ife.

Taiwo was taken into one of the back rooms of the house. His legs were placed in what look very much like medieval stocks, and he was handcuffed. F. then cut four giant snails and rubbed the snail fluid over the patient's head and body "to cool him down." Taiwo was then forced to drink a bowlful of an herbal potion containing *Rauwolfia*, which very soon put him into a deep sleep. It was about 2:30 in the afternoon.

I first saw the patient at about ten the next morning. He was still in coma, lying on the floor in the cool, dark room. He had been incontinent of feces and urine. His muscles were twitching, and he could not be roused.

I returned to see F. three weeks later. On this occasion, Taiwo was conscious, talked rationally, and greeted me in a friendly manner. The handcuffs had been removed, and he was in walking shackles. He gave a good account of his illness, which he said had started about fourteen months earlier. In brief, he had stolen another man's wife; several months later he had begun to have a series of nightmares from which he would awaken shouting and surrounded by the other people in the house, who had to hold him down. After some time, he began to feel very weak and had to hire laborers to work his farm. He began to have a persistent headache and noise in his ears. He also described his psychotic episode:

The night I ran mad, I was hunting and had killed two antelopes. I was searching for others. I had formerly seen some under a certain tree, and I went there and sat under the tree to wait for them. Early in the morning, all of a sudden, I heard someone whistling and calling my name. I looked around, but didn't see anyone. The voice said "Taiwo, get up." I couldn't bear it, and got up, though I didn't answer the voice. I started home, but before I got home strange things started to happen. I seemed to be seeing things in thousands. I don't know how I behaved; I heard people greeting me, but I couldn't identify them. Next thing I remember is some people tying me. I do not know when they brought me here.

Both the doctor and his patient believe that the illness was due to *asasi* (sorcery) and that the wronged husband had been calling Taiwo's soul and had finally succeeded in damaging it. It was clear that the patient was considerably better. He no longer had any headache or noise in his ears, and he was eating and sleeping well.

I visited F. again about three weeks later. He said that he had discharged Taiwo prematurely because neither he nor his relatives could pay any more of the twenty-pound treatment fee. He said that Taiwo was much improved at the time of discharge but that his sickness would probably recur because he had not had enough medicine and the discharge sacrifice and ceremony had not been performed.

THE ORISA CULTS IN THERAPY AND PROPHYLAXIS

Some mention has already been made of the network of *Orisa* cults and of the role of the *babalawos*, the distinctive Yoruba priest-diviners, in linking them together. The full extent of the role of the *Orisa* cults in healing has never been investigated, but the following outline will suggest the relationship among the patient, the *babalawo*, and the *Orisa* cults.

In practice, when a man falls ill, he will first try a home remedy or one purchased from an itinerant medicine peddler.[14] If he does not recover, he may consult a *babalawo* who, after divination, will advise that he make a sacrifice to the witches, his double, his ancestors or one of the *Orisas;* take certain medicines or use certain magical devices for protection against sorcerers, witches, or bad spirits; change his place of abode (because of the witches in the compound) or, more rarely, change his occupation (because he is not fulfilling his heavenly contract); change his character—be less aggressive, proud, impatient, and so forth; take a medicine for disease of the body; become an initiate into one of the *Orisa* cults (generally one's lineage *Orisa* or one that was formerly in one's lineage, although this association may have been forgotten by living members and may be discovered only by divination).

The *babalawo* may suggest more than one (and perhaps all) of these solutions in a series of divination sessions, should his first recommendations not produce the desired effect. A psychotic patient is usually taken first to a treatment center. It is only after there have been several recurrences of the illness that the *babalawo* recommends initiation into one or more of the *Orisa* cults. I do not want to give the impression that the *Orisa* cults are only healing agencies. They are much more than that— they are foci of divine power in the community, power that is used for religious, political, and legal, as well as therapeutic, ends.

Two common kinds of *Orisa* cult are those characterized by "possession" and "masquerade." From superficial observation, it seems that the possession cults are predominantly for women and the masquerade cults for men. It is also of interest that male members of certain possession cults (like Osun and Sango) wear female hair styles and attire on ceremonial occasions: In fact, possessed individuals are often called the "wives" of the *Orisa*. The significance of this male-female division in the cults clearly requires further study.[15] I shall now briefly describe two cults: the first a female possession cult, Sopono, and the second a male masquerade cult, Gelede.

The Sopono Cult. Sopono is the generic name for the family of small-pox spirits. The diseases caused by the *Sopono* family, however, are of much greater range than is included in the Western designation "small-pox." They include many fevers (particularly with delirium), rashes, carbuncles, boils, and psychoses.[16] The *Soponos* usually attack those who have the deity in their lineage; they may, however, attack others who are so rash as to whistle (which attracts the *Soponos*) or to walk in the noonday sun, especially in the dry season. This cult was forbidden by the British government because of its activities in spreading smallpox,[17] but it is still very active in many parts of Yorubaland.

Although the Soponos were blamed for ten of the 101 cases in my series, only three were initiated into the cult as part of their treatments. The others were merely required to sacrifice to Sopono during their stays in the treatment center and received routine treatment for "Sopono madness." I shall briefly describe the initiation of one patient and also a typical annual Sopono festival.

I first saw K. on July 5, 1962, in the compound of a female elder of one of the sections of the Sopono cult in Abeokuta. She was psychotic at the time, disheveled, overtalkative, and impulsive, but she could carry on an intelligible conversation. She was being cared for in a nearby treatment center to calm her down before her initiation. The purpose of her initiation was to prevent further recurrences of her illness.

According to the healer and others present, her illness had started some ten years earlier. She had been taken from one treatment center to another and had spent a six-month period at Aro Hospital and six other native treatment centers. There had been several remissions in her illness, which allowed her to take clerical jobs in Abeokuta for short periods. She had been to school for several years and could speak some English. Her relapses had, on two occasions, been related to childbirth: the first in 1958 during pregnancy with twins (both died) and the second after the death of her child by a healer who had "cured" her and married her.

The patient gave the following account of her illness:

> My father was a member of the Sopono cult, and we also had Sango, Osun and Obatala in the family. My elder sister was an initiate in the smallpox cult, but not because of mental trouble, it was because of an abscess in her leg that wouldn't heal. No one else in the family was mad as far as I know.

> When the trouble first started about ten years ago, when I would go to sleep it would feel as if to say ants were crawling around my head. Something was drawing my heart as if to cut it off. I felt as if my chest was expanding. I couldn't sleep. My body was hot and had a shrinking feeling and my heart beat rapidly. I saw *Egunguns* (masquerade-cult members) in my dreams, and they would be flogging me and driving me. One time I was by the seaside and the *Egunguns* were driving me, and I fell into the sea.

> When the trouble first started though, it didn't worry me too much. It was during my pregnancy for twins that the sickness really relapsed. I got very weak, had stomach pain, a very bad headache and was unable to sleep. The twins both died. I went to several native treatment centers and improved somewhat. I went to Aro Hospital too and received electrical treatment and pills and again improved. Later I had another child, and my sickness came back again after the baby died.

The healer made the following remarks about her behavior since admission to his treatment center about a week earlier:

> When she first came, she was restless, sleepless and talked too much. She was singing and passing feces every minute, so instead of keeping her in the *Orisa* compound I took her to my compound. Before she came she was singing Sopono songs, and they took her to a *babalawo* who said she must be initiated if she was to have a permanent cure.

When I took her to my compound, she was always singing and shouting and trying to grip everyone who came near her. When we chained her, she rubbed her shoulder in dirt; that is why it is cut. She tore off her clothes and was smearing feces over the walls. There has been no sacrifice yet, but she is much better now. I have been giving her *ero* Sopono (medicine to soothe Sopono). She is to be initiated in fourteen days time if her sister comes to pay the money.

The initiation into the Sopono cult takes twenty-one days and, at the present time in Abeokuta, costs thirty pounds. I have not myself witnessed the initiation, which is secret, but I have several accounts of the proceedings, and my interpreter, who happened to have a room in the Sopono compound, witnessed much of K.'s initiation ceremony. Here is his account:

It started Saturday evening about nine o'clock, after they had got everything ready in the shrine. They got the girl to be initiated and while chanting Sopono songs, they covered her with a white cloth. She had to enter the shrine backwards, and sat on a grass mat. They were calling all the Sopono spirits, Jagun, Igbain, Wariwonron, Bale, etc. Then they tied something up in a bundle and put it on her head. She was taken out to the back of the shrine where they buried the bundle, washed her, and brought her back to the shrine. She was evidently carrying bad luck away on her head to bury it, for one of the songs was saying that she was carrying evil away into the bush.

Coming back to the grove she entered the inner room, and sat on a stool painted red with camwood, and they shaved her hair. They were singing songs all the while. Then they placed a small calabash containing certain things upon her head. They called all the different Sopono spirits in turn. These they chanted over and over again for over an hour. Finally the girl was possessed and collapsed, and the calabash fell off her head. The spirit they were calling when she was possessed is the spirit that had "born her." When she was possessed they took her and laid her down. She stayed asleep for about thirty minutes and then woke up.

For the next three weeks, the girl remained in the shrine. Every morning she was washed and painted all over with camwood. During the first seven days she was not allowed to talk, but during the time in the grove she had been taught many songs and dances by the old women. On the third, seventh, fourteenth, and twenty-first days, sacrifices were offered. After the twenty-first day, she was taken about the market by the elders of the cult, dressed in new clothes and adorned in the black beads that are a token of the cult. The people in the market "dashed" her money, and initiation was then complete, and she returned to the community.

It is during the annual festival that members become possessed by the particular spirits that "chose" them on the first days of their initiations. I quote the following extract from my notes to give something of the flavor of the public portion of one of these annual Sopono festivals. It took place in a small village about five miles from Abeokuta on December 13, 1961:

> The people were in festive mood when we arrived and most of the village seemed to have turned out. The main proceedings took place in the center of the village where a bamboo-and-palm roof had been made over an open space among the huts. Many large calabash bowls were laid out for sacrifice. These contained pounded yam balls, solidified pap, pieces of rope smeared with blood, the odd goat's head and some other unidentifiable objects. A pile of black sticks painted with red and white spots completed the array. The cult women, dressed alike in purple print cloth, were bustling about, as were a few male elders of the cult. The drumming had already begun, and there was an air of anticipation which heightened as the drumming became more insistent. One of the cult members went among the people touching their heads with some pap to take away bad luck. The pap was put in one of the sacrificial bowls. There were many children standing about, round-eyed.

> Then the possession commenced. A knot of younger women collected about one tall old woman with a pock-marked face, all singing and moving to the drum beat. One girl stood before the old woman with her arms about her neck. They placed one of the sacrificial bowls upon the girl's head, and the women began to sing louder, calling upon the spirit of the particular Sopono that habitually possessed this girl. The girl's face became vacant, and her eyes focused upon a distant place. Suddenly she fell forward in a kind of swoon; the "mother" supported her; someone else seized the calabash so that it wouldn't fall; others threw water on her feet. In a few seconds she revived a little; they guided her fingers up over the rim of the calabash, and she was drawn to one side, where she stood, somewhat dazed, the "wife" of the god.

> Ten or twelve other girls were possessed in the same way. Then in single file, bearing the sacrifices upon their heads, they commenced a slow dance about a tree in the center of the clearing. Finally they moved out in a procession about the whole village. Each householder splashed a little water and palm oil on the ground, and the possessed girls each dipped her foot in the pool and moved on. When all the bad luck and illness of the village had been collected in this way, the procession moved off, single

file, to a place in the thick forest where sacrifices are deposited for Sopono beneath an ancient tree. The entire proceedings took about three hours.

To return to the patient, I saw her on several occasions during her initiation, and she seemed to be improving steadily. I last saw her on September 30, 1962. At that time, she was neatly dressed and pleasant in manner and conversed normally. She was able to recall some of the details of her illness but seemed reluctant to discuss them. She was then living in the Sopono compound because some of the initiation sacrifices had not yet been completed for financial reasons.

The Gelede Cult. Gelede is a male masquerade cult that protects its members from witchcraft. My own data on this cult are rather scant, but its formal aspects have been very well described by Beier.[18] Men join the cult because of impotence, because their wives are barren, or because of other diseases or misfortunes caused by witchcraft. My informants, the male elders of one section of the cult in Abeokuta, said that, although men do not join in search of defense against mental illness, still if an initiate were to refuse to dance under the mask or were to defect from the cult, he might well be punished with mental illness.

During the annual festival, the men masquerade as women, wearing women's clothes and flaunting prominent bullet-like breasts. Some look grossly pregnant, and others carry wood carvings of children on their backs. All wear grotesquely carved wooden masks, some of which are frightening: The mask called *Ogede,* for example, is about five feet high, a black wooden cylinder, with breasts, straight outstretched arms, long black hair, and a huge alligator mouth. A child is carved on the back. In action, the figure towers some eight feet tall, presenting quite a terrifying appearance, especially at night when the more important parts of the festival take place.

I asked if the men become possessed by Gelede spirits under the masks and received the following reply:

They are not really possessed but immediately they wear the mask, they change in behavior. They are more or less half possessed. Last year one of the men suffered from the severe guinea worm during the festival. He had almost to creep into the enclave to put on his costume. But with the mask on, he danced and behaved as if he didn't have any guinea worm. The spirits of the Gelede will act on them. They don't really remember afterwards what they do during the dance.

During my interview with the Gelede elders, two or three old crones several times poked their heads in the window to correct and scold the men. I had never before witnessed such an attitude of officiousness and

arrogance on the part of women during my interviews with elders of
other cults or with the healers. It seemed to be part of the general picture of the cult as dominated by the "mothers," that is, the witches. As
one of Beier's informants told him, "Gelede is the secret of women.
We the men are merely their slaves. We dance to appease our mothers."

§ Summary of Psychotherapeutic Elements in Yoruba Therapy

The therapy of Yoruba healers is often effective. The relative importance of the magical (or other psychotherapeutic) factors and the
physiological factors in healing is difficult to determine because in
almost all the cases I studied the two elements were intertwined. I did
follow the management of one severe neurotic who received no physiologically active agents, however. The illness was of four years duration
and had been treated by several practitioners, both indigenous and
Western, with no more than temporary relief. After commencement of
treatment by a competent *babalawo*, the symptoms cleared and the
patient remained well for the period I studied him—some thirteen months.
His treatment included several expensive sacrifices, a good deal of
magical ritual, and initiation into the Ifa divination cult. Here is some
evidence then that nonphysiological factors may be of considerable
importance.

The psychotherapeutic elements in primitive medicine have been
discussed by numerous authors.[19] Most of the psychotherapeutic elements
they describe are also present in Yoruba therapy, and I shall therefore
present only a brief summary, elaborating only those aspects that require
further discussion.

SUGGESTION

Suggestion is the most important element in all primitive psychotherapies. We may first isolate certain factors in the healer-patient relationship that heighten the suggestibility of the patient and add power to
explicit suggestions made by the healer:

1. The "omnipotence" of the healer through his dealings with the spirit
world.

2. The healer's impressive performance. During divination the patient does
not even tell the diviner what his problem is; the diviner learns it through

his spirit contacts; the diviner is often a good intuitive psychologist and very much in tune with the peculiar stresses of his culture. He often makes impressive "blind" diagnoses.

3. His use of sacred and magical formulae, gestures, and paraphernalia.[20]

4. The anxiety of the patient, which is often deliberately increased by the healer who may warn him of serious consequences should he fail to follow directions. The patient's anxiety is in marked contrast to the healer's confidence and optimism.

Many of these factors occur in Western healing (in fact in all healing) but, while the suggestive element (when it is recognized) is criticized as unscientific in official Western medicine, it is utilized to the fullest extent in Yoruba medicine.

The patient receives a continuous barrage of suggestions at all levels from the most intellectual to the most concrete and primitive. This strategy of multilevel bombardment is not unlike that employed by contemporary advertising: We are told to buy the product; we hear slogans about it; we are indoctrinated about the good effects of using it and the dire consequences of failure to use it; ditties extolling it persist in our minds; we may even be given a sample taste of it.

Direct Command. Whenever the healer and patient are together—during the administration of medicines, healing ritual, divination sessions, sacrifice procedures, and discharge ceremonies—the patient is given continual assurance that the treatment will make him well. A suppressive element is also prominent, particularly during the treatment of psychotics; for example, after using verbal magic equipment, the healer shouts at his patient: "Stop behaving like a madman!," "Be quiet!," "Don't be rude," "Don't listen to those voices!"

Simile. At times, particularly in incantations, a direct command will be illuminated by a simile: "As the river always flows forwards and never back, so your illness will never return." A simile conjures a concrete image at a level of mentation below that touched by the direct command.

Illustrative Story. This element is particularly evident in Ifa divination and sacrifice procedures. Each *Odu* section in its complete form consists of a verse, a story that enlarges upon and clarifies the verse, and one or two short songs. The *Odus* are really a series of ancient precedents set by individuals who were faced with various problems and who, through sacrifice, solved them. During divination and sacrifice sessions, the complete verse-story-song complex is repeated, and the patient is directed to sacrifice as in the precedent case or suffer the consequences.

Song. Song is also part of the Ifa healing system. During healing sessions, the songs are sung by the healer, his assistants, and the patient himself.

Sacramental Elements. Sacramental elements include rituals, magical gestures, and objects that represent in the material world what is taking place or expected to take place in the spiritual or psychological world. The following example is an illustration:

> A neurotic patient with somatic complaints and "bad luck" with his wives consulted a *babalawo* and was required among other things to carry out the following ritual; he prayed to a cowrie shell that had been specially energized with medicine and incantations that his illness "would go back from him." He then took the cowrie into the bush and recited a prayer saying, "I am paying the money of sickness [cowries were formerly used as currency by the Yoruba], I am paying the money of misfortune, I am paying the money of misery, I am paying the money of death." He then made a ring around his head with the cowrie and flung it as far as possible into the bush.

Sacramental Elements Involving Body Contact. Many procedures of this type have been described. The head is frequently the target of these sacramental procedures; it is probably relevant that the head is the most common locus for somatic complaints. The procedure of shaving, greasing, cooling, and cutting the head is one example, as is the discharge ceremony involving the sacrifive of doves and the bespattering with blood.

Such multilevel communication increases the potency of the suggestion and allows the healer to deliver the same suggestion repeatedly without becoming tedious and losing the patient's interest.

Official Western medicine allows itself the direct command: "Take this and you will feel better," and sacramental elements may also furtively enter into physical examination or other diagnostic or surgical procedures (a syringe full of venous blood for laboratory examination may mean to the patient that a good quantity of black toxic blood has been removed), but on the whole most suggestive elements are regarded as charlatanry. Patent-medicine advertisements frequently use the illustrative-story technique and nonmedical healers make much use of body-contact methods (in chiropractic and faith healing, for example). I know of no use of song in Western healing, but that song has more persuasive power than direct command is suggested by the amounts expended by advertisers upon the "singing commercial."

SACRIFICE

Sacrifice is one of the cornerstones of Yoruba psychotherapy. Sacrificial procedures are complex and diverse, and I can present no adequate description of them here. A good deal of misfortune, including mental and physical illness, is attributed to the effects of conscious purposive agencies or spirits. These spirits have the same propensities and needs as men and can be recompensed and mollified. As we saw from the account of the witches, the sacrifice is sometimes really extortion demanded by the witches in person. At other times, the sacrifice is set out at a place designated by divination, and the witch or spirit is expected to accept it in a spiritual sense.

In almost all sacrifices, there is a sacramental element. The sheep's or goat's head is touched to the patient's head and chest three times, while prayers are offered that the misfortune will pass from the patient to the animal. Sacrifice has a marked anxiety-reducing effect, and many patients have remarked upon their ability to relax and have a good night's sleep following sacrifice ritual.

MANIPULATION OF THE ENVIRONMENT

As a result of divination, a patient may be instructed to move to a new compound "because of the witches or sorcerers in his present quarters," or he may be told to change his occupation because he is not living in conformity with his "heavenly contract."

EGO-STRENGTHENING ELEMENTS

Patients are sometimes instructed to join *Orisa* cults to prevent relapsing into their illnesses. In addition to the abreactive elements operating in these cults, which I shall describe shortly, there are clearly strong supportive aspects. The patient enters a new circle of friends bound together by initiation and joint possession of esoteric lore and secret objects.

The sense of protection and the sense of "being watched over" by one's double, one's ancestors, and one's *Orisa* have, no doubt, profound ego-strengthening effects. It should be remembered, however, that these factors do not increase the patient's inner strength in a mature way. His strength is borrowed strength, and like a "transference cure"[21] it lasts only as long as association with the cult.

ABREACTION AND GROUP THERAPY:
THE ROLE OF POSSESSION AND MASQUERADE

I have described the public possession ceremony of the Sopono cult, which is performed on behalf of the entire community to rid it of misfortune and illness. In all the parts of this ceremony that I have observed, the devotees have evinced a quiet, controlled kind of possession. As far as I could tell, no significant catharsis took place during such possessions. I was told, however, that during the private Sopono ceremonies (and in the public ceremonies of other cults that I have observed—for example, Erinle and Egun) there does occur a wide range of otherwise asocial behavior that has abreactive effects. For instance, women acting in male roles as hunters or drummers and occasionally dressing in such male clothing as the uniform of a sanitary inspector; women who were normally polite and even obsequious to me becoming bold and defiant; women eating dirt, throwing themselves on the ground, climbing trees, and so forth.

Many authors have discussed the psychotherapeutic aspects of possession phenomena in other cultures: Wolf and Kiev in Haiti, Mischel and Mischel in Trinidad, and Leiris in Ethiopia.[22] Mischel and Mischel list the following psychotherapeutic aspects, which I believe also operate in Yoruba possession cults:

> attainment of high status through a cult role (the possessed person also enjoys a degree of control over others never realized in his everyday role);
>
> acting out of aggressive and sexual behavior;
>
> reversal of sexual roles;
>
> temporary freedom of responsibility for actions.

It must be remembered, however, that for the Yoruba, and I believe for most other cultures in which possession occurs, the most significant element in possession is "prophesying." The possessed becomes the mouthpiece through which the spirit communicates with his devotees; and he gives explicit directions about the management of family affairs. I have witnessed this prophesying on only one occasion: at an evening meeting of one of the Christian faith-healing churches. In this case, several women were possessed by the "Holy Spirit," and very personal advice was dispensed to many of the members. It seems that during possession the members can speak their minds about fellow members. It was, in fact, not unlike some kinds of Western group therapy. Perhaps

this group therapeutic aspect of possession is as important as the cathartic effects that have been so much emphasized.

PERSONALITY-GROWTH FACTORS

None of the factors so far discussed involves the patient's insight
into his own deeper motives, with resulting expansion of self-awareness
and personality maturation. Indeed, I have seen very little evidence in
Yoruba psychotherapy of any attempt to change the individual. It is
true that some personal advice is offered during divination sessions and
during some *Orisa* possession ceremonies. But this advice, appropriate
as it often appears to be, is of a very superficial type, comparable to
Western "counseling" but administered in a more highly charged atmosphere. In the abreaction phenomena, there is no attempt to build
the "split off" and unacceptable "spirit" elements into the conscious
personality. The transvestite urges or the masculine-protest elements are
permitted periodic expression in conformity with the principle of "repetition compulsion" but are not integrated into the self in any way. On
the contrary, it is forbidden for a devotee to hear about his behavior
during possession; he "forgets" what he has done during possession or
masquerade. While making a film of the Sopono festival, I had considerable difficulty in obtaining permission from the cult elders to take
pictures of the possessed women for this reason: If a Sopono worshipper
were to see herself while possessed she would die.

Of course the insight and personality-growth functions of psychotherapy are very recent elements in Western psychiatry. I have discussed elsewhere the difficulties involved in doing "insight" therapy with
Yoruba patients.[23] Psychoanalysis and other insight therapies do not,
in fact, have wide appeal outside Western countries. This failure cannot
be attributed to economic factors or to the scarcity of trained practitioners alone; I suspect, rather, that this form of psychotherapy is not
compatible with these cultures and that it does not suit the needs of
their modal personalities.

§ The Future of Indigenous Therapy
for Psychiatric Disorders

The problem of the relationship between Western and indigenous
forms of medicine will assume increasing importance as more and more
underdeveloped countries make significant entries into the modern world.
India and China have already taken steps toward integration of tradi-

tional and Western medicine. Both James and Opler[24] speak favorably of these integrative steps; Gould, however, in an article entitled "Galen in China" views integration as retrogressive.[25]

Two recent studies, both carried out in Ghana, have also drawn attention to the importance of traditional medicine in African psychiatry.[26] Of the various indigenous institutions in Ghana, Jahoda points out:

> Were it not for this extensive preliminary screening . . . mental hospitals would be overwhelmed by a flood of cases with whom they could not possibly deal. The lesson is that any campaign of enlightenment ought to be cautious in condemning traditional healers and similar institutions, because they perform an extremely important social function.

There are, of course, dissenting voices. Margetts,[27] who spent several years as Specialist Psychiatrist in Kenya, is one:

> One hears something of the usefulness of so-called traditional therapy in the treatment of African mental patients. This refers to tribal methods of treatment by medicine men or religious healers, who may define mental illness by concepts of magic, superstition and religion, in addition to or in place of primitive medicine and surgery. . . . There is no doubt that in the very remote areas the native healers do some good (usually on the basis of strong positive suggestion based on fear and faith), but they often do harm too, though perhaps irresponsibly. There is probably no more reason to fit traditional healing into a mental health program in this day and age in Africa than in any other country in the world.

It seems clear that there is no good reason to encourage indigenous healing practices for physical illness in any culture. Western diagnostic technique and Western pharmacological and surgical knowledge far outstrip every other known system of medicine. In addition, Western practices are universally applicable: They are not culture-bound.

Psychological medicine is different, however, in a number of ways. Western psychiatric techniques are not in my opinion demonstrably superior to many indigenous Yoruba practices. I feel confident that investigation of the indigenous psychiatry of other groups will lead to the same conclusion. Psychotherapeutic techniques fit with the cultures in which they have developed and cannot cross cultural boundaries so successfully as can physical therapies. Lambo[28] writes, "We have repeatedly found that in the sphere of psychoneuroses some illiterate patients who have failed to respond to our kind of approach have recovered under the influence of "native psychotherapists at the native treatment centers." Psychiatric ills are not so pressing a public health problem as are many physical ills. They are not killers. The limited resources of underdeveloped countries must be devoted first to such major health problems as malnutrition, infectious diseases, and parasitic infestations. This consideration coupled with the other two make it clear that the mental-health programs of underdeveloped countries should make the fullest use of indigenous psychiatric facilities.

It is only fair to point out some of the less desirable features that exist at least in Yoruba indigenous psychiatry. The most serious defect has an economic base. If a patient incarcerated in a treatment center does not have sufficient financial backing by relatives, the healer frequently withholds proper treatment, and the patient is not adequately fed or clothed. Sometimes the healer will not discharge him, for, as he rightly points out, he has already invested considerable time and money in the patient, and, if he discharges him, he forfeits all hope of recompense. Caught between the neglect of relatives and the legitimate demands of the healer and with no means of appeal, the patient is in a very sorry situation. Although Yoruba family ties are strong, they do not endure long where chronic psychosis is concerned. A spouse loses interest immediately; siblings and fathers hold on somewhat longer; a mother is sometimes remarkably persistent.

A second abuse or potential abuse is the fact that an individual may be deprived of his freedom without official sanction. In Nigeria at the present time, there is the anomaly that, although the law requires a certification procedure before involuntary admission into Western mental hospitals, in native treatment centers a patient may legally be shackled, sometimes for years, without any official procedures. It is interesting, however, that, although I heard many pleas for release from treatment centers, I never once heard the complaint that a patient was being held contrary to his legal rights.

What of physical abuse, neglect, or the use of dangerous drugs? I saw no evidence of physical abuse in any of the treatment centers I studied. I have, on four or five occasions, however, seen scars on patients, the results of beatings in other treatment centers. Shackling is not a very desirable procedure; most healers, however, take pride in the fact that their patients wear shackles for only a few days. On the other hand, if his relatives disown him, a patient may be kept in shackles for long periods—not because of psychotic behavior but to prevent his escaping before his fees are paid—clearly a very undesirable state of affairs. I once saw some severe "bed sores" (or rather earth sores) as a result of prolonged shackling to a log. Some patients receive substances in their eye as part of their treatments; these substances cause severe conjunctivitis (which, to the healer, indicates good results); although I have never seen eye damage as a result of this procedure, I have been told by other Western physicians that corneal ulcers sometimes develop. If they do, these procedures should of course be discouraged.

Finally, I have been told by several Yoruba that patients admitted to some treatment centers are given "poisons" to make their madnesses worse so that the healers may charge higher fees. The existence of this practice was confirmed by a reliable healer. The plant used is *apikan* (a species of *Datura*), which contains hyoscine and scopolamine and probably other hallucinogenic agents. I do not know how common this practice is, but I did see the plant growing in the compounds of two healers. (Of course, drugs with similar effects are used in Western psychiatry, although for different motives.)

These undesirable features do not, it seems to me, warrant total rejection of the indigenous system; on the contrary, they suggest that a liaison with official psychiatry would provide, as a secondary gain, some measure of salutary official control. This paper is not the place for presentation of a detailed plan for such a liaison. But existing Western psychiatric facilities could form centers for networks of native treatment centers, with regular visits by psychiatric nurses. Treatment centers in such a system might receive small government subsidies on a per capita basis. Such support would obviate the one really major defect in the existing indigenous system—neglect of the indigent patient. Subsidies would be cheap in comparison to the cost of total Western psychiatric care. It must be added that the healers themselves would enthusiastically welcome such a liaison.

Notes

1. R. G. Armstrong, "The Development of Complex Societies in West Africa," *Proceedings of the 7th Conference of the Nigerian Institute for Social and Economic Research* (Ibadan: 1960), pp. 20-7.
2. F. Willett, "Ife and Its Archaeology," *Journal of African History*, 1 (1960), 231-48.
3. K. Murray, *The Art of Ife* (London: Crown Agents, 1955).
4. R. A. Dart, "Cultural Status of the South African Man-Apes," W. P. True, ed., *Smithsonian Treasury of Science*, III (New York: Simon and Schuster, Inc., 1960), 887-921; and L. S. B. Leakey, *The Progress and Evolution of Man in Africa* (London: Oxford University Press, 1961).
5. Armstrong, "The Use of Linguistic and Ethnographic Data in the Study of Idoma and Yoruba History." Paper presented at 4th International African Seminar, Dakar, December, 1961.
6. The *babalawo* is one of the important types of Yoruba healer. He employs a form of divination called *Ifa*, which involves the use of a vast body of oral literature, the *Odus*. In the *Odus* is enshrined much of Yoruba religious, historical,

and medical lore, as well as much folk wisdom. Indeed the *Odus* are as remarkable in their way and as unexpected as the Ife Bronzes. Maupoil's excellent monograph in French is the most complete account of *Ifa*. B. Maupoil, *La géomancie à l'ancienne côte des esclaves* (Paris: Institut d'Ethnologie, 1943). English works on the subject include W. R. Bascom, "The Sanctions of Ifa Divination," *Journal of the Royal Anthropological Institute*, 71 (1941), 43-53; Bascom, "Ifa Divination: Comments on Clarke's Paper in the Journal of the Royal Anthropological Institute [69, 235-6]," *Man*, 42 (1942), 41-3; Bascom, "Two Forms of Afro-Cuban Divination," Sol Tax, ed., *Acculturation in the Americas*, III (Chicago: University of Chicago Press, 1952); J. D. Clarke, "Ifa Divination," *Journal of the Royal Anthropological Institute*, 69 (1939), 235-56; and R. H. Prince, "Some Notes on Yoruba Native Doctors and Their Management of Mental Illness," *Proceedings of the 1st Pan-African Psychiatric Conference* (Abeokuta: 1961).

7. Prince, "Curse, Invocation and Mental Health among the Yoruba," *Canadian Psychiatric Association Journal*, 5 (1960), 65-79.

8. Prince, "The Yoruba Image of the Witch," *Journal of Mental Science*, 107 (1961), 795-805.

9. P. Morton-Williams, "The Atinga Cult among the South-Western Yoruba," *Bulletin de l'IFAN*, 18 (1956), 315-34.

10. The European witch cult described by M. Murray (*The God of the Witches* [New York: Anchor Books, 1960]) and T. C. Lethbridge (*Witches: Investigating an Ancient Religion* [London: Routledge & Kegan Paul, Ltd., 1962]) bears a remarkable similarity to the cult among the Yoruba. The similarities seem far too close for independent invention and seem to indicate, as M. J. Field (*Search for Security* [Evanston: Northwestern University Press, 1960]) suggests, that the institution is a widespread paleolithic one. The hand-ax cultures (cf. Leakey, *op. cit.*) no doubt took institutions, as well as material techniques, with them from Africa. Regarding the sexual license of the European witch cults, Murray believes that the cult had the power to increase or destroy the fertility of the soil, of animals, and men—and that the license represented attainment of magical control over fertility. It is possible that the Yoruba witches have the same beliefs, although I did not get close enough to them to verify this point. Murray also believes that one reason for the eating of children at initiation was to cause magical sealing of the mouth of the novice (as a child cannot talk, so the initiate will not be able to talk). Again I was not able to verify this theory from my Yoruba material. The idea finds some substantiation, however, in the confession quoted on p. 92, "Until I took the soup, they said I was the sort of person likely to give away their secrets." Lethbridge alleges that there are still practicing witch covens in England today.

11. S. S. Farrow, *Faith, Fancies and Fetich* (New York: The Macmillan Company, 1926); J. O. Lucas, *The Religion of the Yoruba* (Lagos: C. M. S. Bookshop, 1948); Bascom, "The Sociological Role of the Yoruba Cult-Group," *American Anthropological Memoir*, 46 (1944); Maupoil, *op. cit.*; and E. B. Idowu, *Oludumare, God in Yoruba Belief* (London: Longmans, Green & Co., Ltd., 1962).

12. The *Egunguns* are a male masquerade cult usually included among the *Orisa* groups. I have had very little contact with *Egungun* worshippers, but they are of great importance in the over-all pattern of Yoruba culture, and I believe they play an important role in the management of certain psychiatric illnesses. Some writers like Lucas (*op. cit.*) and H. U. Beier ("The *Egungun* Cult," *Nigeria Magazine*, 51 [1956] have described it as an ancestor cult, but Bascom ("Sociological Role") disagrees. Many informants have described *Egunguns* as messengers of misfortune in dreams. The *Egungun* dream is extremely common among patients suffering psychiatric disorders.

13. A. van Gennep, *Les Rites de Passage* (Paris: Librairie Critique, Emil Mourry, 1909).

14. Beier ("Quack Doctors in a Yoruba Village," *Dokita*, 1 [1960], 57-8), writes of his observations in Osogbo: "By far the largest section of the community, I should guess 70%, receive neither European nor African treatment but fall victim to the itinerant quacks, who walk about with a wooden tray on their belly and cry 'fine medicine, fine medicine.' On this tray almost anything can be found from Aspro to Penicillin and almost any patent medicine is being prescribed for any kind of disease."

15. To clarify the therapeutic functions of these cults, operational study of the active members of each cult, with special attention to the reasons why each individual became a member, is needed.

16. Idowu, *op. cit.;* and Prince, "Some Notes."

17. A. K. Ajisafe, *Hisotry of Abeokuta* (Suffolk: Richard Clay, Bungay, 1924); and Lucas, *op. cit.*

18. Beier, "Gelede Masks," *Odu, Journal of Yoruba and Related Studies,* 6 (1958), 5-23.

19. See A. L. Leighton and C. D. Leighton, "Elements of Psychotherapy in Navaho Religion," *Psychiatry*, 4 (1941), 515-23; M. E. Opler, "Some Points of Comparison between the Treatment of Functional Disorders by Apache Shamans and Modern Psychiatric Practice," *American Journal of Psychiatry*, 92 (1936) 1371-87; A. F. C. Wallace, "Dreams and the Wishes of the Soul: A Type of Psychoanalytic Theory among Seventeenth Century Iroquois," *American Anthropologist*, 60 (1958), 234-48; K. Stewart, *Pygmies and Dream Giants* (London: Victor Gollancz, Ltd., 1955); J. Gillin, "Magical Fright," *Psychiatry*, 11 (1948), 387-400; and R. Sereno, "Obeah, Magic and Social Structure in the Lesser Antilles," *Psychiatry*, 11 (1948), 15-31.

20. Bascom, "Sanctions."

21. O. Fenichel, *The Psychoanalytic Theory of Neuroses* (London: Routledge & Kegan Paul, Ltd., 1955), Chap. 23.

22. M. S. Wolff, "Notes on the Vodoun Religion in Haiti with Reference to its Social and Psychodynamics," *Revue International d'Ethnopsychologie Normale et Pathologique*, 1 (1956), 209-40; A. Kiev, "Spirit Possession in Haiti," *American Journal of Psychiatry*, 118 (1961), 133-8. W. Mischel and F. Mischel, "Psychological Aspects of Spirit Possession," *American Anthropologist*, 60 (1958), 249-60; and M. Leiris, "La possession par le Zar chez les chrétiens du nord de l'Ethiopie," *Mental Disorders and Mental Health in Africa South of the Sahara* (C. S. A. Publication 35 [Bukavu, 1958]), pp. 168-75. These authors also believe that self-inflicted injuries occurring during possession may have a penitential quality. I have not observed any self-inflicted injuries resulting from possession among the Yoruba.

23. Prince, "Western Psychiatry and the Yoruba: The Problem of Insight Therapy," *Proceedings of the 8th Conference of the Nigerian Institute for Social and Economic Research* (Ibadan, 1962).

24. D. W. James, "Chinese Medicine," *Lancet*, 268 (1955), 1068-9; and Opler, "The Cultural Definition of Illness in Village India," *Human Organization*, 21 (1962).

25. D. Gould, "Galen in China," *Lancet*, 270 (1958), 47.

26. Field, *op. cit.;* and G. Jahoda, "Traditional Healers and Other Institutions Concerned with Mental Illness in Ghana," *International Journal of Social Psychiatry*, 7 (1961), 245-68.

27. E. L. Margetts, "The Future for Psychiatry in East Africa," *East African Medical Journal*, 37 (1960), 448-56.

28. T. A. Lambo, "Neuropsychiatric Observations in the Western Region of Nigeria," *British Medical Journal*, 2 (1956), 1388-94.

Stephen Fuchs

Magic Healing Techniques Among the Balahis in Central India

THE BALAHIS are a caste of untouchable weavers and village servants inhabiting mainly the central regions of North India, Madhya Pradesh, Rajputana, and Uttar Pradesh. They form an important low caste, numbering no fewer than 600,000 individuals. The Balahi caste is related to such other untouchable castes of Central India, as the Chamars, Kolis, Doms, and Mahars. The Balahis, however, have also received many additions from the higher Hindu castes—people who, for one reason or the other, have been excommunicated and thus forced to ask for admission into the Balahi caste, which always welcomes members of the higher castes into its ranks.

In family and caste organizations, the Balahis conform closely to the higher Hindu castes, and, although they are untouchables and social outcasts, they are not devoid of a definite sense of social rank and prestige. For one reason, they are well aware of the fact that several castes among the untouchables are socially inferior to their own, and they recognize, furthermore, distinct social grades, even within their community circle. The Balahis thus belong to a definite social group in which they feel at home and secure.

The Balahis are Hindus by religion, although they have certain cults of their own—an elaborate Earth-Mother cult and a worship of clan gods, for example. Apart from these cults, the Balahis conform in all other aspects to Hindu religious beliefs and practices, although they are generally excluded from Hindu temples and cannot take part in Hindu worship. The Balahis have their own shrines and images, in front of which they perform much the same rites and celebrate the same feasts as the Hindus. They even have their own priests, whom they call "Brahmans." The Balahi Brahmans, however, are not members of the genuine

Brahman caste, and they are treated simply as Balahis by the Hindu castes.[1]

With the rural Hindu population, whether cultivators or artisans, the Balahis share a strong conviction of the efficacy of magic, omens, and divination. From earliest childhood, they live in an atmosphere saturated by such beliefs. Ignorant of the true driving forces in the realm of nature, they are inclined to see everywhere the manifestations of mysterious superhuman powers. This trend is strongly nourished by wandering Hindu monks and mendicants, as well as by professional entertainers, who find a source of income in filling the impressionable minds of the simple villagers with Hindu mythology and magic.

Encumbered as they are by serious economic and social handicaps, the Balahis rarely have the opportunity to receive even the most elementary education in schools. Inquisitive Balahis who seek after the causes and meaning of natural phenomena, are therefore easily silenced with mythological explanations, which they are forced to accept implicitly in the name of religion. To question the truth of such explanations would be considered a deplorable lack of religious fervor.

This explains, no doubt, why the Balahis, suspect the machinations of superhuman forces behind every striking event in their lives. Through curious and ingenious magic devices, they try to secure the help and favor of well-meaning superhuman spirits, as well as protection against the tricks and wiles of evil and malignant forces. In their opinion, it is wise to take the spirits into account in all of life's undertakings, for they are inescapable and formidable forces.

This deep-rooted belief in the existence of a magic world and its inherent influence upon their own lives is particularly noticeable when the Balahis fall sick or otherwise become victims of adversity or ill luck. Endowed with ordinary human intelligence, the Balahis too are inclined first to explore natural causes for any striking events in their lives, but their lack of education and their inability to grasp knowledge in its true perspective stand in the way of their discovering these natural causes, and in their frustration they put the blame on unknown superhuman forces.

§ Disease

The Balahis are well aware of the fact that certain diseases have natural causes, and they look first for natural remedies to cure them. When a Balahi falls sick, he first resorts to the usual household medicines, which are readily available and which are indeed quite effective in various ailments. If these medicines fail to cure an illness, friends and relatives lend their advice, and it is believed that no harm will be done if the patient takes several medicines at the same time—if one does not help, the other may, and among many remedies a patient is bound to hit upon the right one. In addition to the medicines offered by well-meaning friends and neighbors, a quack doctor is sometimes called in to treat the patient. In almost every village, a man or woman can be found who is reputed to have knowledge of herbs and healing potions, some of which are quite effective. The Balahis are, however, not yet accustomed to medical treatment by qualified doctors, and in many cases they can ill afford to pay the fees for such treatment.

Mental disorders are generally not recognized as genuine diseases. In fact, cases of insanity among the Balahis are rare. Insane or mentally retarded children are probably not allowed to grow up. The harsh economic conditions and the primitive methods of child care among the Balahis are too unfavorable to allow the survival of children with serious physical or mental handicaps. Furthermore, children born with deformities are considered monstrosities and killed. Children who prove troublesome or unduly different in behavior are neglected at home and die of starvation or of additional illnesses, harmless in themselves but fatal in their undernourished states. The incidence of infant mortality among the Balahis is, in any case, very high and certainly works for the "survival of only the fittest."

Those who become mentally deranged after reaching adulthood are usually left free to wander about as they please. Kind-hearted or superstitious people give them food, in the belief that some spirit has taken possession of them and that the spirit can be served and obliged by giving alms to them.

If an insane person becomes violent, he may be tied to a post by his relatives or even chained and kept locked up in a room of the house. In one village, I was told, a demented young man lived for six years in the house of his parents, chained to a post in the back room. Another harmlessly insane man wanders from village to village, sometimes fairly well dressed, at other times almost naked, with long beard and locks. It is said that his father too is subject to occasional fits of insanity. His brother, however, is a hard-working and intelligent farmer who could well afford to look after his insane brother.

Sometimes, when a patient becomes violent, he is firmly tied, an iron is heated, and the patient is burned on his arms above the wrists, at his ankles, on the neck, and on the back of his head. This rather inhumane physiotherapeutic treatment seems sometimes to produce beneficial results, comparable to those obtained in regular mental hospitals through electroshock and other forms of convulsion therapy.

§ Cure of Disease by Divination

When a disease fails to respond to natural remedies, the Balahis are convinced that a certain deity or spirit has been offended and has sent the illness in revenge. There are two kinds of "medicine man" to effect a cure. One is the *janka,* and the other is the *barwa.*[2] The *janka* works through divination; the *barwa* calls to his assistance a superhuman force. The *janka* is called to find out by divination which god or spirit is responsible for the illness and what offerings must be performed to placate the offended deity. The *jankas* whom the Balahis consult usually belong to their own caste, but *jankas* of other castes may also be consulted if they are available and ready to undertake the cure.

In every village, some men or women can be found who diagnose the symptoms of patients' sicknesses in this manner as a profession. While any success enormously enhances their reputations as healers, failure does not necessarily diminish the people's trust in their powers. It is easy to find an excuse or to blame the stars if something goes wrong with the treatment.

When a *janka* undertakes a cure, he enters the patient's house and touches his feet with folded hands. This greeting is, meant not for the patient, however, but for the deity or spirit that supposedly possesses him and causes the illness. Then the *janka* feels the pulse of the patient with his left hand and pulls the fingers of the patient's hand with his right hand. Each time he does so, he mutters the name of some god or spirit. He knows many such names, but when his memory fails he goes on repeating names after names until such time as he hits upon the god or spirit answerable for the illness. The joints of the patient's fingers often crack in the process of pulling, and it is by counting the number of cracks that the *janka* is able to discover which superhuman force brought about the disease. Some *jankas* practice such other methods of divination as repeated measuring of grass stalks, constant observation of an oil lamp's flickering while reciting the names of gods and spirits, or forming queer figures by winnowing grain on a fan. In addition, they may use certain devices that are usually associated in the West with dowsing and water-divining.

The same methods are applied when the *janka* tries to find out what offerings have to be made in order to cure the patient. The usual demand is for eggs or chickens or even for a goat, but it is always combined with a quota of coconuts and such other things as are palatable.

When this complicated diagnosis is successfully accomplished, the *janka,* along with some members of the patient's family, escorts the sufferer to the shrine of the deity whose wrath has produced the sickness. In the event of the patient's being physically unfit to visit the shrine in person, the *janka* and the relatives go alone to appease the angry god on behalf of the unfortunate sufferer.

At the shrine, the *janka* recites some incantations (*mantra*). These *mantras* are stereotyped formulae that are believed to have intrinsic magic value and are effective provided the *janka* knows them by heart and that certain rigid conditions are fulfilled. These conditions include payment of an appropriate fee by the patient to his teacher (*guru*) for tutoring him properly during the nine days preceding Dasehra.[3] The following incantation is an example: "Allah! Bismillah! Raheman Rahim! Kali! Mahakali! Brahma's sister-in-law! with folded hands I pray: Save! But if you don't cure the patient, I shall dishonor your mother!"[4] The Balahis boldly claim that the latter part of the recitation is equally indispensable for the effectiveness of the incantation, for it impresses the urgency of the case upon the angry god.

After reciting these several incantations, the *janka* makes six or seven knots in a red string. After each knot, he repeats his *mantras,* ending with some hearty curses. At long last an offering is made to the deity; a ceremony of worship is performed; and the red knotted string is fastened around the neck, wrist, or arm of the patient.

A meal is served. The *janka* and the relatives of the patient have a feast, but the poor sufferer is not allowed to touch any of the food served on this occasion. Young women and children too are not allowed to feed. The *janka* then demands his fee and promptly receives whatever little amount is due to him. The gift is placed on the same plate on which the offerings were previously presented to the chosen deity of the day.

After the completion of this ceremony, the patient is expected to improve quickly and soon to be completely cured. If the cure fails, it must be repeated, or other methods must be employed to restore the patient's health.

In diseases of purely physical origins, the treatment carried out by the *janka* may be considered completely worthless, judged according to the principles of modern medical science. It may even prove harmful; for, while the *janka* performs his rites, much valuable time is wasted, and the patient may get worse while being deprived of proper medical treatment. In most cases of illness, however, the Balahis' traditional beliefs about the origins of disease are important psychological factors. It would be wrong to ignore them. The *janka's* performance can thus be regarded as a kind of psychoanalytical treatment of considerable therapeutic value.

The Balahis share with most uneducated Hindus the conviction that physical disease, in one form or other, is caused by the displeasure of some superhuman agency—a deity or spirit. This displeasure the patient may have incurred by a deliberate transgression of one of the numerous rules and taboos that every Hindu—even the untouchable—must observe. Punishment follows even if the transgression is unintentional and also when the transgressor is completely unaware of his offense. A sickness, consequently, often causes anxiety and a feeling of guilt in the patient. This anxiety may be the more troublesome if the patient is uncertain about the precise nature of his supposed transgression. On the other hand, a patient who is conscious of having committed an offense often regards his illness as the result. It may create in him the conviction that no medical treatment will be of any avail and that no cure can be accomplished until he has atoned for his offense and placated the offended deity or spirit by appropriate ceremonies and offerings.

It is consequently the delicate task of the *janka* to conduct his divination in such a manner that the patient either reveals his transgression himself or becomes aware of the precise nature of his offense if he has committed it unintentionally or even unconsciously. An experienced *janka* will prolong his divination until the desired result is achieved. His task is facilitated by the fact that very little remains hidden in a Balahi village. If the patient has committed any action for which he, in his own opinion, deserves divine punishment, the *janka* very likely knows about it before the patient approaches him for consultation. Should the patient suffer from a vague feeling of guilt because he cannot remember any definite wrong action, the *janka* usually has little difficulty in discovering such an action, for the rules and taboos prescribed by Hindu law and custom are too numerous to observe them all.

But should it really happen that no fault can be discovered in the life of the patient, it is assumed that a member of his family has committed it or possibly that the offense was committed in a former life. Like other Hindus, the Balahis also believe in *karma*[5] and rebirth. The appearance of worms in wounds, for instance, is commonly diagnosed by the Balahis as punishment for incest committed in a former life. After a cure has been effected, the patient has still to undergo the purification ceremonies prescribed for a person who has committed incest.

The divination of the *janka* and his treatment of the patient with incantation and sacrifice to the deity are therefore quite in accordance with the principles of sound psychology. After this treatment, the patient is mentally at peace, and all psychological obstacles to his cure are removed. That in most cases no proper medical treatment follows his performance is the *janka's* fault.

§ The Shaman (*Barwa*)

While the *janka* cures by divination, the *barwa* effects his cures by magic. The *barwa* claims to be possessed by a superhuman spirit (*bhut*) or by a deity in whose authority he acts and who speaks through him (or her), while a *janka* uses only natural devices like finger-pulling, measuring with grass stalks, observation of the flickering light, figures on the winnowing fan, and so forth, to ascertain the type of disease from which the patient suffers, the identity of the offended deity or spirit, and the kind and number of offerings necessary to effect a cure.

The *barwas* whom I have had the opportunity to meet were mostly people who themselves quite sincerely believed in their magic powers. The failure of an attempted cure—a fairly frequent occurrence—could not shake their confidence in their own abilities. I have also, however, met a few *barwas* who frankly admitted, after I had won their confidence, that their devices and cures were fraudulent and that they deceived their credulous clients. Some of them knew a few sleight-of-hand tricks, which they used to win the confidence of their patients. These tricks they had learned from their fathers or teachers, and their secrets were zealously guarded.

Most of the *barwas* whom I met appeared to me intelligent men but of somewhat nervous and unstable temperaments, boastful and averse to steady and hard work. Some of them, however, were rather reserved, quiet, and given to fits of depression.

Neither the vocation of the *barwa*, nor that of the *janka* is hereditary, or limited to a particular caste, sex, or age. Anyone taking a fancy to the mysterious and gifted with a certain mental and psychic aptitude may be initiated by an accomplished *barwa* into the ABCs of his art. The future fame of the new *barwa* depends heavily on his success in curing the sick.

A *barwa* recruits his disciples and successors in a most natural and often casual manner. He may find them among his relatives or neighbors, who frequently attend séances and lend him their assistance. At one performance of the *barwa,* one of them may fall into a trance, and from then on it may happen more frequently. Later he may be asked occasionally to take the *barwa's* place. Children are often present at a *barwa's* exorcism, and afterward they imitate in their play the behavior of the *barwa.* It occasionally happens that a boy or girl at play really has a fit and falls into a trance. Sometimes, however, it is severe illness that causes similar fits or hallucinations. The patient himself, as well as his relatives, has only one explanation for these phenomena—that a spirit or deity has taken possession of him. The patient will then consult a *barwa* and ask for a cure or for permission to serve as an apprentice and disciple.

It is evident that the *barwa* induces his state of trance deliberately and intentionally. He does so either by first drinking large quantities of liquor or by inhaling the smoke of hemp or camphor while chanting endlessly the same incantations and magic charms, gazing all the time at the figure of his favorite deity. An assistant beats a rather monotonous rhythm on a drum. After a while, the *barwa* begins to tremble in his whole body, while he rolls his head with incredible speed and vigor. At the same time, a stream of incoherent words pours from his lips. The words are shouted in a high, unnatural pitch. The eyes become vacant and glassy. It is obvious that the *barwa* has lost consciousness. He remembers nothing of whatever happens or is said during the séance. In this state, he is asked questions by his assistants about the condition of the client. Now and then, they catch a clear word from the babbling of the *barwa* and interpret it as an answer of the deity in him to their questions.

Until further research has been conducted by experts in psychology, it is impossible to make definite statements about the true nature of the *barwa's* self-induced trance. It is probable that its character varies, mainly in relation to the causes that produce it. In many cases when it is deliberately produced, it may fall in the category of autohypnosis. For in this hypnotic trance, the *barwa* often inflicts severe punishment on himself without feeling any pain and apparently without subsequent ill effects to his health. At other times, the trance may also be attributed to the heavy doses of alcohol or drugs that he has consumed; occasionally, especially on certain feasts, the trance may be simply a hysterical faint precipitated by a state of nervous exhaustion or an atmosphere heavily charged with intense emotion.

In the opinion of the people, however, an opinion that is shared quite sincerely by the *barwa* himself, it is a superhuman spirit or power that has taken possession of the *barwa's* body, inactivated his mind, and now acts and speaks through him. This familiar now reveals the secrets of the other world when asked by the *barwa's* disciples and clients; he reveals which *deos* (male gods) and *matas* (female deities) are causing the disease or the accident, how they can be appeased, and by what offerings. He also discloses the machinations of witches and gives advice for counteracting black magic; on the other hand, he is also ready to assist when black magic is to be performed by the *barwa*.

Some *barwas* can command the services of familiars even when they are not in trances. A spirit of this type is usually believed to be a *pir* (Mohammedan spirit). He is supposed to fulfill every wish and command of the *barwa* to the letter. He can kill or harm a person in such a cunning manner that no suspicion ever falls on his master. He will furnish any object that the *barwa* desires. With the help of his familiar, it is generally believed, the *barwa* is also able to read another person's thoughts. Often, when a client intends to employ the services of a *barwa*, he first tests him by asking him to read his thoughts. With a little experience in practical psychology, the *barwa* has little trouble accomplishing this feat.

In return for his services, the serving spirit is said to demand a solemn sacrifice once a year at Dasehra. Should the *barwa* omit this sacrifice at Dasehra, the spirit is believed to kill him in punishment for his negligence.

The celebration takes place on the ninth day of the month of Kuar (in September or October), which is also called Nau Durga. The feast is really in honor of Bhawani mata.[6] Nine days previous to the feast, the *barwa* prepares a basket filled with black soil. He sows wheat grains in this soil. Then he carries the basket into a small hut erected at the side of his house, where he keeps the image of his favorite deity. He places the basket at the side of the small brass or stone figure. For nine days he tends the sprouting wheat seedlings day and night and waters them carefully. He guards them anxiously against vermin and worms. In nine days, they grow to a height of about five or six inches.

On the eve of the feast, on the ninth day, the *barwa* performs a sacrifice in the hut, offering lemons, a pumpkin, and red and yellow powders and sacrificing a cock. Then, invoking his familiar, he smokes a pipe of hemp or drinks a glass of liquor to produce the proper mental disposition for the advent of the familiar. Soon he begins to tremble in all his limbs, to roll his head, and to talk in a high-pitched voice—sure signs that his familiar is taking possession of him.

The attendants of the *barwa*, his disciples and relatives, assist and support him when he seems in danger of falling to the ground in convulsions. They shake him and wake him up when he becomes unconscious. They force him to lift the basket with the wheat seedlings on his head and to carry it to a nearby river or pond. They themselves take another basket with the ingredients for an offering, as well as pieces of pumpkin and lemons. While walking to the watering place, they beat a peculiar small drum shaped like an hourglass and covered on both sides with lizard skin.

Several other *barwas*, of the same village or of neighboring villages, of the same or of other castes, with their personal attendants, also direct their steps toward the same river or pond. The crowd of curious villagers, however, keeps at a respectful distance. The various processions, converging at the watering place of the village, keep shouting slogans in praise of Bhawani mata, beating their drums, and throwing pieces of pumpkin and lemon about.

All stop at a huge boulder in the water, which is supposed to be the haunting place of the demon-god Mahishasur (or Maisoba), who was once upon a time slain by the goddess Bhawani. Mahishasur appears in the form of a buffalo and is believed to live under water. He is usually worshipped on the spot where cattle are driven and carts cross over.

On this boulder, each *barwa* offers a pumpkin broken into pieces and a lemon cut into halves. Then the baskets with the wheat seedlings are placed around the boulder on the ground. Often a virgin girl is made to sit near the offerings and is worshipped. She represents the goddess Bhawani, who, as a virgin, slew *Mahishasur*.

After that, the *barwas* take their baskets and carry them into the water. The heavy earth-filled baskets instantly sink to the bottom, while the wheat seedlings float away. All the while the attendants of the *barwas* beat the drums and dance incessantly in a frenzy of emotion. The *barwas* join them in the dance. Some of them stick knives through their cheeks or thrust them into arms and thighs. Or a *barwa* heats an iron chain in a fire, steps into the burning fire himself, and whips his bare back with the red-hot chain without apparently being hurt. It is claimed that not even a scar can be traced afterwards.

After some time, the excitement abates, and calm is restored. The villagers, who have so far been onlookers from a safe distance, now approach, embrace the *barwas*, and wish them well.

Though exhausted and perspiring profusely, the *barwas* gradually recover their normal states of mind. They feel greatly relieved, for the nine preceding days have strained their nerves to the utmost. They have scarcely been able to close their eyes for a short sleep, for fear their seedlings would be damaged or dry up. Had this happened, they would have been prevented from making the sacrifice of cocks or goats demanded by their familiars. And the omission of the sacrifice would have been punished by death or severe sickness. No *barwa* can omit with impunity to pay this annual tribute to the deity for generously bestowing upon him the extraordinary powers of healing and of driving away the evil spirits possessing the sick all through the year.

Female *barwas* (whose familiars are usually *matas*) have their annual feast in the spring. It is called Ganagaur. During their ceremonial procession, in which they too carry baskets of barley or wheat seedlings to the riverside or village pond, the women are greatly influenced by their spirits. They tremble in all their limbs and often roll on the ground in convulsions. Sometimes they fall into fits lasting for days, during which they appear completely paralyzed. In the course of time, they recover without any medical aid.

But such persistent fits, which are obviously of a hysterical nature, are rather an exception. Usually, after the ceremony at the river or pond, all return safely to the village and participate in a festive dinner, which brings the whole affair to a pleasant conclusion.

It thus appears that among the Balahis—as among other castes in the rural areas of northern India—men and women of hysterical disposition and psychic aptitude for hypnotizing themselves easily into a state of trance are generally accepted by the people as in alliance with certain superhuman forces or gods. It should also be emphasized that these people themselves firmly believe that they are "possessed" by their familiars and that it is the spirits who make prophecy, cure diseases, practice or immunize against black magic, and exorcise evil spirits.

We might be tempted to diagnose the case of the *barwa* as that of a "dissociated personality." Whenever he is "possessed," the *barwa* assumes a different personality—that of his familiar, who speaks and acts through him with the authority and behavior of a superhuman force. In psychopathic cases, however, this change of personality takes place automatically and cannot be controlled by the individual patient; the *barwa*, on the other hand, is able deliberately to produce this psychic state.

§ A Magic Cure of Disease

A *barwa* may attempt the cure of a patient through his familiar in two different ways, depending on the nature of the disease from which the patient suffers. If the patient is suffering from a natural ailment, though caused by the wrath of a deity or spirit, the *barwa* employs his

familiar to cure him by his superior powers. But if the illness is due
to the "possession" of the patient by a spirit or deity, the *barwa* must
exorcise this other spirit. The ritual of exorcism is different from that of
a mere magic cure.

When the relatives of a sick man or woman believe that the illness
is due to natural causes, they may consult a *barwa* or a *janka*. If they
have more confidence in the *barwa*, a member of the patient's family
takes a handful of millet grains (*joari*) and a small copper coin (*paisa*)
and passes his fist closely over the body of the patient, from the head
down to the feet. Then he takes the millet grains with the coin straight
to the *barwa* and asks for a séance.

The *barwa* warms water and takes a bath. He spreads a clean sheet
on the floor and places the image of his familiar or favorite god upon it.
In front of the small brass or stone figure, he places a low stool. He
squats down on it. The patient's messenger pours the millet grains and
the *paisa* on the floor within reach of the *barwa*, who now begins to pray
and to invoke his familiar. He burns camphor or hemp over a small fire
in front of him. Holding his hands over the fire and inhaling deeply
the smoke of the incense, he works himself into a trance, swaying gently
on his heels. Three times he passes his hands over his own body from
head to foot. Incessantly he recites his incantations until he passes into
unconsciousness. His whole body begins to shake and tremble, and sweat
pours out of all his pores. He sings and rolls his head from one side to
the other and writhes in convulsions, supported by his attendants.

At least in its early stage, this trance seems to be brought about by
the inhaling of camphor or hemp. This observation is borne out by the
admission of the *barwas* that initially they see those around them much
reduced in size and at a great distance, the usual effect of smoking or
chewing hemp. But later, when the trance is complete, the *barwa* appears
to be fully unconscious and in the possession of his familiar. It is this
spirit that impersonates him and gives instructions for how the patient
can be cured.

As soon as the *barwa* is in trance, an attendant takes a red powder
from a brass tray and, rubbing his thumb from the *barwa's* nose upwards,
paints his forehead with the sacred dye. All present shout *"Jai!"* (Hail!).
They are greeting the spirit or deity that has taken possession of the
barwa.

The patient's messenger now asks, "Deo Baba,[7] of which disease is my
brother suffering?" With two fingers, the *barwa* takes a few grains of the
millet that had touched the patient and throws them into a brass vessel
filled with water. The grains swimming on the surface of the water form

various shapes, which the *barwa* now interprets. He announces the disease
of which the patient is suffering, mentions the name of the deity or spirit
that caused the illness, and enumerates the offerings that have to be
made to ensure a cure.

Now the *barwa* takes a red thread and cuts off three pieces, which
he gives to the patient's relative to be tied around the waist, upper arm,
and neck of the patient. While enumerating the animals that have to be
sacrificed for the patient's cure, the *barwa* allows himself to be influenced
by the patient's economic status. If he is wealthy, a goat will have to be
sacrificed; otherwise only a cock, together with the other usual ingredients like eggs, coconuts, liquor, red and yellow dyes, and so forth. All
these offerings have to be brought to the shrine of the deity responsible
for the patient's illness. The sacrifice is performed by the *barwa* himself,
who afterward may keep part of the offerings for himself.

Finally the patient's messenger asks the *barwa* what the patient may
eat during the period of convalescence and what food he must avoid. The
Balahis are fully convinced that certain kinds of food are detrimental to
the patient's health and, if taken, will retard his speedy recovery. Usually
the *barwa* forbids rice, pulse, cucumber, and food prepared in oil. He
will point out most emphatically that he cannot be held responsible for
any failure to recover if the patient does not observe these restrictions.
Since many Balahis never bother about such restrictions, the *barwa* can
always find an excuse should the patient fail to recover.

Cases of snake-bite are always brought to the *barwas*, who alone can
cure them. *Barwas* who specialise in curing snake-bite must be healthy
and strong men because this treatment requires a great deal of mental
and physical strength. Such *barwas* are said to acquire their magic healing power through abstention from certain kinds of food, especially meat.
They must also avoid "live water," that is, water pouring from the sky
or flowing out of a spring or river on the earth.

It seems that the Balahis, like many other Hindus, are ignorant of
the fact that most Indian snakes are not poisonous. A person bitten by a
harmless snake may perhaps display all the symptoms of snake poisoning
out of sheer fright. In such cases, a *barwa* would be able to eliminate,
through his impressive and convincing ritual, the causes of shock rather
than the effects of actual poisoning. I have questioned a number of eye-
witnesses to cures accomplished by *barwas*, but in no case could these
witnesses prove that the patient who had recovered from snake-bite had
really been bitten by a poisonous snake. On the other hand, I have also
heard of several cases in which the *barwas* had not been able to save the
lives of patients bitten by poisonous snakes.

The ritual of a cure for snake-bite begins when the patient is first brought to the shrine of Hanuman, the monkey-god and protector of the village. The patient is covered with *nim* leaves (*Melia azidirachta Indica*). The usual ingredients are offered to Hanuman—incense sticks, yellow and red dyes, coconuts, and so forth. While reciting his magic incantations, the *barwa* passes his palms over the arms and legs of the patient down to the fingertips and toes. Then, massaging the patient's limbs, he pretends to drive the poison gradually down to the fingers and toes and, by the spell of his powerful magic charms, out of the body. During this exorcism, he appears to be in a trance.

There are some *barwas* who specialize in stilling the pain resulting from a scorpion's sting. Repeating his magic formula incessantly, the *barwa* passes his palm lightly over the arm or leg of the afflicted, thus driving the poison from the heart toward the wound. There the pain is usually felt for several hours. Some of the *barwas*, however, are expert enough to make the pain subside within a few minutes.

The method of healing suggests the cure is effected through hypnotism. This suggestion is confirmed by some *barwas*, who claim that they can conjure the pain of a person stung by a scorpion into another person, who feels it as intensely as if he had really been bitten by a scorpion.

It is obvious that the methods of curing disease adopted by the *barwas* do not differ materially from those of the *jankas*. There is, however, one significant difference: The *jankas* do not fall into trances, their method being that of divination, while the *barwas*, even though they may merely divine, do so in a state of trance. They cure and divine through the power and authority of the familiars that are supposed to "possess" them.

It may also be pointed out that in Balahi society the *barwas* and, to a lesser degree, the *jankas* take the place of physicians and healers and as such fulfill a socially important and useful task. This task is not recognized merely in their own conviction: It is widely recognized and acknowledged by the whole community. Among the *barwas*, there are certainly quite a few who, even in their own societies, would be considered mentally sick. The conviction of their own usefulness and the high reputation in which they are held by their own communities may help them to retain their sanity and save them from slipping into deeper mental disease. It is indeed remarkable how rare cases of insanity are in rural areas. The Census of India, 1931, records only thirty males and seventeen females as insane in the Nimar District of Madhya Pradesh per 100,000 of the population.

§ Exorcism

While the *barwas* attempt the cure of certain diseases that are thought to be merely *caused* by superhuman powers, they are also thought competent to exorcise spirits and deities that are in full possession of the patients. The Balahis, like most of the people in rural areas of India, believe strongly in the possibility and frequent occurrence of such "possession." Not only certain physical diseases like epilepsy but most types of mental illness are ascribed to such "possession." Mental diseases and even moral aberrations may be attributed to "possession" by superhuman and evil forces. People who habitually break the traditional rules of conduct and who frequently contravene the accepted code of morality may be suspected of being possessed by evil spirits. Thus women who have violent temperaments and quarrelsome natures or those who are kleptomaniacs or sexual perverts are often branded as witches.

Such people are generally regarded as dangerous to society, and the exorcism of the spirits possessing them is therefore inevitable. If such exorcism is not practicable for any reason or proves unsuccessful, the life of the "possessed" is often in danger. Cases of murder motivated by fear of harm to the community from possessed persons are quite frequent.

The manner of exorcism varies slightly, depending on the nature of the spirit or deity that is supposed to "possess" the sufferer. The exorcism of a *churel* (the spirit of a woman who has died in childbirth), for instance, is more complicated and difficult than that of any other spirit, because a *churel* is considered to be the most dangerous among the evil spirits. It is the spirit of a woman who has had to die in the prime of her youth and at a moment when she was fulfilling her most cherished vocation, bringing forth new life!

Thus only a powerful and experienced *barwa* is qualified to undertake such an exorcism, for which he may naturally expect a substantial fee after successful performance of his duty.

The *barwa* is called to the house of the patient, who is usually a woman. He squats on the floor in front of her in mute observation. Then he orders a member of the house to bring a burning dungcake. He calls upon the patient to bend over the fire, into which he has poured some spices, and to inhale the smoke. A sheet is thrown over the patient in such a way that it envelops the fire also. Thus, no smoke can escape. Inhaling deeply, the patient soon begins to get giddy and dizzy. This dizziness is the sign for the Barwa that the *churel* is entering the woman's body.

Sometimes the patient is first placed within the iron tire of a cart wheel. It is believed that the "possessed spirit" has no power to harm her so long as she stays within the circle of the iron tire. Should the tire be taken off during the exorcism, the patient will be killed instantly by the *churel*. A few years ago in one village, a Balahi woman, walking within the protective circle of such a tire, was brought to the shrine of the mother-goddess, where the *barwa* intended to complete his exorcism. While she was trudging to the shrine, together with people carrying the tire, a cobra suddenly crossed the path. The men who carried the tire were frightened at the sight of the cobra and almost dropped the tire. But an old Balahi kept his head and managed to kill the snake, meanwhile imploring the men to hold on to the tire. All the people who witnessed or heard this incident were convinced that, had the woman left the protective range of the tire, she would have been killed instantly by the *churel*.

When the patient begins to tremble, the *barwa* recites some incantations to make the *churel* "possessing" her more responsive. Then he asks some questions like: "Who are you? What do you want?" The sheet covering the patient is not taken off until the *churel* in her condescends to answer the questions through the woman's mouth. Paucity of air often makes the patient almost unconscious and faint. She starts coughing and vomiting. But the *barwa* remains adamant. If the *churel* is too stubborn and refuses to answer, the patient is severely whipped with a hair-whip or is made to suffer burns in the process of exorcism.

At last, the *barwa* receives a satisfactory reply and passes on to the next question. He now inquires what conditions must be fulfilled for the *churel* to leave the woman. The spirit is usually reluctant to answer this question, but, compelled by the magic power of the *barwa's* familiar, it discloses at last by what kind of offerings it can be induced to leave the victim. After a series of pleadings and lengthy disputes and exorcisms, the *churel* promises to depart. Such a duel between the *churel* and *barwa's* familiar invariably ends with the victory of the latter, but it is a dramatic battle full of sharp attacks and witty repartee.

For the last act, the *barwa* takes off the sheet that has so long covered the patient. He takes his shoe or sandal and shoves it into the afflicted woman's mouth. By this act, which in general Indian opinion is most offensive, the *barwa* expresses his victory over the *churel*. Holding the *barwa's* shoe between her teeth, the woman is then led outside to a tree. She is ordered to touch the tree with her forehead and at the same time to drop the shoe to the ground. As soon as she has done so, the *barwa* grasps the hair of the woman and drives a nail through the strands into the tree. Then he cuts the lock off near the head. The patient is so excited during this last scene that she falls to the ground in a swoon. When she is aroused from her fit, she is cured. She may suffer for some time from the after-effects of the rough treatment she has received during the exorcism, but she is cured, and there is rarely a relapse into her former illness. At least so the Balahis claim.

There is no doubt that in less severe cases of mental disease, especially in cases of hysteria, such an exorcism can be quite effective. Not only is the ritual most expressive and exhausting, but also the patient, in most cases, is very co-operative. For one reason, the man or woman under treatment personally believes firmly in the possibility of being "possessed" by a superhuman spirit and the ability of the *barwa* to drive it out. Second, the patient positively and often desperately desires to be rid of the "possessing" spirit. Furthermore, the ritual is often a real "shock treatment," and some *barwas* handle the patients with extreme cruelty. Finally, the patient, unless he is already too far gone, must be aware of the great danger awaiting him in the event of the exorcism's failure. The patient might then be regarded as permanently possessed by an evil spirit and consequently a public danger. The superstitious fear of the Balahis and other castes in the rural areas ascribes all accidents and cases of illness occurring in the village to this particular evil spirit and makes it impossible for the patient to live in the village. All these reasons are no doubt effective in making the *barwas'* method of treatment a success.

There is an imperative need for more mental hospitals run on a scientific basis. It is obvious that many mental cases could be cured by proper psychiatric treatment. But as long as these medical facilities are absent, the *jankas* and *barwas* of India will continue their treatments and will bring relief to the patient sufferers of the villages. Fortunately, life in the rural areas of India is still little burdened with nervous strain and mental tensions, so that diseases of the mind are comparatively rare. Furthermore, infant mortality is so high, and conditions of survival in early childhood are so severe that only robust and healthy children can survive. Thus hereditary mental debilities have little chance to develop. The rapid industrialization of India and the general improvement of the conditions of life may promote material progress among the Indian population, but they will also bring in their wake a steep increase of mental disease, for which traditional treatment by *jankas* and *barwas* will be pathetically inadequate.

Notes

1. See S. Fuchs, *The Children of Hari. A Study of the Nimar Balahis in the Central Provinces of India* (Vienna: 1950), pp. 17-80, 223-329.

2. *Janka* means "the expert," literally, "the knowing one." *Barwa* means "shaman," who, in a state of trance, is in contact with superhuman forces.

3. Dasehra is a Hindu feast in honor of the god Rama. It is held in September or October.

4. Literally, "I shall pierce the private part of your mother!" Such threats, as forms of abuse, are in common use among the Balahis and other people of low class in India. The addition of such abuse to a prayer is intended to shock the deity into granting the favor. Similar blasphemies are used in times of drought: Hindu farmers may throw dirt and refuse on the image of the village god. He is supposed to wash it off with a rain shower. The use of Mohammedan and Hindu names for God can be explained by the close cultural and religious relations between Mohammedans and Balahis in the Nimar District of Madhya Pradesh, where this *mantra* was recorded.

5. *Karma* means literally "action." It is the law of retribution for every good or bad action committed in former lives.

6. "Bhawani mata" is another name for Parvati, the wife of the god Shiva. She uses this name in her demon-slaying capacity. In other regions of India, the name "Kali" or "Durga" is used instead of "Bhawani."

7. An honorific title for the spirit supposedly possessing the *barwa*.

K. E. Schmidt

Folk Psychiatry in Sarawak:
A Tentative System of Psychiatry of the Iban*

SARAWAK, the most western of the three Malaysian states in Borneo, is the size of the United Kingdom. Kalimantan or Indonesian Borneo covers the greater part of Borneo, the third largest island in the world. Once the land of the renowned White Rajahs, it is thinly populated by approximately three-quarters of a million people, the largest groups being the indigenous people (the Sea-Dayak or Iban and others), the Chinese, and the Malays.

The following account focuses on the group characteristics, religion, and psychiatric system of the Iban, the largest single group in Sarawak. I shall describe the system of classification and the causes of emotional disturbance within the context of the Iban culture, instead of translating it into concepts of Western psychiatry. The parallels between the syndromes as defined by the Iban in terms of taboo violations and other supernatural phenomena, for example, and as defined within Western culture are clear enough.

§ The Iban or Sea-Dayak

The Iban are only one of the indigenous peoples in Sarawak; most of these groups share common cultural elements—like longhouses and a history of head hunting. In other cultural features, including language, however, they differ. The Iban are found in some coastal areas but

* Thanks are due to the Director of Medical Services of Sarawak for permission to publish this account and to the fifty-three informants interviewed in the course of this investigation.

mainly farther inland. They live along the rivers and inhabit longhouses on stilts. "They constitute a very valuable element in the population of Sarawak, not only from their numbers, but also from their force of character. They are active, hardworking, industrious . . . and in their domestic relations are amiable . . . and when treated with civility and sympathy all their good points come to the surface."[1]

"They are very human . . . they love passionately those who are kind to them, and trust absolutely those whom they recognize as their superiors. They are cheerful, merry and pleasure-loving . . . and the love for bright colors is very marked. They are fond of song . . . of games . . . (and) of dancing. . . . They are . . . apathetic . . . but they are truthful and honest. . . . The Dyak is frugal. He does not as a rule seek to accumulate wealth. Domestic affection is great. Parents will risk their lives for children. An old father or mother need never work unless they like. Their children will provide for them."[2]

Gomes describes their "mental and moral characteristics" in 1913: "The Dyak has no idea of clear thinking, and logic finds no place in his brain, and the most contradictory opinions seem to dwell together in perfect harmony in the turbid stream of his mind. The conceptions of cause and effect are hopelessly muddled, and anything he cannot account for, he attributes to the action of unseen spirits. He cannot distinguish between coincidence and causation, and will argue that because his grandfather died after he had climbed a tree, therefore his death was caused by his climbing a tree, and consequently neither his father nor himself nor his children are to climb trees, if they wish to enjoy good health!"[3]

The Iban personality has an elaborate structure. There is the body (*tuboh*), which contains the mind and soul (*semengat*). The Iban believes that there are seven minds, arranged according to seniority. The youngest stays inside the body, while the other six are about, looking for food, shelter, or water, and listening to warnings (especially about spirits—*antu*).

It is believed that the seventh mind also leaves the body during sleep, sickness, and "madness." A famous *manang* (native healer) stated that bad dreams are more likely to occur in a physically weak individual. The dreams are sent by spirits who seize the chance to approach the *semengat* (mind-soul) when it leaves the body temporarily during sleep.

Iban men are beautifully tattooed and used to wear long hair flowing down their backs, although the latter practice is fading. They used to wear the *sirat*, a loin cloth with long ends hanging down between the legs like an apron in front and a tail at the back. Their women used to wear only ankle-length skirts. Today the men often dress in shorts and shirts and the women in Malay dress.

In general, they are short people, averaging between five feet and five feet, three inches tall among the men and a little less among the women. Their skin is hairless and has been described as coffee-colored. They are lean and nimble and live by their tribal laws (*adat lama*—customs of old), which, in their conservatism, they are loath to change even with increasing penetration of their communities by government and other races and religions.

The Iban wear a kind of short sword (*parang*) continually, as do all the indigenous peoples, for it is a necessary implement in the dense jungle they inhabit. They are skilled in the manufacture and use of blowpipes with poisoned darts.

One can still see today the heads of slain enemies strung to particular posts in the longhouses. Heads meant power and wealth and standing: the more slain enemies, the greater the man. The custom has been successfully suppressed since the 1920s.

According to Gomes, in the old days no Dayak chief of any standing could be married unless he had procured the head of an enemy. Heads were necessary for certain ancient ceremonies like the *Gawai* by which the mourning period *ngetas ulit* is ended. It was customary in some tribes to bring home heads as offerings to the spirits when a new village was to be built. Although the presumption was that a man who had secured a human head was necessarily brave, in fact the head of a woman or child served the purpose. The Dayak value the heads, hang them over fireplaces, make offerings to them, and believe that the souls of their slain owners will be their own slaves in the other world.[4]

§ Iban Religion

The Iban believes in a deity called Petara (Almighty God), from whom are derived other deities like Singalang Burong, the god of war and of brave men, and Pulang Gana, the god of the soil and rice farming. Some people believe that every person has his own *petara* or guardian angel. The difference between *petara* (god and angel) and *antu* (spirit) is at times a little vague. Crudely, *petara*, is a good spirit, usually rather aloof, always benevolent, providing such boons to man as the use of iron, fire, and the (poisonous) tuba-root for fishing; it gives guidance and is called to feasts as an honored guest.

Antu are of several kinds and, in the case of ancestral spirits, may also be benevolent; they appear in many shapes to lead man out of trouble. There are also, however, many mischievous and even bad ones who may inhabit animals, floods, or certain trees or may assume absurd shapes like that of the giant Girasi. All varieties of spirits demand respect.

Because he is surrounded as it were by *antu* in all forms and shapes, the Dayak lives in continual fear of the unknown. He frequently tries to ascertain his fate to the minutest detail both for himself and his tribe by the reading of omens,[5] mostly those obtained from interpreting the flight of birds or from the inspection of the liver of a pig. The Dayak agriculturist plans when the impulse and the omen move him. Among the Dayak, the sense of the supernatural is extremely keen, and its impact pervades every action of his daily life. Spirit voices point out where he should build his house and warn him to turn back from ill fated expeditions.[6]

This view reported by a Christian missionary is meaningful in the light of Schaerer's statement that "the divine idea [*Gottesidee*] is the center of Dayak culture from which everything else is determined and back to which everything else is related" and that "the thinking [of the Dayak] is encompassed by the [religious] beliefs and in this dependency it stands, as all religious thinking does, apart from causal logical thinking."[7]

According to A. J. N. Richards, the longhouse community of several *bilek* families is supported by its special relationships with such "unseen powers" as the gods, the dead, and the evil and mischievous powers of the hills and forests. These relationships are maintained by the proper conduct of ritual "festivals" (*gawai*), offerings, and "magical" efforts. The determination of the specific ritual required is made by consultation with the gods, the omen-birds, or the examination of a pig's liver. Sometimes guidance is received in dreams from a tutelary spirit or ancestor. These various rituals are designed to ensure a proper balance among the people, to propitiate the spirits of evil, and to satisfy the gods and ancestral spirits.

As A. J. N. Richards has written: "Any disturbance of the balance must be corrected without delay, or the entity which is the community or family will be damaged or perhaps destroyed. Everything has value, whether tangible or not. The value is not in money but is capable of expression in terms of physical objects of ritual worth: for instance, words uttered or things done which embarrass another or put him in fear may be valued in certain kinds of plates, or in token articles of iron. Restoration of balance in this sense is secured by furnishing a 'fine' (e.g. *pemalu, chakap, pepat, nusi rita bulak*), by making good the loss with something of equal ritual value.

"The fine in such cases is more than a mere apology to allay personal feelings of anger or desire for revenge, it is a restoration of the balance within the group, made so that the group can continue to exist and preserve its relationship with all the powers.

"An 'offense' against custom (*adat lama*) is therefore a disturbance of the balance within the community, an encroachment on its property, whether tangible or not, and the significance of 'payment' of a fine lies in its magical or ritual effect of restoration and not in its causing the offender to suffer punishment and loss."[8]

Understanding of the psychiatry of the Iban is incomplete without scrutiny of the role played by taboos. A taboo (*mali*, elsewhere called *penti*) is usually established by the meeting of man and spirit. This meeting may be between an *antu* and a man's *semangat* while the latter has strayed away from the *tuboh* during sleep. It may however be a daytime encounter between a man and a spirit in the form of an animal. The mouse-deer or *pelandok* is especially favored by *antus*. This peculiar animal has the features of both a deer and a mouse and stands about a foot high. The animal will often lead a man out of the jungle if he has lost his way. It may be safely assumed in such a case that the good *antu* in the form of mouse-deer was in fact the soul of a forebear. After such an event, the man may be told in a dream that he and his descendants must not kill and eat *pelandok*.

The Iban are also firm believers in charms.

§ Iban Views of the Causation of Mental Illness

In Iban society, all mental illnesses (*gila*) are attributed to super-natural agencies (*gila laban antu*), as indeed are all illnesses (*sakit*). The varieties of *gila* are presented in terms of native categories of causation rather than in terms of the clinical entities utilized by Western psychiatrists.

VIOLATION OF TABOOS

The commonest cause of mental illness is *gila laban muli penti pemali*, violation of a taboo. Robert Graves writes in *The Greek Myths*, in a note about the madness of Orestes (who was pursued by the Furies after he had murdered his mother): "Erinyes (the Furies) were personified pangs of conscience, such as are still capable, in pagan Melanesia, of killing a man who has rashly or inadvertently broken a taboo. He will either go mad and leap from a coconut palm or wrap his head in a cloak, like Orestes, and refuse to eat or drink until he dies of starvation, even if nobody else is informed of his guilt. Paul would have suffered a similar fate at Damascus but for the timely arrival of Ananias (Acts IX, 9 ff)."[9]

Since taboos belong to families, an individual runs the risk of insanity if he violates a taboo established by an ancestor.

In some cases, the animal protected by a taboo may be a monkey or a python and, in others, a variety of bird. Once a major chieftain told the writer that his family is bound by such a law because his grandfather, at the age of thirty, dreamed that he must not kill, eat, or even touch a kind of bird called *burong tiong*. He therefore ordered that all his descendants obey the same command forever. The chieftain's brother-in-law did not accept the ban and shot this bird and took it home. At 2 A.M. the next day he became insane. He refused to talk and became aggressive and threatening.

In another case, a twenty-five-year-old Iban woman was admitted to the Lau King Howe Hospital in Sibu. She was complaining of a headache and could not sleep. She heard a voice talking to her and had been observed talking to herself. She had been laughing and crying unaccountably, had been restless, and was out of touch with reality. She was said to have met a ghost who disturbed her. She told a staff member of Sarawak Mental Hospital in Sibu that his voice abused her. The patient had recovered a normal warm affect a month later, when she was visited by the writer. By that time, she had received two electroconvulsive treatments and chlorpromazine medication.

Her story was that she had been married to an Iban policeman about a year before and that the marriage had broken up approximately nine months later because he accused her of seeking adventures whenever she returned for visits to her longhouse for periods of one or two weeks. She finally left him and returned to her longhouse. Her husband, she alleged, had in the meantime been dismissed from the Sarawak constabulary because of misappropriation of money. He also had remarried and was currently working as a rubber-tapper.

The patient said that she had been *gila* (mad, insane) for one month prior to the breaking up of the marriage. When asked what had made her *gila*, she said that she was under the influence of an *antu* (spirit) whom she had met in the jungle and who wanted to marry her. He appeared in the form of a young Iban. She heard and saw him for two days and nights and said that her mother also saw him. She refused him intimacy. She was quite certain that it was a spirit who, she alleged, "always wants to make me die." No *pelian* ceremony was held to free her of this spirit, partly because the nearest *manang* lived an hour away and partly because her family sent her relatively quickly to Sibu Hospital.

The reason, she stated, why she became *gila* was that she thought it likely that some cobra meat was served in a meal she had taken with some friends and that she had broken a taboo. In her family cobra meat was forbidden, a taboo handed down from the ancestors. The alleged sequence of events follows:

She ate cobra meat, thus breaking the family taboo.

Her *semengat* was then vulnerable to an *antu* who wanted to marry her.

He appeared to her in due course, but she refused him.

He therefore snatched her *semengat* "from her head" during sleep.

She did not know where he took it but thought it had since been restored to her by the *ubat* (medicine) she had received.

BEING MISLED BY SPIRITS

The more general idea of a spirit having turned into an animal and then misleading a man is a recurrent theme. A *penghulu* (chieftain) reported a case in which an evil spirit had turned into a deer and, while pursued by an Iban, had turned into a fairy at midnight. The Iban followed this fairy during the night and "married" it in the jungle. When he returned, he was locked up for fear that he would get lost. While he was on the whole well oriented, his talk was irrational, and at times he was destructive, tearing up his clothing and destroying his mat. He recovered gradually after some time.

FAILURE TO FULFILL AN ANTU'S COMMAND

A person may learn from the spirits of the dead, who sometimes appear in dreams, where to find a charm to protect him against the sword of an enemy. In return, he must hold a feast to honor the spirits of the dream or be punished by insanity. Along these lines, a man dreamed of traveling in a flying boat and attending a feast. There he was instructed to hold seven feasts (*gawai*) on successive days, sacrificing one white pig and one white fowl at each feast. His brothers, however, refused to help him. Two weeks later, without having held a feast, he became restless with fever (*selap*) and in three days became irrational and threatening and aimlessly wandered into the jungle. He dug holes in the river bank, saying that there were plenty of fish there. In six months he died.

In another case, a man of thirty-five years, after finding the highly regarded tooth of a wild pig, dreamed that he should sacrifice a fowl in thanksgiving. Failure to do so resulted in his admission to Sarawak Mental Hospital in 1955, at which time he exhibited incongruity of thought and affect and talked irrationally. Every month, at the time of the full moon, he still becomes aggressive, withdrawn, and mute.

A case of *gila laban antu* is of interest here since it demonstrates "the constant fear of the unknown and of unexplained events which even today govern the daily life of the Iban." A woman and her daughter paddled in a canoe up the Batang Lupar toward their longhouse. Both saw a long-haired baby afloat in the water, which they recognized as a spirit (*antu*) called *genalz,* the spirit of the water. They had been "passed by a spirit" (*pansa antu*) or "touched in the head" (*pansa untai*). When they came home and related their experience, people told the younger one to give a *gawai* and make offerings in order to avoid disaster. A few days later as she was washing her clothes by the river, they suddenly disappeared. She then "became insane," wailing and shouting, appealing to the *antu,* crying "don't take it." She was restless, and her talk was disconnected; she became sleepless, refused food and drink, and died after one or two weeks in the longhouse. The people concluded that the *gawai* had been held too late to save her life. This case of noncompliance involved a tradition that demanded a feast immediately after the encounter with a spirit in order to appease him.

In the same category fall those cases of psychiatric abnormality in which the cause is said to be the refusal by an Iban of a command given in a dream to become a *manang* or the refusal of a *manang* to become a *manang bali*—that is, one who wears woman's garments, talks, walks, and behaves like a woman, and who is said to be a very powerful healer.

SPELL-CASTING

Spell-casting plays some part in the causation of mental illness in Iban opinion, although some Iban believe that the practice may have been learned from the Malay. It is said that an Iban who wishes to learn the art of casting spells may fail to master it fully and is then in great danger. Charming is not usually employed for revenge but to make a person respond to the love of another. A spell is usually not cast directly upon an individual but on something belonging to him—a garment, for example. Charming is an application of sympathetic magic with

elements of both homeopathic and contagious magic.[10] Since charms play
a considerable role in the life of the Iban, they have to be looked after
properly. It is believed that lack of reverence toward them may lead to
misfortune or insanity.

An ancestor of one Iban family was given a special sword (*nyabor*)
by Bunga Nuing (an auxiliary god of war in the following of Kling,
the leader of the heroic world on Panggau somewhere between heaven
and earth). This gift made him and his descendants very powerful in
warfare and gave them prosperity. No reason for the gift was known
to my informant. One of the descendants desecrated the blade by using
it as an ordinary knife, failing to honor it as a gift from the god. The
family has declined since then. Two of the children (a boy and a girl)
became so abnormal mentally that they wandered off aimlessly into
the jungle, committed incest, and lived like the birds without permanent home. The family was fined for this transgression in the *penghulu's*
court but was unable to pay. The chieftain (a relative of the informant)
put the money down, taking part of their land in return. That family
is now landless.

Heads of slain enemies also have a power quite their own; they
are surrounded by the magic of charm and demand the same attention.
One outpatient at the Kuching Clinic *suffers* from symptomatic epilepsy
as punishment for not having shown customary reverence to the heads
taken by his ancestors and hung on the veranda of the family's *bilek*.

TRESPASSING

Walking under spirit-offerings, over a burial ground, or on a forbidden plot of land believed to be an abode of the spirits sometimes
causes mental illness. This condition is called *bumai tanah mali*. One case
of this sort involved a woman, many years ago, who suffered from a
mental abnormality called *djukat*. After she died, everyone avoided her
grave because her spirit had become an evil *antu* called *koklir*, which,
it was believed, would appear as a beautiful young woman, lead men
astray, and castrate them, producing death or insanity. Among the Malay,
this type of spirit is called *pontianak*.

There is a particular kind of tree called *kayu kara* or *kayu ara* in which
antu commonly live; walking under it produces mental illness.

BREAKING TABOOS IN PREPARING FOR MANHOOD

This offense may lead to insanity. To walk under a woman's garments
(perhaps hung up to dry) is forbidden, for example. The abnormality

may take the form of blood-shot eyes "from too much concentration"; the afflicted person will withdraw from his companions. Such mental abnormality is called *gila isin* from *isin,* meaning "tough"; elsewhere, it is called *gila urat* from *urat* meaning vein. In one reported case, an Iban joined up with a *guru* (teacher) to learn the art of self-defense. He learned all sorts of techniques for spell-casting during this training. When he finally left the *guru,* he went home to his longhouse and fell in love with a girl whose parents objected to the association. He therefore applied a love charm, which was successful. The parents employed another spell-caster to counteract the charm, and the suitor, who had abandoned his teacher prematurely, became mentally ill.

OTHER CAUSES

Frustrated love of a girl for a man is considered to be another cause of mental illness. The role of inheritance is disputed as a cause of *gila.* Some Iban maintain that, for mental illness to occur in two subsequent generations, the member of the second would have to meet with an *antu* himself, but that an increased tendency to do so would have been transmitted in his mother's milk. In the descendants of mentally ill people there is an increased tendency to break the same taboo again and duly to suffer the same consequences. Inherited mental illness, when recognized, is called *gila beturun* (*turun* means "to come down").

If children have too little work to do they may become lazy and insane due to poor blood circulation. Economic failure or social disgrace is another recognized cause of the condition *gila bendar,* "true madness." It has also been said that a person may become insane if he leaves the Iban *adat lama* (old custom) and becomes a Christian.

The Iban also recognize a few physical causes of mental illness, including contact with a promiscuous woman, anemia, plethora, and a retained placenta (insufficient blood in the afterbirth).

§ Descriptive Nomenclature of Varieties of Mental Illness

Gila bendar (true madness) is a term for any condition involving violence by a patient. It may be caused, some say, by agents other than spirits—economic failure or social disgrace, for example.

Ngamok (running amok) to the Iban clearly is caused by an *antu's* telling the victim's *semengat* to run loose. The word *ngamok* means "fighting." Running amok is, of course, a condition not peculiar to Ibans. It also occurs among Malays and some Islamic groups, and identical behavior patterns occur in other parts of the world. Suffice it to say here that a very large spectrum of underlying conditions may cause it. The cultural setting determines its form and direction.

Gila besi (*besi* means "iron") is a phenomenon probably similar to *ngamok* and characterized by sudden unprovoked attacks on others with a piece of iron, usually a *parang*.

Gila urat (*urat* means "vein") has already been mentioned in connection with men who attempt to become supermen (*gila isin*). Its special significance appears to be that a strong man's enemies can sometimes have his veins calcified by magic. He will become weak and babble like a child.

Gila ketawa (*ketawa* means "to laugh") is a condition in which a person talks and laughs to himself, wanders about aimlessely, and cannot sleep.

Gila kejubong (*kejubong* is the name of a fruit) is a descriptive term for a patient who laughs to himself, tears off his clothes, and dances by himself. The *kejubong* is said to have been prepared in a certain way by the spirit to produce this behavior pattern. The condition is said to be curable by *belian* (holding a *pelian*). It is also preventable by destruction of the fruit so prepared.

Gila ngaransi (*ngaransi* means "angry") describes a patient who throws his belongings away and destroys his property.

Gila nganu (*nganu* means "to address," "to scold") describes a state in which a patient scolds and hits others.

Gila nyadi (*nyadi* meaning "active," here it means "violent") is the term for a state of continuous violence, presumably equivalent to chronic mania.

Gila bejako (*bejako* means "to talk") is an even more circumscribed term, denoting autistic talk as the predominant feature.

Gila laban muai penti pemali denotes insanity caused by a broken taboo.

The condition of *gila untak* (*untak* means "brain") is said to arise from too much study.

Gila babi refers to epilepsy and is attributed to supernatural causes.

Gila isin (*isin* means "tough") describes a person who, having failed to become a strong man, may be quick-tempered and sometimes physically violent.

Mamau is clearly equivalent to senile dementia and occurs only in the elderly. Some say that it may also be caused by a broken taboo. It may be a sequel to *gila laban muai penti pemali*.

Jugau refers to people who are dim-witted and foolish.

Tuyo occurs in the young; it is characterized by autistic talk, some withdrawal, and odd behavior. It probably covers both arrested childhood-schizophrenia and mild hebephrenia.

Djukat covers both toxic-infective delirium and puerperal psychosis.

Jayau, which is also called *mamau laban jayau,* is characterized by lack of sleep, loss of appetite, and a tendency to suicide and is said to be caused by love-charms, frustration in love, and revenge for rejection as a lover.

§ Native Healers

AIMS OF TREATMENT

Of the three means by which any *antu* may affect the *semengat* of a person (disturbance from outside, possession by the *antu,* and removal of the *semengat* by the *antu*), the healers list the last as the most common. The depth of the psychosis depends on the distance to which the *semengat* has been removed by the spirit.

Individual phenomena like visual hallucinations are therefore explained by such statements as "the heart of the patient is not in its proper place." This displacement affects the brain; vision becomes unclear and disturbed. The aim of treatment is to restore the soul-mind to its place in the body and to reintegrate the patient into the group once the bad spirits have been defeated and new taboos given as safeguards against the relapse. The *manang* aims at integration into the family group (*pelian—ceremony*) while the *lemembang* aims more at a harmonious longhouse-community (*gawai—*ceremony).

There are four types of healer that deal with mental illness: *manang, lemembang, dukun,* and *bomoh.* A *dukun* is a practitioner who sells *ubat* (medicine), a type of herbalist. A *bomoh* is a Malay who works charms. Both these categories are not of Iban origin and are losing more and more ground to the hospital-assistants (male nurses), who are trained in the government hospitals and staff the government dispensaries.

Of the native healers, the *manang* is the one to whom people come with all ills, including mental illness. The following description of the Land Dayaks applies to the Iban *manang* as well: "The performance of the manangs were much more lively, making up in melodrama. . . . These two practitioners diagnosed, prognosed, invoked deities, danced in semi-trance consulting their deities in person, derived power from special objects in their possession, demonstrated superhuman qualities and caught souls. But the most important way in which they differed in their practice from the others was that they actually treated the patient, either by sucking or pulling the sickness out of him, or by using mysterious medicines, or both. There were other people in the village who gave herbal medicines, but only these practitioners did so as part of a spiritual treatment."[11]

This spiritual treatment consists of a *pelian* or ceremony in which the *manang* attempts to find the cause of the mental illness by reading it from his stone of light (*batu karas* or *batu ilau*). He locates the place to which the *antu* has taken the *semengat*. He then demonstrates to an awed audience his hazardous journey there through many rivers and over mountains and the ensuing fight with the spirit for the *semengat*. If he is successful in recovering it, he restores it to the patient by blowing or breathing it back into his head out of his hands where he is carrying it. To prevent relapse, several taboos are introduced—for example, crossing the sea for one month; wearing a black ribbon on the head; eating *ikan sembilan* (a sting fish), papaya, or gourd. The kind of *pelian* conducted by the *manang* always depends on the assumed cause rather than on the clinical picture.

A trance usually precedes the diagnosis, after which the *manang* is asked whether or not he can cure the condition and what the price is. Should he fail in one *pelian*, another or several more may be necessary. The *manang* calls on his own "secret helper" or guardian spirit (*yang*). In the case of an ordinary person, the guardian spirit is called *tua*.

The consultation fee of the *manang* can be announced by him only after the reading of the *batu karas* with which he first determines where the *antu* has taken the *semengat*, the distance he must go to get there, and which *pelian* to hold. He then calls the *antu* and battles him with a *parang*. This fight is usually carried on in a dark room by the *manang* alone after he has described in his incantations the adventurous journey of his own *semengat* to meet the *antu*. If the *antu* is killed, blood will appear on the *parang*, and a newly killed animal, which harbored the *antu* will be found nearby.

The trance indicates that the *manang's* body is without his *semengat*, which has left to go after the *antu* that led the patient's *semengat* away.

If a *manang* fails repeatedly to restore mental health by *belian* (holding a *pelian*), a *lemembang* is called in as a sort of consultant theologian. While the *manang* fights the *antu* for the *semengat* of the patient in the family-centered *pelian* ceremony, the *lemembang's* priest-like function is to invoke the good spirits, especially the great *petara*, to help in the *gawai* ceremony.[12] This ceremony involves the whole longhouse community. The *gawai*, which is held in order to cure sickness and mental abnormality is called *gawai sakit*.

During the *gawai*, the *lemembang* reads the important features of the case from the liver of a recently killed pig. The important diagnostic feature is the length and angle of the blood vessels of the liver. The *lemembang* calls all good spirits as guests from their abode in the Panggau River where departed heroes live. He then sings and leads communal singing. At dawn, when the good spirits finally come, there is eating and dancing on the *tanju* (drying platform of a longhouse). A chicken is waved at the celestial guests, who are told of the problem. Food and drink are offered to them, along with prayers.

RATES OF FAILURE AND SUCCESS

Failure to cure mental abnormality is attributed to failure of the *manang* to get the good spirits to help and his inability to make the *antu* let go of the patient's *semengat*. Failure may also be due to the fact that the spirit is too powerful or has run too far away with the patient's *semengat*. In addition, the spirit may have devoured the *semengat*, destroying it altogether and making a cure impossible.

Relapse rates after these methods of treatment are difficult to determine, since relapse depends on whether or not the taboo is broken again or whether or not another dream is disobeyed.

The rate of cure has been given variously as 50% to 90% by one *manang*, while several others have estimated a cure rate of one or two of ten cases of mental illness.

TRAINING, REWARDS, AND POWER

While *manang*ship is handed down from father to son, apprenticeship may also be served. Uusually a spirit appears in a dream and commands a man to become a *manang*. The spirit of the dream is usually the *yang* or personal guardian spirit who assists at subsequent crises. Manang Jalai, for example, while disabled by a fractured leg, dreamed that he walked up a mountain and came upon a *gawai*. From the assembled crowd an old man rose and told Jalai that his foot would heal if he would study to become a *manang*. He thereupon entered an eight-year apprenticeship, during which time the wound gradually closed.

A *manang* must undergo an initiation ceremony called *bebangun*. First, however, he must endure *bertama* (to enter) *ginti* (hook) in which an iron hook approximately one-half-inch long is implanted under the skin of the lower leg. From time to time, a *manang* must also submit himself to a *betimba* (ceremony of ladling water). It is believed that his body is saturated with fragments from the ills he has treated, which must be removed. At this ceremony, fellow *manangs* apply *ubat* (medicine) to him as a protection against the ills of his patients and against the *antu*.

A *manang* is thought by many to take a great risk of becoming ill, both mentally and physically, although some Iban believe that a *manang* will never become mentally ill.

Payment of a *manang* is usually in the form of household utensils and rice. The fee varies according to the difficulty of the journey the *manang* or his *semengat* must undertake in order to reach the abode of the *antu* that has taken the patient's *semengat*.

§ Comparison with the West

Whether or not the native healer has advantages over his European psychiatrist colleague in the management of mental illness is, of course, a difficult question to answer. Clearly, the native healer needs no expensive hospital nor the concomitant costly and time-consuming transport there. He needs no fulltime professional nurses and no expensive imported drugs, nor does his method of management require complicated legal and administrative machinery. Most important, the patient remains part of his family and tribal community, while, at present, long journeys are necessary for the Iban to reach medical or specialist facilities. The danger of breaking family bonds is then very great indeed.

Furthermore, the healing method itself involves the family and neighbors in a *pelian* and the whole longhouse in a *gawai*, ceremonies that tend to strengthen bonds.

The general belief among Ibans is that, where strong beliefs form the background of *gila*, the native healers achieve much good, often more good than European psychiatrists. As a last resort, however, a patient is always sent to a government medical institution.

The longhouse community of the indigenous ethnic groups of Sarawak is the form of communal life that, to a psychiatrist, appears closest to ideal—and to that extent is probably unique and rarely achieved elsewhere. It is generally a larger community than the extended family of Africa. Unfortunately—again from the psychiatrist's point of view— it is in the process of breaking up into villages (*kampongs*) with their own numerous new problems. It is difficult to avoid the conclusion that the apparent low incidence of mental illness among the native ethnic groups is due to the protective function of the longhouse and to role assignments for those who are afflicted. This writer believes that, while a longhouse leaves much room for improvement, especially in physical hygiene and farming methods, it is unsurpassed as a form of community. This point becomes especially clear in contrast to the capital, where high blocks of flats are occupied by people who no longer form communities.

In general, the psychiatric phenomena encountered among the various ethnic groups of Sarawak fit well into the reference framework of European diagnostic categories. All phenomena carry of course some local color, depending on the extent of Westernization of the group. But there is no essential difference between paranoia observed in a Kenya girl in Long Jawi, the highest and most remote longhouse-group in the upper reaches of the Balui, a branch of the mighty Rejang River, and the same phenomenon in a European visiting the country. The three classical criteria of the sensitivity-reaction (*sensitiver Beziehungswahn*) are present in both, even if the implications in the second example are much wider and not easily dealt with by the native healer in the communal setting of the longhouse.

The more one moves outside the capital, however, the more varied is the psychiatric scene that emerges, and the more frequently does the Westerner encounter unusual syndromes.

Among the indigenous people, many short-lived explosive psychoses occur. While a good proportion of the victims relapse at some later stage, many are never heard of again. Running amok is only one such syndrome. *Latah* is another common condition. It is characterized by an irresistible urge to imitate movements, gestures, words, and sentences and appears to be a state of increased suggestibility observable both in an hysterical setting and in encephalitis.

Among the Chinese, a high prevalence of mental disorder, in comparison with the Malays and all indigenous people, is striking, measured in numbers of admissions to both Sarawak Mental Hospital and the outpatient clinics. A great many of these patients, highly significant statistically, are in fact explainable geographically, for the Chinese have easier access to psychiatric institutions clustered as they are in the urban areas.

Among the Malays, cases of pure schizophrenia are rare, and the incidence of psychiatric disorder in general is even slightly lower than that of the indigenous tribes. Most of the endogenous psychoses encountered in Malays can be termed schizo-affective disorders, which are often present with hypomanic symptoms. One distressing feature is the relatively high prevalence of neurosyphilis among Malays, amounting to almost half the cases of admission to Sarawak Mental Hospital.

The chaos of languages in Sarawak constitutes the main difficulty for anyone concerned with mental health in this country. Among its bare three-quarters of a million people, at least twenty-one different languages (not dialects) are spoken. This situation obviously militates strongly against hospitalization, which is avoided as much as possible, since even normal people are unable to converse freely with one another.

Notes

1. The Rev. J. Perham, quoted in The Rev. E. H. Gomes, *Seventeen Years among the Sea Dayaks of Borneo, P. I.* (London: Seeley, Service & Co., Ltd., 1911).
2. Gomes, *The Sea Dayaks of Borneo* (Westminster: Society for the Propagation of the Gospel in Foreign Parts, 1907), p. 60.
3. Gomes, "Mental and Moral Characteristics of the Sea Dayaks," *Empire Review*, London, August, 1913.
4. Gomes, *Seventeen Years*, p. 72ff.
5. C. Hose and W. MacDougall, *The Pagan Tribes of Borneo*, Vol. II: *Animistic Beliefs* (London: Macmillan & Co., Ltd., 1912), Chap. XV.
6. E. Green, *Borneo, the Land of River and Palm* (London: Borneo Mission Association, 1911), p. 64.
7. E. Schaerer, *Die Gottesidee Der Ngadju Dajak In Sued-Borneo* (Leiden: E. J. Brill, Publisher, 1946).
8. A. J. N. Richards, "The Ibans," T. Harrison, ed., *The Peoples of Sarawak* (Kuching: The Curator, Sarawak Museum, 1959), p. 14ff.
9. Robert Graves, *The Greek Myths* (New York: George Braziller, Inc., 1959).
10. J. G. Frazer, *The Golden Bough* (London: Macmillan & Co., Ltd., 1949), Chap. III, p. ii.
11. W. R. Geddes, *Nine Dayak Nights* (London: Oxford University Press, Ltd., 1957), p. xiv.
12. Gomes, *Sea Dayaks.*
13. E. Kretschmer, *Der Sensitive Beziehungswahn* (Stuttgart: Thieme Verlag, 1929).

Michael Gelfand

Psychiatric Disorders as Recognized by the Shona

THIS ACCOUNT deals with the mental disorders of the large Shona group, which comprises more than two-and-half million Africans in the greater part of Southern Rhodesia. Included in this group are at least four major tribes, but there are no important differences among them in their outlooks toward disease. Indeed, the conception of disease among the Shona is not very different from that of most tribes of Southern Africa.

The Shona are a pastoral and agricultural people—both aspects of their life are important. The tribes are divided into clans, each with its own totem and each ruled by a subchief with lesser chiefs under him. Among the Mashona tribe, however, there is no paramount chief, but instead each major clan in the tribe is ruled by a chief. Every major clan is supposed to have been founded many hundreds of years ago in the region it now occupies, and the successive ruling chiefs are all believed to have been descended from the original founder. In addition, the spirit (*mudzimu*) of the founder still lives as the clan or tribal spirit, to which the clan turns for advice on all matters of communal welfare. The tribal spirit or *mhondoro* is especially concerned with rain, crops, and succession to the chieftainship and is particularly upset if incest is practiced. The *mhondoro* will then show its displeasure by allowing no rain to fall.

The *mhondoro* makes its presence known by selecting a particular person as its medium; whenever the clansmen wish to know something of concern to the group—the possibility of drought, for example, the medium is approached. Under the influence of music, he falls possessed, (a hypnotic or dissociated state) and the spirit speaks through him and usually answers any question put to it.

Each clan lives within its defined boundaries, ruled by a subchief, and is further divided into many units or villages, each composed of the kinsmen of a particular family group. In the Shona villages, the characteristic mode of life can still be regarded as traditional for the most part. It is true that in some areas the inroads made by Christianity and Western civilization have been so great that many older customs have disappeared, but in most villages the basic features still remain.

The Shona village or *musha* is essentially a family affair, for, though there may be one or more strangers living in the family group, the rest are relatives. In a Shona village, the grandfather and father are held in the greatest respect. Women have lower status than have men. Most authority is vested in the man, and, when his wife or daughter brings him food, she kneels before handing it to him. No woman is allowed to come and sit at the *dare,* a small clearing in the village yard where the men and boys congregate for their meals. The wives and daughters eat their food separately in the huts with other females. No woman is allowed to sit on a seat, log, or stone but only on the ground. In sex matters, the man can always ask or demand relationship with his wife, and the wife may never refuse. She is subservient to him in all matters pertaining to sex, and after the act is over she must clean his genitals with warm water.

The duties of the two sexes are clearly defined. The girl performs certain tasks, as does the boy. For instance, cooking and preparing beer are only performed by women. The milking of cows falls to the male, who looks after the cattle in the cattle pen, where no woman may assume any responsibility. The tasks of making baskets and utensils fall to men, but only women make clay pots. The erection of buildings is a prerogative of the male, except for smearing the floor with cow dung which can be done only by women.

Fetching water from a well or stream is women's work—no man collects water. Firewood for cooking in the hut is gathered by women, but that for making the fire at the *dare* is collected by men. Hunting and fishing also fall strictly to the men, but certain aspects of fishing, like poisoning the pools, can be done by women.

Both men and women participate in growing food. They help each other with planting, weeding, and gathering of the crops. There is an almost equal division of agricultural pursuits and endeavors. Each adult has his or her own small plot of land, and all help one another, although the husband's plot does receive first consideration. The crops are stored in separate granaries, but the first call is made on the food supplies of the wife.

The wife prepares the food, which is of a relatively simple basic pattern. With almost every meal there is a stiff porridge called *sadza* prepared from a cereal, as well as relish, which consists mainly of cooked vegetable leaves, monkey nuts, or occasionally meat and fowl.

The three important events—birth, marriage and death—in the cycle of every individual follow approximately the same pattern that is seen in other African tribes. We need pay little heed in this account to the birth of the Shona child, but marriage is important. Usually, especially among the traditional Shona, there is a period of secret or private engagement between the couple, when the girl gives her lover a token of her affection and loyalty. Nowadays this article may be a handkerchief, but formerly it was often something very private that she had worn on her body—we are told this token or *nhumbi*, as it is called, might have been some of her pubic hair or an article of clothing that had touched her genitalia. This token is really a promise to marry him, but should the girl change her mind and should he feel that he has been let down, he may refuse to return the *nhumbi* or pledge and place a spell on her instead, causing her to become sterile. In other words, a Shona girl is careful to whom she promises her hand in marriage.

The marriage ritual is fairly complicated, but essentially it consists of the transfer of cattle to the girl's father by the parents of the man soon to be married. While most of the details of marriage have been modified today, the principle of *lobolo* still exists. The wife and her off-spring become the property of the husband. When a son tells his father that he wishes to marry, the father sends a go-between (*munhai*) to the village of the girl to negotiate the marriage, sending with him the first payment, the *rutsambo*. The girl is called in first by her father and asked if she wants to marry this man. After she gives her consent, the *munhai* returns and reports to the man's father the number of cattle (*danga*) expected in addition to the *rutsambo*. A few days later, the bride's father arrives to collect his cattle and takes them back to his village. One of these cows is reserved for the girl's mother.

After another interval, perhaps of several weeks or more, the bride is fetched amid much celebration and excitement and leaves for her husband's village, accompanied by an aunt and her own sisters. The bridal party is welcomed in the new village. After several days of cele-bration with beer, the newly wedded couple meet for the first time in their own hut. In former days, although not today, he would have been asked the next morning whether or not he was satisfied: whether or not the girl had been a virgin. If not, she would have been put through an important ritual amounting to punishment for her social offense. It is cus-tomary before the wife leaves her own village that she be inspected by an elderly woman in order to determine whether or not she is a virgin. If the young husband were to announce after the wedding night that he was not happy, the go-between would be sent back to the girl's village carrying a blanket with a hole in its middle. A fine would then have to be paid by the girl's father.

If she is a virgin, as is more likely, the man's family must then provide a beast for his parents-in-law. This ceremony is known as the *masungiro*. I have purposely stressed the importance laid by the traditional African on virginity.

The cattle that the girl's father has received as the bride's wealth are now used to enable his own son to "purchase" his wife. The cow given to the girl's mother is important—should her son-in-law fail to make this payment, she would be most upset; after death, her spirit would certainly bring untold unhappiness and illness to the descendants of this daughter whose husband failed to honor her.

It is believed that the spirit of a married person, especially if there are offspring, continues to exert a tremendous influence on the living dependents. No one dies, for the spirit (*mudzimu*) lives on and protects the family, the most important spirit being that of the grandfather. At the burial, special care must be taken to bury the body in the correct manner; the grave is to be constructed in the traditional manner, and the implements of the deceased are to be placed on the surface of the grave. The precincts of the grave are to be swept. Any omission will anger the spirit, which means trouble and sickness for the family, even many years later.

Death is cruel, and the Shona are always greatly upset at the loss of a relative, especially if the person is young. Death is natural only for the aged, when it appears to be an act of the creator. Otherwise it is perpetrated by a *muroi* (witch) or sometimes by the anger of a dead person whose spirit (*mudzimu*) is offended and has elected to punish the family in this way. It is imperative for a person who is sick—and equally important to the survivors if he dies—to consult the diviner to learn the reason for the illness or death. Otherwise the anger or wrath of the departed relative or of the witch will continue unabated, and more unhappiness will come to the family. A very large part of the witch doctor's duties are concerned with divination.

The death rituals vary greatly in detail from territory to territory and even from district to district, but an account of those in Mashonaland demonstrates the main principles of African burial. There is first that of *kuriga* (the burial); second that of *Gata*—the determination of the cause of death and the carrying out of the instructions of the *ngange* in order to prevent further tragedy. Third comes the ceremony of *kurova guva*, usually held six months to a year later.

A few days after the burial, a small delegation of the deceased's relatives seek the witchdoctor to learn why he died. Even though they may have been told before death the reason for the person's illness, confirmation must be sought after death, in case the spiritual world has not been appeased or the witch discovered.

After a person's death, his belongings are collected in a bag and kept by someone like the *vatete* (aunt or sister of the deceased) until the ceremony of *kurova guva*—generally a year after death, when all the relations and friends gather again at the village and proceed to the grave to pray, offered beer to the spirit, and sweep the surface and precincts of the grave. The spirit is then settled and at peace.

The Shona have a clear idea of what constitutes madness (*kupenga*). They recognize a person as mad when he does not talk sense or when he performs foolish or amusing acts without realizing what he is doing. He may be restless at times, sometimes violent, and quiet on other occasions.

The Shona are well aware of man's liability to psychological disturbance, and, although most of their *nganga* (witch doctors) treat all kinds of complaints including mental disorders, a few claim to be specially skilled in the latter. The Shona appreciate the serious nature of a mental disorder, but at the same time they know that a great number so affected recover completely, even permanently, and it is therefore easy to understand how a certain *nganga* who happens to treat a mental subject receives credit for a recovery that would have happened regardless of his efforts. The *nganga's* reputation is enhanced by such a recovery, his failures are forgotten or overlooked, and the word soon spreads that he is particularly skilled in the treatment of mental disease.

There can be no doubt that a *nganga* can be of assistance in a patient's recovery from a mental breakdown, especially when an external or exciting factor is largely responsible for it. The *nganga* in his highly colorful dress creates a deep impression. He stands out as one endowed with a special mystical or supernatural power, which his family has inherited for untold generations. He understands his own people in a way that no European, however skilled, can ever hope to equal. There is no doubt that the *nganga* instills more confidence among the traditional Africans, who still constitute the majority on the continent, than the Western doctor—especially when the complaint is a neurosis or an anxiety state.

In this setting, the medicine man has a very big part to play, for he is not only the medical practitioner but also the go-between for the spiritual world and the individual. Since disease has an essentially spiritual basis, he is the diagnostician as well as the priest. Indeed he is the consultant for all problems affecting an individual. He can tell not only why a person is ill, which of the ancestral spirits are offended, and what will placate the spirits but what has happened to a lost article and who stole it, whether or not a long journey will be successful, and so on. The medicine man consequently is an essential figure in this society. When a state of tension exists in a family, quick recourse can be made to him and an answer soon received. While one common cause of illness or death is the anger of a departed relative, the other is the machinations of a witch. One of the main duties of the medicine man is therefore to tell whether or not witchcraft is responsible for the upset. The medicine man discovers the spiritual cause of an illness through the procedure commonly called "divination." To divine, he usually throws his set of wooden "bones" (*hakata*), each of which has special markings on it, and according to their lie he can tell which spirit is offended or if a witch is responsible. Not all *nganga* divine with bones. For instance, a woman practically never throws *hakata* but divines with her healing spirit; she falls into a kind of trance or state of possession, and in this way reveals the cause for the illness or death.

The *nganga* is the keystone or main figure in African medical practice today, and it is therefore relevant to discuss briefly the mental make-up of the Shona *nganga*. Paul Radin stresses the neurotic make-up of the *shaman*, to whom the Shona *nganga* corresponds.[1] Each is required to pass through a period of acute mental strain during initiation, and only after it is over are they ready to start treating patients. The Shona *nganga* also passes through an interesting period of illness before people come to recognize he is being troubled by a healing spirit, but there are no definite characteristics of this illness, although at times it may take the form of mental confusion. In contrast to those who become *shamans*, no special type of person is destined to become *nganga*. Nor have I been able to detect a neurotic personality in the make-up of the Shona *nganga*. In fact, I have always been impressed by their normal, stable personalities.

On the other hand, the mediums for the tribal spirits (*mhondoro*) responsible for rain and the general welfare of the Shona tribe almost invariably become mentally disoriented in the period before they are accepted as mediums. It is necessary at this juncture to give a few more details about the tribal medium of Mashonaland, for he is intimately concerned with spirit possession. Mashonaland is divided into a number of districts, each under its tribal spirit (*mhondoro*), whose function is to bring the rain and to guard the well-being of the community as a whole. Each tribal spirit is supposed to select one person as its medium or host through whom it makes known its views and demands to the people.

As he becomes possessed, the medium begins to shake vigorously and behaves as if he is in a trance or hypnotic state. There can be no doubt that a possessed individual is in an abnormal frame of mind. Possession is hastened by appropriate music and is preceded by extensive muscular contractions with rapid to-and-fro movements of the head and limbs. The medium is said to be incapable of recalling what he says during this trance. When possession is complete, all the preliminary contractions cease, and the medium behaves normally, although every now and then he may grunt or emit long sighs.

When the spirit leaves, the medium again begins to shudder, yawn, and stretch out his arms as if in flight. Occasionally, these actions are so intense that he falls to the ground in a state of exhaustion. I have never seen a medium take alcohol during or before possession. Nor does he fast before the ceremony, as has been suggested, in order to induce a state of hypoglycemia. Possession is so frequent an occurrence that it can be expected at almost any ritual ceremony—among both men and women. It is a form of mental reaction that deserves the serious consideration of psychoanalysts practicing in Africa.

When one attempts to analyze the rationale of the treatment meted out by the medicine man, one encounters certain difficulties. The principles adopted seem to be the same whether the disease is gastric, respiratory, or mental. There are, however, a few special procedures for mental illness.

One will often be able to detect which particular remedy is employed through its symbolic features, what is often called "sympathetic magic." For instance, to give a patient strength, security, and steadfastness, the shell of the tortoise is administered; to restore the strength in the patient's back, a portion of bone removed from the python's back.

All witch doctors also practice contagious magic, in which the power or "magic" is transferred to the victim through an intermediary agent. For instance, a person can procure some article of clothing that his rival or enemy has worn close to his body and take it to the witch doctor, who then can pronounce a spell on it and cause the victim to fall ill.

But it is not always possible to detect symbolism, for herbs or portions of animals or insects or their excretions are also given. Most of the remedies employed probably have little scientific validity. Usually the size of the fee charged by the *nganga* depends upon the difficulty of obtaining the particular root employed.

Exorcism is practiced by all witch doctors and is frequently employed in the handling of mental disease. The object of this method is to drive out the spirit causing the illness. Usually the medicine man waves an animal tail over the patient, while at the same time sprinkling a medicine on him. Another popular method employed for mental disease is to transfer the spirit from the patient to an animal—a sheep or fowl, for example—which is then driven into the woods, taking the curse with it. A similar idea underlies the practice of taking the patient to a crossroads where the spirit is exorcised by pronouncing special words. The evil spirit leaves the mad person and remains at the crossroads to be picked up and removed by some passer-by.

In order to understand the causes of mental disease among the Shona, we must examine briefly the factors they recognize as responsible for disease as a whole. They believe that any spirit can bring about any disease. They also believe that disease may be due to natural causes. The death of an old man does not evoke surprise, for it is part of life that everyone should die. No fear or alarm results if a man passes away after an accident, as people can understand clearly how that happened. It is not considered natural for any child or adult up to middle age to become ill or die, especially if death is sudden or inexplicable. Death, even after a chronic, troublesome, and painful illness, necessitates recourse to a *nganga* who can divine its cause.

Four important groups of spirits are believed to cause sickness, the two most frequent being the spirits of the parents or grandparents (*vadzimu*—spirit elders or ancestral spirits) and the witches (*muroi*). The *vadzimu* are more often considered responsible for sickness or death than the *muroi*—about twice as often according to my experience. The *ngozi* or angered spirit is related to those of the *vadzimu* but is the angry spirit of one who died an unnatural death through murder, for instance. The Shona believe that these spirits can all cause mental as well as physical sickness, but they recognize that there are other factors that lead to mental disorders, factors like incorrect use of magical medicines, ghosts (*chipoka*), worry, strain, and improper development of the brain.

Although the Shona have no difficulty in knowing when a person is mentally disturbed, it is extremely doubtful that a *nganga* can differentiate between neurosis and psychosis, except that he may recognize which is the more serious. He cannot diagnose an anxiety state that manifests itself in such visceral symptoms as abdominal pains. He can only attribute it to a disorder in the abdomen. He knows when a person is mad, behaves in a peculiar manner, and cannot be reasoned with, but he certainly cannot classify the different psychoses, although he appears to recognize certain mental syndromes that he invariably attributes to an offended spirit.

§ Witchcraft (*Kuroiwa*)

In interrogating *nganga*, one notices that witchcraft is one of the most frequent causes given for mental breakdown. Further, there are certain types or patterns of mental disease that the African attributes to witchcraft.

It is quite likely that an African who is depressed will confess to being a thoroughly wicked person and a witch. This reaction can be expected among people who associate or link badness and evil with witches. In the same way, a European in the throes of depression would mention his utter badness but would not use the word "witch." Many *nganga* claim to have cured people who admitted to being witches, while a Western doctor would have said the patients were suffering from a form of melancholia.

In common with other African tribes, the Shona believe that madness may be caused by a spell cast by a witch. One *nganga* described how an enemy or witch might procure a small portion of the victim's stool or urine, place it in a container, and hang it on a tree. When the wind blows in the victim's direction, it is believed that a curse descends upon him from the tree and that he loses his mind.

There are many different ways in which people can be bewitched. One example, described by a different *nganga*, is that of a woman who went to a more fortunate neighbor's hut to borrow a little salt or some other food substance. The neighbor refused to lend it to her. This refusal angered the poorer woman, who decided to procure a medicine with which to make the child of the selfish woman mad. This illustration serves to explain that it is unwise for anyone to display signs of selfishness lest they bring down upon them the wrath of someone endowed with the powers of witchcraft, for tragedy can ensue. The person so affected with madness becomes possessed at times with the spirit of one of the ancestral spirits, which speaks aloud through him and says, "I am mad because you did not give your neighbor salt, and that is why I am like this." This story provides a good example of delusion that may be attributed to spirit possession.

An interesting feature of African mental disease is the large number of mentally disturbed people living alone in the woods or wilds. Many have been there for a very long time. They are greatly feared and are referred to as *gandanga.* These people were either driven away from their villages when they first evinced madness or ran away themselves and disappeared into the woods. Some of them could not bear to live with others or were frightened by their weapons. In the woods, they had to fend for themselves and feed themselves, and so they became the wild men of the forests. They were known to be dangerous and to have killed people. It is quite possible that every *gandanga* was driven out by villagers who could not cope with his affliction. Ostracism may have been the only way of dealing with him, unless he were tied up or confined to a cave, where he would die of neglect and starvation. The mental disorder of the *gandanga* is said to be bewitchment, and his illness is referred to as *chisara chisara.*

The Shona understand mental backwardness in a child but often do not recognize the differences between the congenital form and that developed by a normal infant or child after a brain infection like meningitis. All forms of idiocy and mental retardation are included in the term *rema* and are attributed to the action of a witch upon the fetus. Most *nganga* believe that nothing can be done for this form of mental disorder.

Kupenga kwechitsiko (menga ra mumba) is probably an anxiety state or hysterical disorder and is characterized by the display of mental imbalance in front of others that improves when the victim is alone or leaves the village. It is said that he has been bewitched by someone in the village who dislikes him but that he recovers when removed from the influence of the witch.

Old or elderly people are often linked with the practice of witchcraft, and when an old witch dies his body must not be deposited in a grave without proper ritual ceremony to "fix" or drive away the evil spirit. If this ceremony is not performed, the spirit's evil influence will continue and return to cause mental breakdowns among his descendants or even among strangers. A special ceremony called *kupfukirwa* is therefore performed to drive off the spirit. A *nganga* takes a black fowl, administers a special medicine, and then allows it to run away into the woods where it is lost. It is believed that this ceremony ensures that the witch will never return.

The Shona recognize certain special features in mental disorders. For instance, a person who eats mud (probably geophagy) or other "dirty" matter is said to have a particular form of mental aberration caused by a witch. In a disorder of a similar nature, the victim continually repeats certain movements or actions. An example is the drummer who cannot stop drumming. This disorder is possibly a form of obsession, but among the Shona witchcraft is held responsible.

A person who suddenly starts talking nonsense or even performs senseless acts but in his more lucid intervals is able to carry out his normal duties is *ebenzi*. *Ebenzi* is believed to be caused by *varoyi we masekati*—the witch who performs his nefarious tasks during the daytime and plants poisonous objects along the paths of his victims.

Perhaps related to kleptomania is a thief's disorder resulting from bewitchment by the person whose belongings he stole. The man goes mad but continues to steal, and his constant thefts are now attributed to the bewitchment, which has produced an illness called *zuwanda* in which the sufferer imagines that something is continually moving over his body.

Another interesting mental disorder is that in which the patient mimics a particular animal, whose selection depends on the preference of a witch. For instance, if the *muroi* employs a snake to bewitch his victim, the victim crawls on the ground like a serpent. This type of mental disorder is known as *mamhepo* and is said to afflict those who are mean and selfish and refuse to help others. For instance, the woman who owns many dresses or plenty of salt, milk, sugar, and bread but refuses to share it when asked risks developing *mamhepo*, which comes in bouts or spasms during which it may be difficult to restrain the sufferer. As many as four people may be needed to hold her, but between the attacks she is apparently normal. *Mamhepo* is probably a form of hysteria or a sequel to epilepsy, for unless the *mamhepo* is cured the patient may develop convulsions and die.

A person who is struck down by paralysis in one or both limbs and is at the same time mentally disturbed may also be bewitched, in which case recovery is not expected. It is said that a patient with such an affliction usually dies within a year. This disorder is apparently associated either with grave cerebral disease like a tumor or with a vascular accident.

Benzi mazurazura, also attributed to witchcraft, is a mental disorder in which the subject strikes others without realizing what he has done but later discovers it. In another form of *benzi* called *benzi rema kuhwa*, the cause of which is not clear but may also be witchcraft, the sufferer continually tells lies. At first, people believe what he says, but they soon realize that nothing he says is true. It is possible that such a victim suffers from hallucinations that are not recognized as such.

It is believed that the witch generally plays with owls, which she keeps in gourds stored in the ground. These owls in themselves are considered dangerous even to their owner, for should she make a mistake when using them she or her children may be destroyed by them. The witch may send an owl on one of her wicked errands to bewitch a victim, who then develops a disorder called *kuvanda*, in which the neck becomes stiff and twisted, resembling a severe form of Forticollis.

Mental breakdown caused by a witch is held to be much more serious than that produced by the ancestral spirit (*mudzimu*). When the *mudzimu* is responsible for the illness, the patient may still be able to comprehend what is said to him and what is happening around him; he may even be able to stop unnecessary or foolish acts when asked. When, however, he does not realize what is happening around him, his illness is said to be due to the *muroi*. The *nganga* obviously does not realize that in one instance he is dealing with a neurosis and in the other a psychosis.

The richer and more fortunate Africans are most liable to attack by witches or sorcerers. It is believed that they are subject to these disorders because their fortunate positions arouse envy in the minds of others. Since witches are abnormally jealous individuals, individuals blessed or singled out above their fellow men would be obvious targets for their witchcraft.

Although a witch is evil and harms others, there are special men endowed with the ability to punish them when they have harmed innocent people. They are said to be possessed with the spirit known as *chikwambo* and may be likened to the white witches of Europe, who, by punishing or eliminating the guilty, fulfill a useful purpose in society. They are really a type of *nganga*. Let us imagine that someone has stolen valuable property or borrowed money and refused to return it. All efforts to recover it have been futile. In desperation, the aggrieved person seeks a *nganga* with the *chikwambo* spirit, for he knows he will then be able to recover his property. It is believed that to settle this score the special *nganga* sends a living animal— perhaps a hare, baboon, dove, or tortoise —to the guilty person's hut. There it suddenly appears and starts to speak to him, demanding that he pay his debt. If he drives the animal away, the *chikwambo* sends another, until he becomes so frightened that he and his family hasten to settle the debt. It is quite possible that the African does not recognize a hallucination as such but attributes it to a spiritual cause; when an individual sees one in the form of an animal, his friends and family thus believe that he has actually seen one sent by the *chikwambo* spirit.

§ The *Mudzimu* (Ancestral Spirit, Spirit Elder) or *Ngozi* (Angered Spirit)

The ancestral spirit, that is the spirit of a departed grandparent or parent, if annoyed, may punish one of its dependents, especially a grandchild, with illness. A mentally disturbed person is sometimes said therefore to be suffering from the wrath of one of its ancestral spirits.

Several forms of mental disorder are attributed to the ancestral spirits. One example described to me is that of a man, child, or young adult found wandering in the woods. The illness is due to the anger of its dead parents who were living as strangers in a certain village and neglecting the child. The child becomes mad and disappears into the woods to become what is termed a *muranda*. A *nganga* is consulted, and the villagers are told that the child's *mudzimu* is upset. To appease the spirit, it is given a black goat or a fowl, which is chased out of the village and allowed to run into the bush where the original *muranda* was first found. The child will then recover.

Mental Defectiveness (*rema—dull person*). The birth of a child with a low intelligence may be attributed to the anger of the spirit of a very distant forebear, which has selected one of its descendants to bear the brunt of its wrath.

If several members of a family become mentally confused or mad, their illnesses are likely to be attributed to an angered ancestral spirit (*ngozi*) not of the patient's family but of the family harmed by his people. After the death of a victim—for instance, in a murder—the angered spirit or *ngozi* strikes at a member of the murderer's family. One after another, the members of this family become ill until the case is recognized and full compensation made.

Another mental disorder called *Musare we Ngozi*, also attributed to the angered ancestral spirit, is one in which the patient behaves as if he were having a fit, uttering nonsense.

Kutanda Botso. When a man or woman wears old slacks, rags, and pieces of blanket around the waist and moves from village to village begging for food, people realize that he is suffering from *kutanda botso* due to the spirit of his dead mother angered because, when she was alive perhaps many years ago, he was unkind to her and beat her. At each village, the penitent picks up a little earth with a small piece of calabash and blows it away saying, "Grandmother, you left your snuffbox." These words express his guilt. The villagers all make fun of him but give him a little millet, which he collects in a large calabash. He continues in this way until he has about three basketfuls of grain and then returns to his home, where beer is brewed with the grain and a ceremony held. The son with the *ngozi* spirit asks his mother's forgiveness, saying, "I have done everything for you, Mother." An ox is killed for the angry spirit, and all the members of the village eat its meat. As the *ngozi* is now placated, the patient recovers within a few days. *Kutanda botso* may be a form of schizophrenia.

Madness Caused by Magical Medicines. An important cause of madness is the incorrect use of medicine with certain magical powers. One such popular medicine, known as *divisi*, is employed to increase the productivity of the soil, but the farmer must burn it in the center of his field if it is to be successful. If he burns it in another part of his field, the magic reacts against the farmer, who loses his senses.

The madness known as *kupenga kufukirwa* is another in which the victim has been harmed by magical medicines. When a man has practiced as a witch for many years and has brought about the deaths of many people of whom he was jealous, his magical medicines turn against him in his old age, and, they induce him in his confused state to confess all his previous practices.

§ The Importance of Strain

The *nganga* I have questioned also recognize that severe worry and strain can result in mental breakdown. There are many instances of this type of disorder. For example, a person who has stolen something begins to fear that he will be discovered, and the continual worry leads to his breakdown. Similarly, an adulterer's fear that his wife will discover his peccadillos may bring the same results. Strain may also follow when someone wants something so badly that he can think of nothing else and finally breaks down mentally. He may want cattle, children, or a girl friend. Envy and jealousy are bad traits often responsible for nervous disorders. When a man is rejected by his girl friend after spending all his earnings on her, he may become so upset that he procures a medicine to win back her affection. If it fails, he is so distressed that he becomes confused.

The Shona also know that a person with a mental disorder may complain of hearing voices. To them, however, these noises are due to ghosts (*chipoka*) that approach and beat his ears. The sufferer is continually rubbing his ears and is liable at times to jump up, seemingly without cause, and onlookers find it difficult to understand such behavior. It is believed that some *nganga* may remove the influence of *chipoka* by sprinkling a special powder (*mbanda*) on the person with an animal tail, which is part of his equipment. The same powder is also burnt in a *chayenga* (piece of broken clay pot), and its smoke is inhaled by the patient. It is believed that when the ghost sees the smoke it moves off and leaves the patient in peace.

In another mental affliction caused by ghosts (*chipoka*), the subject disappears suddenly every now and then. One moment he is seen with someone, and the next moment he is missing. His family or friends have to search for him and bring him home. This type of disorder is given the name of *masaramusi* and is found in adults of either sex.

Kupenga kuvumuka is probably a form of hysteria or perhaps a variant of epilepsy. The subject suddenly jumps up or talks without stop. The suddenness of the episode in some ways resembles an epileptiform seizure. This disorder may suddenly affect a person of either sex, and no age group is immune.

§ Treatment

The different measures adopted by the *traditional* Africans to control the mentally disordered are interesting, although much of what happens still remains a mystery. There is evidence that, when a patient becomes difficult to manage or a danger to others, he is tied up in the village precincts against a heavy object like a log of wood, so that he is unable to run about and harm others. He cannot remain there for long. From what I have learned, there seems to be no doubt that, when a mad person is difficult to control and is not likely to become more manageable, he is confined to a cave, where he probably perishes from lack of food and water. More usually, even today in the more remote parts of Mashonaland, the subject is driven from his home to take refuge in the woods where, as already mentioned, he is known as *gandanga*. There he lives on what he can find in the forest and roams about, injuring anyone who tries to obstruct his path. The well behaved or manageable patients are tended by their own families until they recover, as many do, aided by the suggestive therapy of the witch doctor (*nganga*).

As can be expected, the *nganga* uses many different curative measures. Many are based on similar principles, and they cannot all be described in this paper. I think it best to describe only those used by one *nganga* from Rusape. Although the reader may wonder about the meaning of some of his remedies, the suggestive aspect of the *nganga's* efforts cannot fail to impress him.

Much thought and argument are usually devoted by the *nganga* to the causes of madness, for, as we know, if they can be recognized and treated, the patient will recover. The African *nganga* has the same purpose as the Western doctor, and he too sets out to find the cause, which he believes is usually a spiritual one. By removing the influence of the spirit concerned, he believes that he will effect a recovery.

Ngozi (angered ancestral spirit). The *nganga* collects the leaves of the *zumbani* tree, some of the grass left in a dead person's hut, and the leaves of the small tree *mufandichimuka*. He stamps all these together on a grinding stone and burns the mixture to ashes. The burning ash is given to the patient, whose head is covered with a blanket so that he can inhale its smoke. This smoke induces the *ngozi* spirit possessing the patient to speak through him, divulging its name and explaining why it is seeking revenge. After the *ngozi* has spoken, the *nganga* takes the patient and a black hen to a pool (*Nziwa*). Here he looks for a *Mukute* tree, which grows near the water's edge, and orders the patient to sit under it. He cuts off the fowl's smallest toe and then makes a small incision (*nyora*) on the front lower part of the patient's neck and on the lowest cervical spine. He then dips the hen's toe into powder and rubs this powder, which now contains the blood of the toe, into the cut he has just made. The *nganga* next dips the hen into water, rotates the patient's head, and says, "*Ngozi,* leave the patient alone and come to the hen." The patient is then instructed to step into the pool and wade to the other side without looking back. The hen is left at the crossroads and disappears into the woods where it is soon lost and with it the spirit that had entered it. The *nganga* returns to the patient's house with him and mixes some roots of the *Mukuyu* tree with water from a pond that is known never to become dry and gives the patient the water to drink for about a week.

Madness Caused by Witchcraft. The *nganga* collects any item blown by the wind before it reaches the ground and mixes it with the seeds of the *mufuta* tree, the roots of the *mupatamhora* tree, the roots of the *muroro,* and a little of the patient's urine. He ties them together in a bundle, which he hangs from a branch of any tree and leaves it there for two days. Then he takes the patient and two ground nuts to the tree. He asks the patient to sit under the tree and close his eyes; he then cuts the string of the bundle so that it drops down on the madman's head. Immediately afterward he throws the two ground nuts onto his head and orders him to return to his home. Finally, the *nganga* makes another medicine by cooking roots of the *murungu* tree with those of the *mukwa* tree in a pot on the hearth, placing three pieces of the mushroom called *howamuwanga* on top of the hearth as well. The medicine is taken in the form of thin porridge.

Incorrect Use of Medical Remedies. For the type of madness resulting from the incorrect use of a magical medicine like *divisi,* this *nganga* collects a portion of the root of any tree that crosses a path and a piece of the root of any tree growing at the source of a river. He stamps these together with a grasshopper and one seed of every known African cereal until a fine powder is obtained. This powder is mixed with porridge and taken by the patient morning and evening each day for seventeen days. If this treatment is not successful, the *nganga* procures the leaves or bark of any portion of a tree that has fallen into water. He then finds a vegetable called *derere* (a type of marrow), but, if it is not available, a certain fish called *ramba* serves equally well. He mixes these elements together and adds them to a thin porridge, which the patient drinks at noon for twelve days.

Mental Disease Due to Improper or Poor Brain Development (*musoro watenderera*). This type of illness is discovered by the diviner when he throws his bones to find out why a person is mentally disturbed. To treat it, he cooks together some of the fat and the heart of a sheep with the root of the *mupetzaikono.* This soup is then consumed by the patient each day for five days. If this method fails to achieve a cure, the *nganga* cooks the root of the *muchecheni* tree with the roots of the *muonde, muveneka,* and *mutoto* trees and the heart of a brown cock. The patient drinks the mixture each day for ten days.

§ Conclusions

1. The Shona recognizes that mental disease may manifest itself in different forms, which he has tried to classify according to the type of spirit afflicting the individual.
2. While each spirit can cause a variety of mental breakdowns or symptoms, illnesses caused by witches are on the whole the most serious, protracted, and least likely to be cured. Mental backwardness caused by the ancestral or family spirits can also carry a bad prognosis, however.
3. The Shona recognizes that at times the individual recovers completely, relapses, or never improves, but he does not appear to distinguish between neurotic and psychotic disorders.

4. Shona treatment is based entirely on suggestion, which is an important feature of every technique adopted.
5. Visual or auditory hallucinations are thought to be real and sent by spirits.

Note

1. P. Radin, *Primitive Religion: Its Nature and Origin* (New York: Dover Publications, Inc., 1937).

J. Robin Fox

Witchcraft and Clanship in Cochiti Therapy*

§ Introduction

ILLNESS, both "mental" and "physical," though based on universal psychobiological factors, is in its expression highly culturally patterned. One becomes "sick" or "crazy" in a well defined, culturally delimited way.[1] What is defined as illness differs from culture to culture. Behavior labeled as "sickness" in one culture may count as religious ecstasy in another. The sociocultural system of which the individual is a member provides the stresses that cause the illness; the medium of expression of the illness; a theory of disease (spirit possession, soul loss, witchcraft, or attack of gods, ghosts, or germs); the basis for mobilization of help for the patient; a cure; and, in varying degrees, insurance that the cure will be permanent, that is, that there will be no relapse. In many primitive societies, fine balances have been achieved among these factors. Personality traits, cultural traditions, and social groupings combine both to cause and to cure disease. In many societies, however, there are considerable hiatuses among these factors. The society provides the stress but fails to find a cure, or, if it finds a cure, it fails to provide continuous reinforcement. Our own culture sharply dichotomizes the "hospital" and the "society," and, in the case of mental illness, the society is often directly or indirectly hostile to the patient and the hospital. Primitive

* The research on which this paper is based was carried out mainly in the Pueblo of Cochiti, New Mexico, 1958-1959, and was made possible by the Social Science Research Council and the Laboratory of Social Relations, Harvard University. A grant from the British Academy assisted in writing up the material. The help of Charles H. Lange, Evon Z. Vogt, Dell H. Hymes, John W. M. Whiting, and the late Clyde Kluckhohn is acknowledged. A portion of this material appeared previously (J. R. Fox, "Therapeutic Rituals and Social Structure in Cochiti Pueblo," *Human Relations*, 13 [1960], No. 4, 291-303), and acknowledgment is made to the editors of *Human Relations* for permission to incorporate it into this report.

societies and religious healing groups often have the edge on hospitals in that they more often incorporate the sick person into the society and indeed often *utilize* the sickness in some cultural sphere.

Kilton Stewart gives a detailed account of one type of hypnotherapy, practiced by the *negritos* in northern Luzon (Philippines).[2] Here the shaman induces a trance in the patient and instructs him to fight and overcome the "demon" that is attacking him and causing the complaint. Having mastered the demon, the patient demands from him a dance and a song. The shaman then ends the trance, and the patient is told to perform the dance and sing the song just learned—while the whole band witnesses the performance. The important thing about this type of cure is that all the aesthetic life of the band is derived from it. That is, all the songs and dances of the *negritos* are originally learned in such therapeutic trance conditions. These songs and dances are then regularly performed before the whole band, each person doing a dance-drama, in which he illustrates how he ovecame his illness (the demon), and receiving the support and applause of the band. He in turn appreciates and applauds the dance-dramas of his fellows. The likeness to certain types of group therapy is striking, but with the difference that, among the *negritos,* a large slice of the total culture—the aesthetic and recreational—is involved, indeed is derived, from the therapy. Reinforcement is built into a continuing cultural process in which all participate. The group therapy involves the whole social group acting in a whole cultural area; it is not divided between clinic and "outside."

In the American Southwest, the home of the Cochiti, the Navaho Indians have an ethnographic reputation as curers *par excellence.* Their "nine night sings," involving complex rituals and the assembly of thousands of Navaho, have a Durkheimian grandeur. Certainly such a huge effort to achieve a curing success is bound to have a supportive influence on the patient and therefore helps to effect a cure.[3] But the cure does not necessarily last. When the guests have packed up and gone home, the cure is over. Cochiti cures are less spectacular but are, I think, more subtly successful, especially in reinforcement.

Before describing them in detail I shall offer a brief résumé of Cochiti culture and society.

§ Culture and Society of the Cochiti

The Cochiti Pueblo (population approximately 300 in 1958) is one of the Eastern Keresan group of Pueblo (village-dwelling) Indians in New Mexico.[4] These villages lie near the Rio Grande between Santa Fe and

Albuquerque and take water from the river by means of elaborate irrigation ditches. The villages were traditionally compact but, of late, have spread out. The houses, often of two stories and closely packed together, are built of adobe (sun-dried mud and straw) and plastered with mud. Agriculture is the basis of the economy, but recently work for wages has become important.

Cochiti is one of the more acculturated and "liberal" of the Keresan villages, which are notorious for their conservatism and secrecy, but it retains a major part of the traditional culture. As in all the pueblos, this culture is largely concerned with ceremonialism. The indigenous religion was polytheistic and animistic, with the sun, the earth-mother, and a pair of hero twins as its major deities. There were many cults, and the "work" involved in them was divided among various social groups and roles. The main aim of the religion was to achieve fertility of persons, crops, and animals and harmony in society. This entire aim was expressed by saying that "the ceremonies were for rain."[5] Rain in fact symbolized goodness, health, fertility, happiness, and so forth. It came from the clouds, which were identified with the souls of the dead and with certain of the deities, the *shiwana*. The major cult, that of the *katsinas,* was concerned with these deities. There were numerous *katsinas,* and in the rituals men especially chosen from among initiates into the cult performed masked dances in imitation of the *katsinas*. During the dances, the dancer was in fact the embodiment, the essence of the god he represented. Other cult groups performed rituals concerned with hunting, war, and the curing of disease. Most important aspects of Cochiti life had their ritual counterparts.

The tribe was divided into moieties, called *kivas* (*chitya*) after the semiunderground circular chambers used for ceremonies. These *kivas* also had charge of rituals, primarily the public rituals. The most famous is the "corn" or "rain" dance—one of the few ever seen by non-Indians— in which each group dances in turn throughout the day.[6] Two "clown" groups, the *koshare* and the *kwirena,* are important in "managing" the ceremonies. The former represent the dead and the winter season, while the latter represent life and the spring and harvest.[7]

The government of Cochiti was essentially theocratic. The *cacique* (the "chief" of the tribe) and the main medicine men constituted a ruling elite, but their positions were not hereditary, and a show of reluctance was required of those chosen for office. The *cacique* was concerned with the spiritual welfare of the tribe, and his complement was the war captain (priest or chief), who was responsible for discipline. He and his assistant are named after the two war gods, Masewi and Oyoyewi, mythical hero twins.

The coming of the Spanish (c. 1542) and their final firm establishment after the Pueblo revolt (1680) changed much of the outward way of life.[8] A new form of government was imposed, including the office of "Governor," but the new officials were in fact the nominees and puppets of the old priestly hierarchy. Catholicism was accepted but not incorporated into the old religion. The two were allowed to run side by side, with a few minor calendrical adjustments. Economic life changed with the introduction of ploughs, horses, and sheep. The coming of the Americans (c. 1830) changed few of these arrangements, and the pace of change has rapidly accelerated only since World War II.

Cochiti society is characterized by a great complexity of groupings. Like all the Rio Grande pueblo societies, it has the dual-division (moiety) system. In Cochiti, there are two *kiva* groups, Pumpkin and Turquoise. Membership in the *kivas* is patrilineal for males, and women join the *kivas* of their husbands. The *kiva* groups are not exogamous, and roughly 50% of the women marry men of their fathers' *kivas*. The *kivas* are ceremonial corporations, complementing each others' functions and providing dance teams for the big public ceremonials. Each has a head and a group of officials, all male, and an all-male drum cult. The role of women in *kiva* affairs is limited to maintenance work on the structure and the provision of food and dancing partners at the ceremonies. It is possible for a man (but not a woman) to change *kiva* voluntarily, but it is a serious and rare step. Patrilineal membership for males and the enormous amount of time spent in *kiva* affairs means that the father-son-grandson bond is quite strong in this ceremonial context. A small group of consanguineally related males and their wives constitutes a kind of informal subgroup of the *kiva*.

The next most important group in the formal structure is the matrilineal clan (*hanuch*). Exogamous, nontotemic (but named) dispersed clans number about thirteen (it was impossible to obtain complete clan rosters). Some are large, (like the Oak, with more than 100 members); others are near extinction. Their place in the social structure has puzzled investigators, who see their functions now largely in terms of exogamy. Previously they also served as economic units of a kind, co-operating in harvesting, for example.[9] The eldest male was *nawa* or headman and, together with the eldest female, exercised some authority over members but not much. The clans apparently had no governmental functions and little ritual apart from curing. These characteristics set them off from the clans in the "western" pueblos (in Eggan's sense)[10] which play a larger part in social life, but this difference should not lead us to think too readily in terms of the "decline" of the Cochiti clans. They have remained stubbornly in evidence in Cochiti social organization throughout the period of investigation, even though in 1890 Bandalier thought them a "mere survival." They are simply one way of organizing kin for particular purposes, tending in large part to lie dormant in the structure and coming to the fore on certain occasions—marriage, baptism, and curing.

The clans are in theory not internally segmented, and no wide span of segmentation is recognized. Indeed, the Cochiti show little interest in genealogy, and it is rare for relatives to be remembered for more than four generations. The place of the father in procreation is not denied; it is simply not regarded as very relevant. The "unity" of the clan is thus not very apparent. Yet clanspeople think of themselves as "close" relatives, and the clan of the father is regarded as important.

The larger clans are, of course, internally divided *de facto*. The largest, Oak, has at least five distinct lineages. If lineages could be traced back far enough, no doubt most of them would be found to be related, but several may have originated in "foreign" women who intermarried from other pueblos. Each of these lineages has some of the unity that the clan as a whole lacks. In fact, any unity the clan has is derived from the unity of its lineages—each of which is internally strong—linked in a loose federation. The lineage is the unit of most significant interaction in the field of matrilineal relationships. As opposed to the basic alliance of the *kivas* (fathers and sons), it is based on the alliance of mothers and daughters. Two or three old sisters, their married daughters, and their grand-daughters form the typical grouping. The males of the group are the "brothers" of these women but are now becoming detached. Indeed, this detachment would constitute the most important change in the social structure of any matrilineal society. In Cochiti, it may be a situation of long standing, dating from the move into the Rio Grande area.[11] As long as the males were firmly attached to the core of women in the lineage, then the lineage was strong. When they became relatively detached, it was bound to lose its cohesion and wane as a major social group.

This detachment has to be seen in terms of the twin influences of household and family. Tradition presents the older household as a classical matri-uxorilocal set-up. The female core of the lineage resided together, and the males regarded this residence as "home" and were but loosely attached to their wives' households. This system has now com-pletely collapsed (if it was ever predominant) and has been replaced by neolocal residence—very often in a house built by the husband. This change and the Catholic prohibition on divorce have strengthened the bonds of marriage. The lack of a specific "house" to return to on divorce or separation has made the man more willing to stick to his wife and home. As the woman is still firmly attached to her sisters and mother, the man becomes attached to this group as well. A maternal extended family group is thus becoming the "domestic" unit in Cochiti, as the paternal extended family group is to some extent a "ritual" unit—both within the field of kinship. In terms of role relations, the husband-wife relationship has been strengthened at the expense of the brother-sister relationship. The lineage, while still existing conceptually, lies dormant most of the time, but its core and strength, the group of women, remains active.

Since Cochiti is a small pueblo, everyone is ultimately related to everyone else by ties of consanguinity, affinity, and ceremonial kinship. A "web of kinship" therefore exists, and from it two groupings emerge that are concentrations of families linked in various ways. The division between these two groups is not sharp. It is rather that the clustering of important bonds is more intensive in two areas of the total network. The two networks are the basis of recruitment to the baseball teams, which are deadly rivals.[12] Kroeber, who stresses the dichotomy between "kinship" and "clanship" in Zuni, and Forde, in his study of Hopi land tenure, see the importance of this "bilateral" web of ties.[13] Eggan tends to overstress the importance of the lineage and clan, two elements better regarded as part of the "formal" organization of the pueblo life.[14] In terms of the existence of actual decision-making groups, other principles than those of matrilineal descent can be important or even predominant.

The "medicine" and "managing" societies are associations of which membership is voluntary. The former are sometimes related to the latter in terms of membership and complementary functions. Two managing societies, Koshare and Kwirena, are linked to the two *kivas* respectively and help to arrange and supervise ceremonies. A third, the Shrutzi society, manages the Katsina cult. The medicine societies have both curing and governmental functions, in that they nominate the "secular" officers of the village. Membership in all these groups is falling off, and some are near extinction.

The secular officers ostensibly form the most powerful group in the pueblo. The governor and his assistant and the war captain and his assistant are the most powerful men in secular and ceremonial affairs respectively—although it is often hard to separate the two functions. The religious head of the tribe, the *cacique*, has very little real power but a good deal of influence. Together with the council of *principales*—past officials—these men govern the pueblo.

Among informal groupings, the factions are probably the most important, although the virulence of factionalism is abating in Cochiti. The "progressive" faction favors changes, while the "conservatives" stick to the "old ways." The ex-servicemen in the pueblo are doing much to pull these two together in a constructive way.[15]

This breakdown by no means exhausts the groupings in the pueblo (one important group, for example, is the Katsina cult), but it presents some of the most important and gives some idea of the structural and organizational complexity of the village. The society can be seen as based on the double division of the two *kivas* cut across by the clans, extended families, medicine societies, and so forth—although this point of view is not the only one possible. There is considerable overlapping of group membership as a result of the large number of groups and the small population, and this overlapping in turn helps to provide internal unity despite a high degree of conflict.

§ Cochiti Therapy

TYPOLOGY OF DISEASE AND CURE

The distinctions in Cochiti thought between various types of disease and their appropriate cures are not always easy to see. My own data were not collected with this question in mind and therefore show annoying gaps. It seems, however, that there are three main types. First and simplest are "natural" diseases (burns, fractures, and so forth), which are largely curable by natural means—herbal treatments, elementary first aid and sometimes treatment by the United States Indian Service doctors. Then come illnesses caused by witches, which are treated either by a member of a medicine society or, in severe cases, by an entire society. Each society specializes in certain types of cure. The various diseases treated in this way are characterized by some informants as "sharp" (*tsiati*): They are generally sudden illnesses that "seize" patients and are always considered the result of witchcraft. These illnesses are contrasted with "dull" illnesses (*tsatsi tsiati*, literally "not sharp")— those that, in the words of an informant, "just go on and on and don't seem to get better." For these illnesses, the society cures are considered too drastic and "clan cures" are employed. While not able to verbalize the distinction between these two types of disease very clearly, the Cochiti "know" one kind from another and can demonstrate details. In practice, the drawn-out "dull" diseases are not treated as though they had been caused by witchcraft, although it is impossible to pin the Cochiti down to a coherent theory of the causation of disease.

CURING SOCIETIES AND WITCHCRAFT

There are in the literature many details of curing ceremonies gleaned from informants, but no observer seems to have attended a cure. Some of the societies and their methods are common to all the Keresan pueblos.

I shall concentrate on Cochiti, but much of this material is true for all the Keresans.

There are societies proper and "degrees" within societies. In the important Flint society, its two degrees of Snake and Fire are now inextricably merged. This society is powerful because of its associations with the Koshare managing society and because the *cacique* is chosen from it. It also nominates the war captain and his assistant. The Giant society is next in importance, and its head is first assistant to the *cacique*. This society, which nominates the governor and his assistant, is also closely associated with the Shrutzi society and the management of the Katsina cult. The Shikame society is loosely associated with the Kwirena and nominates the *fiscale* and his assistant. The medicine societies are thus intimately bound up with the ritual and political life of the tribe, and form a theocratic hierarchy of government as well as an agency of medical and spiritual well-being.

Recruitment to the societies is voluntary, by "trapping," or by cure: One can join as a result of vocation, of being "trapped" through entering a forbidden area during a ceremonial, or of a desire to perpetuate a cure. There is an elaborate initiation, often lasting many years and involving abstentions, fastings, and retreats.

There are three primary functions of the societies: curing, rain-making, and government. The last is largely delegated to the "secular" officials, and the medicine men concentrate on the first two. In general, they are the guardians of tribal well-being, ensuring its continuing fertility and health, although they function only in a context of immense communal effort in this direction. While sacrifice and prayer, mainly through dance and ritual, are required of all Cochiti, the medicine men are, in Bandalier's words, the "chief penitents of the tribe." They continually fast and pray on behalf of the Cochiti and indeed of all Pueblo Indians. Most of their time, however, is spent in curing. There is evidence of some division of labor among the societies. The Flint society was "considered primarily as doctors, curing illnessses, setting fractures and helping the people combat witchcraft."[16] They were called on to preside at births and deaths and were particularly proficient at curing wounds. The Snake society cured snake and other bites, while the Fire society specialized in burns and fevers. The Giant society also treated fevers and was perhaps preferred for births. The societies collectively led communal fasts and purifications.

In their general role as "penitents," members of societies fast, pray, and make "prayer sticks" in seclusion, thus gaining the good will of the tribal deities and ensuring rain, fertility, and good health. To understand their specific curing methods, one must understand the nature of witch-craft and its place in the theory of disease. Some diseases are to the Cochiti obviously "natural." The medicine men have considerable knowl-edge of first-aid measures and herbal cures for these illnesses. Others are not so obviously due to natural causes and are attributed to the super-natural malevolence of witches. In Cochiti thinking, witches are almost exclusively concerned with causing disease. In Pueblo cosmology, there is an uneasy balance of forces in the universe. The forces of good—the *shiwana* and the various other deities and spirits—are only precariously in control. Even they have to be compelled by elaborate rituals into pro-ducing rain and health. The witches represent a vast conspiracy of ill defined but definitely malignant beings that seek to destroy Pueblo civili-zation by attacking the health of its members.[17] They are of various types, appearing as humans, animals, and birds (especially owls) or as fireballs. Living humans can be witches by being born with two hearts, one good and one bad. Practically everyone is suspected by someone at some time of being a witch or of practicing sorcery. This distinction is not made in ethnographic writings or in Pueblo thinking, but a person actually prac-ticing sorcery (as opposed simply to "being" a witch) is by definition himself a witch or "two-heart." Persons found indulging in sorcery would, in the old days, have been clubbed to death by the war captains after a trial before the pueblo leaders. Such evidence would be required as the proofs of possession of owl feathers or other sorcerer's devices. Witch-craft mythology is riddled with inconsistencies, and it is often difficult to know whether an accused person is simply a "passive" witch, an active sorcerer, or an ordinary human in league with the witches. Witchcraft accusations are rarely specific as to the nature of the witchcraft or the identities of the victims. The accusation is simply that "he is a witch." Such an accusation can only gain sympathetic hearing if feeling generally is roused against the accused on some issue. Accusations have to be made with care because the strong notions of matrilineal heredity make them, by implication, indictments of the accused's matrilineal kin.

It is against this terrible conspiracy of evil that the people, helpless in their lack of ritual knowledge, seek aid from the medicine societies. The societies possess the knowledge, paraphernalia, and courage to com-bat the witches—the sources of their great power in the pueblos.

The witches cause illness by two basic methods. They either steal the heart of the victim, or they shoot objects into his body. To cure him, the medicine societies must suck the objects from the body or recover the heart by fighting the witches. To understand the nature and effective-ness of this curing process, one must enter sympathetically into the

Cochiti imagination. For most of the time, they feel that there is an uneasy balance in the universe. The enormous ritual efforts of the tribe and the vigilance of the medicine men are keeping the universe on an even keel and the witches at bay. But threat is always present. When someone falls very ill or behaves oddly, violently, or erratically, it means that the witches have broken through, in the same way that a drought means that the *Shiwana* have withdrawn—usually because of faulty ritual, which can itself be the result of witchcraft. The terror of mind produced by the feeling that one is in the grip of the witches—that is by being ill —is profound and real and is accentuated by the fear of those around. It is equivalent perhaps to the real medieval terror at feeling irredeemably damned. The fact that this conspiracy of evil has allies in the pueblo and even among one's own relatives is doubly terrifying. Even the doctors can be suspected, and the Katsinas themselves are not above suspicion. Sometimes people fear that they may be unconsciously guilty of witchcraft, for example when their "bad thoughts" about someone seem to result in his death or illness. The over-all atmosphere in the face of sickness or violence or anything completely untoward is one of real, helpless fright. Into this situation step the medicine men. Their curing method consists of accentuating the terror almost to breaking point and then, by triumphing over the witches in a fight, recapturing and returning the heart or removing the objects from the body. Here is White's matter-of-fact summary of the process:[18]

> When a person is ill he may ask to be treated by a medicine man or by a society. If the illness is not severe, one medicine man only will come. But if the patient is very ill, or wishes to become a member of the curing society, the whole society will come. The father of the patient summons the doctor (or society) by taking a handful of meal to the doctor selected or to the head man of the society.

> When one doctor only comes to treat the patient, the procedure is simple. He smokes, sings, mixes medicine in a bowl of water, puts ashes on his hands and massages the patient's body, and sucks out any objects that he locates. But when a whole society comes, there is an elaborate ceremony in which considerable paraphernalia is used. Usually a society spends four days in its house in preparations before visiting the patient. Then when they go to his house, the medicine men smoke, sing, and pray over the sick one for three nights, and on the fourth have their final curing ritual. But if the condition of the patient is critical, they will perform the curing ritual at once. . . . A meal painting is made and paraphernalia laid out. The chief item of paraphernalia is the *iarriko*, the corn-ear fetish. Each doctor receives one at initiation. It is returned to the head man at death.

It is the badge *par excellence* of the medicine man. Stone figures of *Masewi, Oyoyewi, Paí yatyamo, K'oBictaiya,* and of lions, bears, and badgers, etc. are laid out on the meal painting. The medicine men do not possess power to cure disease in and of themselves; they receive it from animal spirit doctors (the bear is the chief one, others are mountain lion, badger, eagle, etc.). Meal lines are drawn on the floor from the door to these stone figures; when the songs and prayers are begun, the spirits of the animal medicine men come in, pass over the "roads" of meal, and invest the stone images. Medicine bowls, skins of the forelegs of bears, flints, eagle plumes, rattles, etc. are used. A rock crystal (*ma caí'yoyo* or *ma coitca'ni*) is used to obtain second sight.

The medicine men wear only a breechcloth. Their faces are painted red and black, and they wear a line of white bird-down over the head from ear to ear; songs are sung, the headman tells the people present to believe in the medicine men that they are doing their best, etc.; water is poured into the medicine bowl from the six directions, each doctor puts some herb medicines into the bowl. The doctors rub their hands with ashes, and massage the patient. When they find some foreign object they suck it out and spit it into a bowl. The rock crystal is used to locate objects in the body and to "see witches." Witches gather about a house during a curing ceremony; they wish to harm the patient further or to injure the doctors. They have been heard to rap on the door (at Cochiti) and call to the doctors, defying them. The War Captains and their assistants always stand guard outside the door during a curing ritual. They are armed with bows and arrows since rifles would not hurt a witch.

Frequently the doctors decide that the heart has been stolen by the witches. Then it is necessary to find it and bring it back. This almost always means fighting with the witches. They go out armed with flint knives; they wear a bear paw on the left forearm, a bear claw necklace, and a whistle of bear bone. The War Chief's guards try to accompany the medicine men when they leave the curing chamber, but the doctors travel so fast it is impossible; sometimes the medicine men leave the ground entierly and fly through the air.

These combats with the witches are occasions of great moment. Cries and thuds can be heard in the darkness. The witches sometimes tie the queues of two or three doctors together and leave them in a tangled mass on the ground. Or, a medicine man might be found lying on the ground bound with baling wire, his knees under his chin. The witches try to overpower the doctors by blowing their breath, the odour of which is unbearable, into their faces. Sometimes the doctors have to seek refuge in the church, when the witches "get too bad."

But sometimes the medicine men capture a witch. He is usually man-like in shape and about a foot and a half long (although he may be as large as a man, or he may be in the form of some animal). Often he looks like a Koshare. He squeals when they bring him in. They place him before the fireplace and then call the War Chief in to shoot him with a bow and arrow. The medicine men frequently return smeared with blood or "black" after a fight with witches. Often, too, they fall into a spasm or lose consciousness upon their return.

The medicine men come home with the heart (*wi nock*). This is a ball of rags with a grain (or four) of corn in the center. The patient is given this to swallow.

When the ceremony is over and everyone has been given medicine to drink, food is brought out (stew, bread, and coffee). The medicine men eat first, then the people. Baskets of cornmeal and flour are given to the medicine men in payment for their services. They gather up their paraphernalia and go home.

This account seems to fit pretty well the experience of both doctors and patients in Cochiti. The sequence of a full-scale cure is interesting. The doctors spend four nights preparing, and it is a pretty exhausting preparation. They do not eat or sleep during this time, and they smoke a lot. They can be heard chanting in the society house. Witch phenomena (fireballs, owls, and so forth) increase during this time, and everyone gets keyed up. Then the doctors go to the house where the patient has been waiting—an agonizing wait—and repeat the performance. They manipulate the paraphernalia, invoke their spirits, smoke, chant, and build up more tension. By the fourth night of this ceremony (the eighth in total), the tension is almost unbearable. The witches are gathering to thwart the efforts of the doctors. The doctors maintain that they can only do their best and that the issue is still very much in doubt. Then a final supreme effort must be made. The monotonous rise and fall of the chant, the near-darkness with the flickering fire, the hideous make-up, the cries in the night and rappings at the door and windows, the elaborate precautions—all these elements build up until the doctors, worked into a controlled frenzy, dash from the house to do battle. Patients describe how they have been nearly mad with fear by this time, unable to move or to cry out and convinced that they are to die. Then comes the terrible battle in the darkness. The doctors claim that, although of course they do a lot of the "business" themselves, it is the witches who get "inside them" and make them do it. They do indeed roll in convulsions and lacerate themselves. One explained, "We are more scared than they are [those in the house]. The witches are out to get us. They get inside us and make us do these things until we don't know what we're doing. We run to the church sometimes." Finally, exhausted, they return. Those in the house are by now at screaming point. "Sometimes we think the witches have got them [the doctors] and that they will come for us." The doctors reappear and enact the ultimate horror. They come in the semidarkness, huddled together fighting with something in their midst that screams horribly. It is the witch who stole the heart. Then, by the firelight, the war chief shoots it, and it disappears. The effect on the patient can be imagined. The incredible relief and tears of joy and gratitude leave him "feeling like all the badness has gone out." The "heart" is returned to the patient. Then, almost nonchalantly, the doctors and people eat stew and drink coffee. Life returns to normal; the universe is on an even keel again.

There is no doubt that much Cochiti illness is psychosomatic. They do not distinguish formally between physical and mental illness. All "illness" is abnormal. Belief in witches provides a cultural medium through which illness can be "expressed." Also, in many cases, a pathological fear of witches can itself bring on illness. Any Cochiti who suffers from certain illnesses will believe himself bewitched, but not all Cochiti are so afraid of witches that the fear drives them to sickness. In the more markedly paranoid individuals, intense fear of others is expressed, indeed felt, as witch fear. The paranoiac traits and the cultural beliefs in witches obviously reinforce each other. When a person feels ill, he suspects witchcraft, which in turn accentuates the illness. But the sociey has, in the medicine man, a cultural mechanism to deal with this situation. Terror of witchcraft is utilized to provide a kind of shock therapy. The patient is put through a terrifying experience, "saved," and his "heart" restored. His relief is so great that, in many psychosomatic cases, this ceremony suffices as a cure. He does not have to join the society that cured him, but he may do so out of gratitude or to help perpetuate the cure.

Cures of this type have usually been of illness among men. The complaints are various but mostly seem to be abdominal pains, rheumatism, and respiratory troubles, as well as anxiety and erratic behavior, insomnia and vomiting. At least two men described as having recurrent "fevers" appeared to be mentally abnormal, and the "fevers" (rises in temperature) were accompanied by violence and hallucinations of such ferocity that they had to be restrained and were shaking and sweating with fear. The hallucinations were, of course, mostly about witch phenomena. The witch theory accounts neatly for all symptoms.

CLAN CURES

The other type of cure involves the clan rather than the society as curing agent. The question arises, How is it decided whether a clan or society cure should be employed? This point has never been pursued by other writers, and again data are scarce, but several striking facts emerge. The most obvious is that, in cases where a clan cure is selected, no mention of witchcraft is ever heard as the cause of the sickness, and it is not called upon to effect the cure.

The clan cure is a variation of the clan adoption ceremony. Clan adoptions are performed, for example, for anyone coming to live in the village who does not have a clan. His head is washed by a woman who becomes his clan "mother," and from then on he is a member of her clan. He is given a new name, and feasting takes place among his new-found clansfolk. Tewa wives are usually treated in this way, in order that their children may have clans, the Tewa being bilateral. A man can be adopted, but it is not so important that he should be. Since the clan organization is matrilineal, it is necessary that the woman should have a clan to pass on to her children. For a man, membership in one of the moieties is more important.

The whole notion of adoption in Cochiti is interesting because it too is bound up with the preoccupation with health. A child is often adopted into a clan or clans other than his own as a kind of insurance policy. The child may be perfectly healthy, but it is thought good for his future health that he should acquire some "extra" clans. He does not become a full member of these clans (for example, a girl does not pass on membership in her adopted clan to her children), but he does stand in a very special relation to their members. They "care for" him in a spiritual sense. Clanless immigrants are believed to enjoy better health as a result of being adopted. One does not have to be ill in order to benefit from adoption, but such benefit can help those who are suffering from certain illnesses. I was able to trace the case histories of some of the patients cured by this method, of one in particular. I shall outline this case, reserving further general discussion until later.

CASE HISTORY

The patient, whom I met in 1958, was a woman of forty years. Her immediate family at that time consisted of her father, a man of seventy-five years who had gone blind in about 1945; her sister, three years younger than herself; and her illegitimate son aged sixteen. Her life history revealed that her mother had died in about 1930, when the patient was twelve. Her father than remarried. (His second wife was a Cochiti woman who had married a man from Zia Pueblo. After her husband's death, she had returned to Cochiti, bringing her son, who married a Cochiti girl.) Neither the patient nor her sister was considered attractive

by the men of the village, and neither ever married. The patient, however, had borne a son in 1942. Three years later, her father began to go
blind. Her sister then got into trouble with the pueblo council for giving
information to outsiders on some ceremonial matters. Her father was
totally blind by 1948, and the cure took place in 1951. Shortly after the
cure, the stepmother died following a long period of declining health.

Early Life. The patient's early family life had been overtly secure
and happy. The mother had been a beautiful, energetic woman and the
father an important ceremonial official. The patient, while of below
normal intelligence, was a serious and conscientious girl who looked after
her younger sister with her mother's help. Then, when the patient was
about eleven or twelve, her mother died. The running of the household
and the care of her sister were thrust upon her. She evidently took the
death of her mother very hard. Her relatives say it was useless to console
her. Her father's remarriage did not help. While it is difficult to ascertain
the relations between the patient and her stepmother, they were evidently
strained and distant. This state of affairs was attributed to the patient's
"queer" behavior, which began shortly after her mother's death.

Symptoms. The first symptom was apparently insomnia. She would
wander about at night and complain constantly that she could not sleep.
Then during the day, she was too tired to do anything, and simply sat
around. She was censured for this behavior at first, but then it became
worse. Her sister describes the symptoms, "She used to put on her best
clothes in the morning and just sit on the step combing her hair. Then
she put on her jewelry, all of it, and sat there all the rest of the day. She'd
cry and moan and she was always sick around the place. She had pains
in her stomach and couldn't eat anything. She sat and talked to herself
all the time, crying and talking." She had vague fears, but "not about
anything in particular"; she simply "acted scared" all the time. Fear of
relative strangers and inability to recognize people were also in evidence.
The pains and vomiting became acute, and she was taken to the Indian
hospital. She was better for a while but was discharged without being
fully cured. "Them doctors couldn't do anything for her, she was sick
in her mind."

The content of her "talk" consisted almost entirely of complaints
about her lack of a home. Her father's rapidly failing sight made him
utterly dependent on his daughters and relatives. Under the old matrilocal system of residence, a man was always dependent on his wife's
mother for a house. This man had never had a house of his own but
had always lived in a house supplied by his affinal relatives. At the time

of the onset of his daughter's serious symptoms, he was living in a house owned by the son of his second wife, his stepson. This house had been built by the stepson for his mother on her return to the village, and it was legally his. As the stepson was himself living in a borrowed house at the time, the two sisters and their father were under threat of a possible eviction. This threat was not so great as long as the stepmother was alive, but she was a fragile woman whose health was progressively failing throughout the period. Under the matrilineal system of inheritance and the institution of female house ownership, the two sisters should have received their mother's house at her decease. But in this case, as in many others, rules and practice did not coincide. Houses are not infinitely divisible, and the house that could have come to the patient in the female line in fact went to the children of her mother's mother's sister. As the recent Pueblo preference for neolocal residence has grown stronger, it has become less common for sisters to share houses, each preferring a house of her own. The onus of providing a house thus in most instances falls on the husband, unless his wife is senior of a group of sisters and inherits her mother's house. The father of our patient was unfortunately caught between the two systems, and his sight began to fail before he could adapt himself to the newer system of male house-ownership.

The result of this potential housing problem was to create actual insecurity for the patient, who was already subject to emotional insecurity. The situation was by no means tragic, for it is doubtful that the stepson would ever have turned them out (in fact, evidence suggests the contrary), but the patient seized upon the uncertainty of the housing situation and used it to express the deep feelings of abandonment and insecurity consequent upon her mother's death. The house that she fretted over should have come to her from her mother, and that it had not done so was a reinforcement of her anxieties over the discontinuance of the mother's love.

There is some evidence that, for all its outward calm, the early life of the patient may have contributed to these feelings. Her sister, three years younger than herself, took her place as the spoiled "baby" of the family, and there was some resentment on the patient's part at having to play nurse to her younger sibling. During the mother's illness immediately prior to her death, the patient had both to look after the unruly child and attend the sick woman. It was during this period that she first became sullen and withdrawn. To understand the patient's fright at the thought of her mother's death, we must appreciate the nature of the mother's continuing relationship with her daughters. This relationship lasts as long as the mother lives. All advice and help in personal and family matters that a woman may need are obtained from her mother. Particularly in the matter of marriage and childbirth and the rearing of children, the mother plays a crucial part, being constantly at her daughter's side. Even today, when there are very few matrilocal households left in Cochiti, this bond remains as firm as ever. Mothers will trudge miles and ford the river in order to help daughters and *vice versa*. It is not simply a matter of practical help but of emotional dependence of an intense nature. With initiation, the boy is to some degree weaned of this dependence, but the girl remains at home with her mother all her life—in feeling if not in fact. Bearing this relationship in mind, we can appreciate the acute anxiety that the sickness and death of her mother must have aroused in the patient. All informants agreed that the "spells" became worse during her own pregnancy and after the birth of her child. She was assisted in childbirth by her mother's mother's sister's daughters—one of whom owned the disputed house. The fear of going through the first birth without the help and emotional support of the mother has been noted in a number of other instances. It is one of the reasons why girls refuse to go to hospital for the delivery. (This prejudice is breaking down in the present generation). Shortly after the birth of her son, the patient's father began to go seriously blind, although his sight had been bad for some time. At this point, the patient was taken to the hospital as previously described. Since she was essentially a dependent person, the responsibilities of a blind father, a sickly stepmother, an irresponsible younger sister, and a "fatherless" baby, coupled with the lack of a home of her own, were too much, and she broke down completely. She failed to give milk properly just before leaving for the hospital, and this function was handed over to a female relative, as is the Cochiti custom.

Mobilization of Help. The situation was growing progressively worse, and after her dismissal from the hospital the girl's relatives decided to take some more positive action. To understand what was done, we must examine the network of extended family and clan relationships surrounding the patient (Fig. 1). The relatives are indicated with the patient (P) as reference point. In Generation 1, there are two sisters who own a house. In Generation 2, two brothers married the daughters of these two sisters, one brother being the father of the patient. The house went to the wife of the other brother, as she was the elder of the two cousins and married first. Finally, it went to the patient's second cousin (her mother's mother's sister's daughter's son), who was also her father's brother's son. The patient's mother died, and her father married a woman from the patient's own clan—Oak. The patient's father's sister's daughter married the patient's stepbrother. It was this stepbrother who had built the house for his mother in which the patient, her father, stepmother, sister, and son were living.

The surviving relatives who could be considered to have some responsibility for the fate of the patient and her family were her maternal second cousin (who was also her father's brother's son); her father's sister's daughter; and the latter's husband, who was also the patient's stepbrother. The first move was made by the cousin who had the house that was ostensibly the cause of the trouble. He made a deal with his father's brother, the father of the patient. The latter owned some land that was suitable for house-building, and the cousin agreed to trade the house for the land. The patient and the other members of her household were thus able to move into a house that was indisputably theirs; they had a home. This solution, however, was not in itself a cure. A fuller cure was arranged by the patient's stepbrother. It had to be a clan cure as, according to my informants, that was the only type that would fit the circumstances. Meanwhile the cousin's own stepmother had provided him with a house until such time as he could build his own.

To arrange for the clan cure, the stepbrother had to take several factors into account. He had first to find someone who would be willing

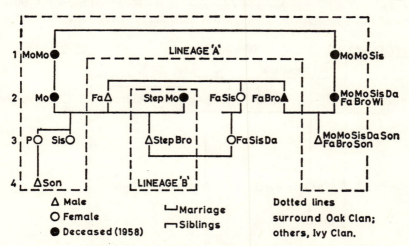

FIGURE 1. The patient's extended family and clan relationships.

to bear some of the expense, and it had to be someone who knew the cure. Ironically enough, the person best qualified to do the cure—the one who knew the ritual best—was the patient's own father. But it was impossible for him to carry out the cure on his own daughter. Central to the idea of the clan cure is the acquisition of new relatives, so that it is obviously a disadvantage to use as curer someone as closely related as a father. The Cochiti did not rationalize it in this way, however—they simply said that it would be "unthinkable" for a patient to be cured by her own father or mother. A complete outsider to the network of relatives would probably be unwilling, however. In these circumstances, the stepbrother turned to his mother's brother for help. This man was under no obligation to undertake the cure, but he nevertheless agreed that he and his wife should do so. The relation of curers to the patient is outlined in Fig. 2.

This arrangement raises some interesting problems. The clan system as an effective form of social organization is breaking down in Cochiti, and the authority of the mother's brother is no longer a reality. But when a matter demands a solution that involves the old basis of grouping, the old patterns seem to repeat themselves. In this case, the stepbrother was right to consult his mother's brother as the proper adviser on clan matters, and the mother's brother was right to help his nephew out. If, however, the central part of the cure is the adoption of the patient into two other clans than her own (the clans of the curer and his wife), then half this advantage of the cure was consciously being foregone in this

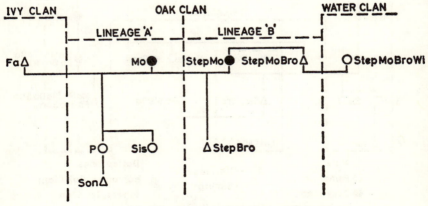

FIGURE 2. Relationship of patient and curers.

instance. This compromise has occurred in other Cochiti cures and is largely due to diminishing willingness to undertake the cure. People have to look more and more to an immediate circle of relatives and also to the numerical dominance of the Oak clan over the others. There is no indication that the patient's father deliberately chose his second wife from the Oak clan, but as this clan is very large the chances of his drawing a wife from it were quite high. The problem arises, however, of how the cure will proceed if one of the curers is of the same clan as the patient. How can the patient be adopted into her own clan? Informants say that, "You just go ahead with the ceremony anyway, like she wasn't an Oak." I think the clue to this apparent anomaly lies again in the gap between theory and practice. Although in Cochiti, there are many people with the title of *ha'panyi* (Oak) and although they are members of the same clan and so theoretically related, the actual relationship is in many cases either very tenuous or nonexistent. More cases of endogamy occur within the Oak clan than within any other, and there is apparently little censure of such marriages. One other clan cure known to me involved an Oak patient and a curer of the same clan. It seems then that, with regard to Oak participation, it is accepted that there may be overlap in membership and that, as long as the curer is of a *lineage* that is not related to the lineage of the patient, the common clan is overlooked. There was in this case no known relationship between the stepmother's lineage and that of the patient. This kind of compromise has to be effected on many occasions in a small community carrying the burden of an archaic social structure intended for a much larger community. The other clan involved in the cure, that of the stepmother's brother's wife, was the Water clan. Initiation into this clan was especially beneficial for the patient, for it contained important medicine men.

The Cure. The stage was thus set for the cure. It took place at the home of the sponsor (the patient's stepmother's brother). An announcement was made four days before, properly relayed with a pinch of cornmeal to all the clan members concerned (Oak and Water). The Water clan and the members of the Oak lineage B were present. The patient's lineage gathered at her home, along with members of her father's clan, Ivy; everyone feasted, and then the patient was conducted to the curer's house where all present joined in washing her head with *amole* suds, the traditional method of sanctifying adoptions. (It is also the method used to indicate and sanctify any significant change in status, such as that undergone at initiation.) All the others brought presents for the patient, including food like melons, rabbits, and corn. Then the patient was given new names, and returned to her people at her own house. The curer's wife and her sisters and all the women of her clan would be henceforth "mothers" of the patient. Similarly, the women of the stepmother's lineage (B) would be "mothers" and would be addressed as such by the patient. One of Lange's informants describes the status of a patient after such a cure: "If an Ivy is cured by Sage and Oak, he is still Ivy but also he is a little Sage and a little Oak. Later if a Pumpkin asks the Sage or Oak to be cured, then the Ivy who is a little Sage or Oak goes along to help out."[19] The cure is unlike an adoption, however, in that the patient's children will not inherit her "little" clans.

This cure took place in 1951, and shortly afterward the patient and family moved into the house that had been given up to them. Since then, the patient has never had a "spell," shows no organic symptoms, and behaves normally. Before the cure, I was told, she was "wasted away to nothing" and "she was pretty near dead sometimes." There may be a tendency to exaggerate in such a case, but opinions were sampled and, as far as independence of opinion could be assured, they were agreed on the symptoms.

We can see how the institution of clanship is utilized to effect a cure and to help maintain it. Our patient is now a member of the Water clan and a different lineage of the Oak clan—she is a "little" Water and is dependent on continuing membership in the Water clan for her continued good health. By becoming a member of this clan she is cured, and by continued membership she stays cured. She acquires a relationship of dependence with a previously unrelated set of people. What is more, her faith in the efficacy of the cure is reinforced when she goes along to participate herself in cures conducted by the Water people. Clan, or rather lineage, membership is also of practical importance in mobilizing help for the patient. The clan system is thus an anchor on to which therapy can fasten and by which continuous reinforcement of treatment can be assured.

I have no other case recorded in such detail, but in three of the other cases (all involving women), the data do suggest a striking similarity in the total syndrome: a hiatus in the mother-daughter relationship leading to considerable anxiety and consequent illness. In all cases, the physical symptoms were vague and the traits of insomnia, erratic behavior, withdrawal, and amnesia were predominant. In other cases, the data were sparse or showed no conclusive evidence of mother-child problems. But it should be remembered that the adoption-cure is thought to be generally effective in ensuring health and is not specifically confined to the type of illness based on problems of maternal deprivation.

§ Interpretation

We have then an interesting problem. There are two kinds of cure for two types of illness. In one type, an illness thought to have been caused by witches is cured by an elaborate shock therapy. In the other type, an illness not associated with witchcraft is cured by adoption into a social group.

Interpretation is bound to be speculative, for we have no proper clinical data for these people, but some conclusions, however tentative, may aid in sorting out the problem.

WITCH ILLNESS

We have suggested that paranoia may be at the root of the witch illness complex. This analysis excludes, of course, the purely "physical" illnesses, to the degree that there are such things. In any case, even if the primary cause of the illness is "physical," the fear of witches engendered by it produces secondary "mental" symptoms that serve to intensify it. An individual is either to some degree paranoid, with stress inducing physical illness, or he is physically ill, which induces a state of acute paranoia. In either case, the paranoia must be dealt with, and the witch theory offers a medium for the expression of the illness, an explanation of its cause, and, through the societies, a means for its cure. Elaborate shock treatment attacks the "cause" of the disease and, by conclusively eliminating it, restores the patient, even if only temporarily. There is no provision in Pueblo cosmology for the final overthrow of the witches.

The sources of paranoia in the culture are hard to trace without clinical data. In a sense, the elaborate witch fears are a kind of "customary" paranoia. But we cannot imagine them persisting unless a good many individuals were motivated by exaggerated fear of others and the world generally, independent of the cultural beliefs about spirits, witches, and so forth. As we have suggested, the two are mutually reinforcing. Various theories of paranoia suggest that its cause may lie in homosexual tensions,[20] general sex anxiety, or projection of hostility as a result of socialization anxiety over aggression.[21] We find some of these factors present in Cochiti to some degree. I have little evidence regarding homosexuality, but certainly aggression problems are rife. The child is indulged initially by a body of female socializers and later is partially rejected in favor of a younger sibling. Even without this rejection, it would be impossible for the degree of indulgence the child receives initially to be sustained, and a perception of rejection is inevitable. Over-indulgence has given him no training in self-control, and he is ill prepared to restrain his aggressions later. Restrain them, however, he must. Aggression is the cardinal sin in Pueblo eyes. At times, the society seems to be geared entirely to reducing, controlling, and repressing it. Pueblo institutions stress co-operation and friendliness, but this stress is a counter to aggressive tendencies, rather than a channel for acting out of harmonious ones.[22] Individuals driven too hard by this child-rearing system will probably develop real paranoia, but most individuals will have a streak of it. This deep motivational aspect of paranoia is reinforced by the stories and experiences of witchcraft with which the child is fed and frightened as a disciplinary technique.[23] Conscious and unconscious learning develop in harness.

Here, unless we are wildly wrong, is the basis provided by the society for its "typical" illness. The witch illness complex illustrates the whole cycle of the society, providing the strain that causes or aggravates the illness, giving it a culturally approved and patterned mode of expression, and using this mode of expression as the basis for a cure by a social group—the medicine society, which, we may note, the patient can then join.

CLAN CURE

The clan cure and its associated types of illness should be seen against the background of the adoption system and its ideology and the ideology and sentiments respecting the clan or, more particularly, matrilineal descent. Why does it seem sensible and successful to the Cochiti to adopt a child into a clan for the sake of its future health or an adult to restore its lost health? For the former, the Cochiti have the readier explanation. The most terrible thing that can happen to a child, they say, is to lose its mothers—its own mother and her female matrilineal relatives. The adoption gives it a set of reserve mothers in the case of the loss of its own, and in any case one cannot have too many mothers. The clan is matrilineal, which means that, for any individual, its pivot is his mother, through whom he acquires his clan relatives. The clan is strongly identified in the Cochiti mind with the mother herself and therefore with nurture and security. When the loss of a mother is feared, or actually occurs (through death, estrangement, or remarriage), the breach is healed by adopting the patient into another clan—by giving him or her new "mothers," who perform such symbolic acts of nurture as washing the head, giving food, and renaming. All these acts are associated with a ritual of change in status (initiation) and symbolize the shedding of an undesirable personality and the acquisition of a new and "healthier" one. At initiation, it is the status of "child" that is shed; at the clan cure, it is the status of "motherless person."

The Cochiti do not verbalize it in this way, but they do express sentiments that are revealing. "We get our clans, like ourselves, from our mothers." "Our clans come from our mothers like all good things." "Why do we have clans? Because we have mothers." "My clan is my mother's name." The idea of uterine kinship is the most popular in explaining the notion of clanship. Clansmen ultimately come from the body of the same woman. If we couple this sentiment with the already mentioned extreme dependence on the mother herself—especially in women—we can begin to see both the sources of the nonwitch disease and the basis of its cure. As in the case of the witch disease, the society provided the strain—the mother-child (particularly daughter) relationship and its imminent breakdown; the ideology—of matrilineal descent and the sentiments associated with it; the mobilization of help—the clan and lineage; and the means of cure—adoption into a clan and the acquisition of "mothers" and maternal nurture. Even in cases where the source of the disease is not the same as the source of the cure (mother-child relations), maternal nurture is still thought to be effective. We must note that the acquired clans do not "do" anything material for the patient. The whole process is symbolic. What they "do" is spiritual. They restore lost security by accepting the patient as one of themselves.

The whole complex of "mother" symbolism is interesting. What Eggan says of Acoma is in general true of Cochiti.[24]

One important pattern at Acoma, which is characteristic of Keresan villages generally, and which contrasts with the Hopi and Zuni to a considerable extent, is the emphasis on the concept of "mother." In the Origin Myth we have seen that the central figure is Isatiku, who is the "mother" of the people whom she created and whom she receives at death. The corn-ear fetishes represent her and have her power; the cacique is her representative and is referred to as her "husband" in the mythology. In the kinship system the term "mother" is widely extended, and recent changes have extended it still further. In ritual relations the wife of the "ceremonial father" performs many of the ritual functions performed by the ceremonial father's sister among the Hopi and Zuni. In the Scalp Dance it is the mother of the twins who dances rather than their sister or aunts.

In Cochiti, the *cacique* is in fact referred to as "mother," as are the medicine-society heads. The fetishes of the medicine men are also their "mothers," and in the ritual addresses both to them and by them the concept is elaborated at length.[25] Although the sentiment and symbolism are more elaborate among the Keresans than in Hopi or Zuni, I suspect that a strong element of maternal identification is present in all these societies. Whiting has suggested that identification occurs with the sex-typed role of the parent who mediates the major resources in the child's life, a resource being anything the child wants.[26] Undoubtedly among the Keresans and in the western Pueblos, this person is the mother. The child thus grows up with a strong female-maternal identification (this fact may, of course, be a source of homosexual tensions). In boys, initiation may well serve to sever this identification to some extent, but in girls it persists. It is noticeable that among the Keresans, where the mother sentiment is so pervasive, the initiation ceremonies are neither so universal nor so fierce as in Hopi and Zuni.[27]

It may well be that the strength of the identification or sentiment is a reason for the persistence of the clan ideology and some associated practices (exogamy, curing) even after the economic and social bases of clan organization have disappeared. In other words, when it ceases to have any other *raison d'être,* the clan may continue to survive because it serves to reduce the identity-dependency drives—especially in its role as healer.

What is striking in this role of the clan is the unconscious cultural insight that "sees" that the motivations involved in the clans' persistence and those involved in much nonwitch illness are the same. The neurosis of our patient was based on a breakdown of those sentiments and social relationships on which the clan system depends in large measure for its effective persistence. The breakdown was repaired by restoring the disrupted relationships (by adoption) and so reinforcing the shaken sentiments. Durkheim and Radcliffe-Brown have argued that ritual serves to emphasize and reinforce those sentiments on which the social structure depends for its continuation,[28] and here we have an example of the truth of this assertion. The cure is "built into" the social structure.

§ Conclusion

Cochiti culture provides the sources of its people's illnesses; it provides the media of expression for them; it mobilizes help for the patients; it effects the cure, and it ensures reinforcement. It distinguishes the illnesses that require dramatic shock treatment from those that require more peaceful nurture treatment, and in each case it utilizes the motivational source of the illness as a means of cure. This system is not the result of individual insight but rather of the slow working-out of cultural patterns over the centuries and the achievement of a kind of adjustment that, given the cultural premises, is very successful.

Already, however, these patterns are changing. The medicine societies are becoming extinct, and American education does not encourage confidence in "witch doctors." The clans are ceasing to function effectively even in their limited spheres, and changes in household composition are complete. All these forces affect the efficacy of curing techniques. They affect the causation of illness more slowly. The Cochiti therefore face the prospect of a persistence of traditional illnesses without the benefits of traditional cures—a situation that necessarily faces many primitive societies in transition. Those concerned with health and sickness in these societies would do well to take some hard looks at the relations among sentiments, culture, and social relations before doing anything to upset their often delicate balance. In many cases, the hospital and the physician are but indifferent substitutes for the society and the shaman on which the patient has learned, and is moved, to depend.

Notes

1. Ari Kiev, "Spirit Possession in Haiti," *American Journal of Psychiatry,* 118 (1961), No. 2.
2. K. Stewart, *Pygmies and Dream Giants* (New York: 1954).
3. A. H. Leighton and D. C. Leighton, "Elements of Psychotherapy in Navaho Religion," *Psychiatry,* 4 (1941), 515-23.
4. C. H. Lange, *Cochiti: A New Mexico Pueblo Past and Present* (Austin: 1959); and E. S. Goldfrank, "The Social and Ceremonial Organization of Cochiti," *Memoirs of the American Anthropological Association,* 33.
5. R. Benedict, *Patterns of Culture* (Boston: 1934), Chap. 4.
6. D. H. Lawrence, "The Dance of the Sprouting Corn," *Mornings in Mexico* (London: 1927); and Lange, "*Tablita,* or Corn, Dances of the Rio Grande Pueblo Indians," *Texas Journal of Science,* IX (1957), 59-74.
7. A. Bandalier, *The Delight Makers* (New York: 1890).
8. E. Dozier, "Rio Grande Pueblos," E. H. Spicer, ed., *Perspectives in American Indian Culture Change* (Chicago: 1961); and D. Aberle, "The Pueblo Indians of New Mexico: Their Land, Economy, and Civil Organization," *Memoirs of the American Anthropological Association,* 50, No. 4, Part 2.
9. Goldfrank, *op. cit.*
10. Fred Eggan, *The Social Organization of the Western Pueblos* (Chicago: 1950).
11. K. Wittfogel and Goldfrank, "Some Aspects of Pueblo Mythology and Society," *Journal of American Folklore,* 61 (1943), 17-30; E. Reed, "Sources of

Rio Grande Culture and Population," *El Palacio*, 61 (1949), No. 6; and Dozier, *op. cit.*

12. J. R. Fox, "Pueblo Baseball: A New Use for Old Witchcraft," *Journal of American Folklore*, 74 (1961), No. 291.

13. A. L. Kroeber, "Zuni Kin and Clan," *Anthropological Papers of the American Museum of Natural History*, 18 (1917), Part 2; and C. D. Forde, "Hopi Agriculture and Land Ownership," *Journal of the Royal Anthropological Institute*, 61 (1939).

14. Eggan, *op. cit.*

15. Fox, "Veterans and Factions in Pueblo Society," *Man*, LXI (1961), 173-6.

16. Lange, *Cochiti.*

17. L. W. Simmons, *Sun Chief: The Autobiography of a Hopi Indian* (New Haven: 1942).

18. L. A. White, "A Comparative Study of Keresan Medicine Societies," *Proceedings of the 23rd International Congress of Americanists*, (1928), pp. 604-19.

19. Lange, *Cochiti.*

20. S. Freud, *Collected Papers*, 3 (London: 1924), 387-470.

21. J. W. M. Whiting and I. L. Child, *Child Training and Personality* (New Haven: 1953).

22. Fox, "Pueblo Baseball."

23. Goldfrank, "Socialization, Personality, and the Structure of Pueblo Society," *American Anthropologist*, XLVII (1945), 516-83; and Dorothy Eggan, "The General Problem of Hopi Adjustment," *American Anthropologist*, XLV (1943), 357-73.

24. Fred Eggan, *op. cit.*

25. Father N. Dumarest, "Notes on Cochiti, New Mexico," *Memoirs of the American Anthropological Association*, VI (1919), 139-236.

26. Whiting, *Resource Mediation and Learning by Identification, Ms.*, Laboratory of Human Development, Harvard University, 1959.

27. Whiting, R. Kluckhohn, and A. S. Anthony, "The Function of Male Initiation Ceremonies at Puberty," E. E. Maccoby, T. M. Newcomb, and E. L. Hartley, eds., *Readings in Social Psychology* (New York: 1958).

28. E. Durkheim, *Les formes élémentaires de la vie religieuse* (Paris: 1912); and A. R. Radcliffe-Brown, *Structure and Function in Primitive Society* (London: 1952).

Part Three

The role of culture becomes increasingly clear in primitive societies that are coping with the impact of modern social patterns. Native practitioners, mobilizing elements of shared traditions, are usually more effective than Western doctors in meliorating the resulting deviance, psychopathology, and failures at acculturation.

Bert Kaplan and Dale Johnson

The Social Meaning of Navaho Psychopathology and Psychotherapy

IN ANY CULTURE, ideas about the nature and causes of mental illness, the actual illnesses that occur, and the method and theory of their treatment and cure may be said to form a single, interrelated, and interdependent system. It is obvious that, where some conception of the etiology of psychopathology exists, therapeutic process will be organized on the basis of this conception and aimed at removing the causes, or remedying the conditions from which the patient is understood to be suffering. What is perhaps not so obvious is that the illnesses themselves will be oriented to and shaped by these conceptions. This paper is devoted to demonstrating and illustrating this thesis. We shall utilize data collected during a three-year field study aimed first at describing Navaho psychopathology and second at analyzing the meanings of psychopathology and other forms of deviance in Navaho society. One of the main theses of the study was that these meanings are not limited to descriptive effects on social functioning but that there is an important and perhaps primary sense in which psychopathology and deviance have a positive or functional significance in the social system.

It is not necessary to present a detailed description of Navaho culture in this paper since it is probably the best known of all American Indian groups. Certainly it has received more attention and study in recent decades than has any other Indian culture.* With about 85,000 members, it is the largest of the American Indian tribes. The Navaho entered the Southwest as part of a migration of Athabascan speakers from the North in relatively recent times. The exact period is a matter of con-

---

* For a general description of the culture the reader may turn to Kluckhohn and Leighton's *The Navaho.*

jecture, but it was certainly considerably before the seventeenth century, when their presence as predators of the Pueblo groups was noted in Spanish historical accounts, and perhaps as early as A.D. 1000 when dated Pueblo sites give indirect evidence of the arrival of an alien group. Linguistic and kinship analysis suggest that these migrants from the North came into the Southwest in a number of separate bands, perhaps at different times and by different routes, and settled in different areas. They were known collectively as the Apache but separately as the Mescalero Apache, the Jicarilla Apache, the Lipon Apache, and, most important for our interests, the Navaho Apache. These Athabascan speakers were apparently quite simple and culturally undifferentiated. They were nomads, had no agriculture, and were relatively warlike. While there is an almost complete absence of archaeological remains, anthropological speculation is that they were a rather typical hunting and gathering society.

It seems likely that in the seventeenth century one of these Apache bands, the Navaho (who themselves seem to have comprised a series of separate bands) came into extensive contact with the Pueblos. One type of contact was raiding, but it appears that, as a result of Spanish intrusion, a considerable number of Pueblo people came to live for a period among the Navaho. Whatever the exact circumstances, it seems safe to say that in the sixteenth, seventeenth, and eighteenth centuries a quite profound Pueblo influence shaped Navaho religion, Navaho agriculture, and Navaho kinship structure in its present form.

We have hypothesized, therefore, that, as a result of this experience, Navaho culture comprehends two historically distinct traditions, one based on the Apache hunting and raiding past and a second based on comparatively recent Pueblo contact. Each tradition has its related set of values, which not only are different from each other but are in important respects opposed and conflicting. Our undoubtedly oversimplified formulation is that the central principle of the earlier tradition is concern for personal and magical "power," while maintenance of social control and harmony is the central principle of the second. The reader will undoubtedly understand that what the second tradition seeks to control is the "power" of the first and that such "power" is exercised mainly in upsetting the order of the second. While we can speculate that, in earlier times, a balance between the two existed and that institutionalized patterns for the expression of both were present, in the present era, with hunting and raiding virtually extinct, there are no vital institutions for the expression of the Apache tradition.

It seems to us that a number of recent descriptions of Navaho values (for example, those by Kluckhohn and Romney and Ladd[1]) have fo-

cused almost exclusively on values associated with the second or Pueblo
tradition. While this focus may be interpreted as involving a one-sided
view of Navaho culture, the more probable explanation is that the later
tradition has come to dominate Navaho conceptions of normality and
that the values associated with the earlier tradition have been excluded
from what is officially regarded by Navahos as normality and virtue. Normality has thus turned its back on important elements in Navaho identity.
Although this rejection is not the subject of this paper and is mentioned
here only as background for what is to follow, it demonstrates one factor
in our thesis that the Apache tradition and its associated values find their
main expression in patterns of deviance and in psychopathology. Deviance
and psychopathology thus have important social functions and are, in
an important sense, contributors to the equilibrium of Navaho society.
This equilibrium is not merely a product of the harmony and cohesion
embodied in the second tradition; it is a delicate balance of two opposing
principles, a balance that we believe lies at the heart of Navaho culture.
Our own opinion is that, if this balance is upset and the second tradition
is too successful in pushing out and suppressing the first, Navaho culture
as we know it will be in serious danger. The tension between the two
provides, perhaps more than any other factor, the heart of what is specifically Navaho. The maintenance of this tension is, in our view, a condition for the maintenance of Navaho culture.

§ Navaho Conceptions of Personality and Action

Basic to an understanding of Navaho conceptions of mental illness is
what Father Berard Haile calls the "soul concept." The following analysis
is partly based on his paper, "Soul Concept of the Navaho."[2] All natural
phenomena, including human beings, are believed to have outer forms,
that can be seen and inner forms (be'gisti'n, "one who lies within it" or
the "inner form of it"). The inner form is believed to exist independently
of its outer shell and to control the latter. It is apparent that this conception is very close to the philosophical position known in Western
society as "Platonic idealism," which holds that the world of appearances
is merely the emphemeral manifestation of a reality that lies behind it—
the world of essences.

"That which stands within" human beings is the wind or wind-soul.
According to Haile, there are seven winds: white wind, blue wind, yellow
wind, dark wind, small wind, left-handed wind, and glossy wind. "By

these winds their living is done." The winds become "that which stands within" human beings and that "by which they have life" and "by which it breathes" and "by which it moves." Our informants in the Ramah area give a somewhat less differentiated account of these winds, mentioning only four: the good wind, the happy wind, the mean wind, and the bad wind. But the situation is much more complex, and a specific "wind" does not seem to be completely identified with any particular characteristic. Rather, certain combinations or relationships seem to be important. When the winds are assigned their proper sequence, the results are benevolent, but when this sequence is disturbed, as for example when preference is given to the dark wind, malevolence and witchcraft result. What is important for our analysis is that the winds that come within a person at birth and give him life also determine what kind of person he is going to become. Four of those that Haile mentions appear to correspond to the good, bad, happy, and mean winds described by Ramah informants. The Navaho say, "His soul is without meanness" or "His soul has meanness," and they believe that a person with a "sunwise soul" is apt to be good and kind, while a person with a "sunward soul," in which the winds travel counterclockwise, will be destructive of property and will steal, rape, and so forth.

Although Haile suggests that the wind, once dispatched into the human body by the supernatural, remains constant, our data contain many indications that certain events change the deployment of the winds. Our data are admittedly not completely clear on this point, but they contain so many references to foreign powers that can affect a person that it seems very likely that something corresponding to a change in winds or possession by alien winds is believed to occur.

We believe it is in this notion of possession, subtle and vaguely stated though it is, that the core of Navaho conceptions of mental illness is to be found. We believe further that this notion has the greatest significance for the nature of Navaho mental illness, it symptomatology, its social treatment, and its cures. This assertion will be developed at greater length after we have described the curing ceremonies. We may note here, however, that attributing illness to a power that possesses one, whether a devil or unconsciousness, rather than to oneself, is the typical mechanism of hysterical illness. Without developing this point or presenting any evidence here, we can state that Navaho mental illnesses do tend, in general, to fall into this class. While they are not hysterias in the Freudian sense and there are few cases of conversion symptoms, the most characteristic illnesses do have as a central element abdication of ego control. Navahos do not say explicitly, "It is not me who is acting this way but

the spirit that is possessing me." Nevertheless, there is a strong feeling
that the patient is helpless to control his behavior. Perhaps even more
to the point, there does not seem to be a bifurcation of the psyche in
which the ego can establish goals or standards opposed to the expression
of unconscious tendencies.

Father Berard states that, while a Navaho may admit that the wind-
soul within him is the "means by which he has life, movement, speech,
dream and thought," he and his language never refer directly to such
dualism. In his language, at least, the Navaho expresses the conviction
that the union of his body with the wind-soul results in the being that
is he. One cannot help thinking, however, that the implicit dualism does
have profound consequences, as do dualisms in Western society. At least
one of these consequences seems to be matter-of-fact acceptance of one's
own and other people's transgressions. While it is socially important that
restitution be made, the fact of transgression itself seems to be of little
importance.

§ Conceptions of the Etiology of Mental Illness

There is an astonishing variety of recognized causes of mental illness among the Navahos; in fact, mental illness can be a consequence
of so many different behaviors that we are led to suspect that it has a
cultural importance far out of proportion to its actual incidence. A brief
survey of these causes may be of interest, and our findings will yield
some clues about this importance. It should be clarified at this point
that mental illnesses are not always clearly distinguished in Navaho
etiology from diseases in general and that much of the Navaho theory
of disease and curing is applicable to mental illness. There are, however,
a large number of quite specific behaviors that lead to mental illness.
This group suggests that mental illness is simply a dire consequence, a
kind of bogey used as a sanction against culturally undesirable behavior.
The best and clearest example of such behavior is incest, but it is not
obvious why many other behaviors are regarded as undesirable. For
example, "in the old days the rim of a water bottle was not finished in a
false braid 'but was just like the rest of the basket.' The old people
were afraid to finish the other way for a water jug—afraid they would
lose their minds"; or, "Baby's ears are not going to be pierced. Would
make him crazy"; or, "You're not supposed to leave a poker pointing to
the fire. If you do that, the old man used to say you'll get crazy . . .

you'll get crazy if you stir food or stir fire with an arrow." If a pregnant woman sees an eclipse of the sun or moon, her baby's mind will supposedly be affected, and the baby will either be crazy or have convulsions. In most of these instances, the people seem to be obeying rules that do not have any personal or social meaning whatever.

Another major class of causes for illness has to do with relations to animals. The animals mentioned as especially dangerous are the bear, the deer, and the coyote. The most spectacular of these conceptions involves the bear. Contact of any sort with a bear is dangerous. For example, "If you go up in the mountain where the bear is bedded down . . . (and) . . . you bedded down there, it will get you that way . . . make your head go wrong"; or, "Sometimes if you cross a bear's path and pick up some ants the bear rolled over, or slept on, you are liable to have mental troubles." The breath of a bear is also dangerous: "They say that if you get the bear breath you will go crazy or goofy or something." Other animals can cause the same results, and there is a Navaho term for "frightening with the breath." "Fright or shock comes from the breath of such an animal [deer, bear] from a distance. It affects the heart. From close it makes you weak. Happens with other animals also, buffalos, antelope."

The most dramatic effects, however, come from "eating bear meat." For example, "Some time ago a person from here with some education went to Gallup and in a restaurant had some bear meat. He returned and became so violent that people had to call the Fort Defiance police, and he broke the handcuffs, and the police had a hard time taking him. A whole lot of policemen barely could hold him, and they straightjacketed him and kept him at the Fort. After, they hired a hand trembler who diagnosed that he had gone to Gallup and needed a sing because of bear steak"; or "My girl friend said [the informant is a woman] let's order bear meat, and we did. First I took a little bit of it, then I ate it all. Nothing happened to us. I just wanted a taste of it. I told my grandfather about it. He said you're going to get mean and get hair all over."

Burning certain animals is also dangerous. "If you [burn] snakes, porcupines, or toads, or many other things, it can affect your mind. Whites do not understand why Navahos fear a fire near a snake or something. Medicine man can cure this." The coyote is another dangerous animal (probably because of its connection with witchcraft): "As the leaders of the dance were approaching the final place, a coyote crossed their path. Shortly after this I fell down and some of the other women began to shake. Also a dog went crazy at that time." So is the deer: "When a man is out hunting, he may get sick from the deer. He loses his head and has pains (any place on his body) like a knife sticking in him. If you look where the pain is, you will find a deer hair sticking in the skin." Being struck by lightning or being near where lightning strikes can cause mental illness. So can any contact with the dead. "I think a few things make you *di'gis* [crazy]. If a man died and you dug the grave and if you have a wife or if you are single, you have to stay in one place for four days with singing by medicine man. . . . if on the same day you bury him, if you went home and then fool around with your wife or any girls, then about ten or five or two years you 'twist'—*di'gis*. Or it might get worse and worse each time, and pretty soon twist you and you get crazy."

Prenatal experiences are especially connected with mental illness. Any contact with the dead is especially bad. "When parents of an unborn child see a dead human being [Navaho only] the child will be affected. Any person might get this from seeing dead Navahos, but with mother it is worse"; "One other thing is before they were born maybe father or mother saw skeletons from old cliff dwellers or from enemies or maybe from another Navaho than Ramah. In this they use enemy way [to cure it]; if they see a dog go crazy while their mother was pregnant, or see a white man or a man from some other race go crazy . . . if they see a person with a spell having water coming from their mouths, their babies will have spells"; "Or if you see cracked or ruined dolls, cracked head or eyes missing, it is the fault of the parents then." "Seeing crazy animals during pregnancy" or "seeing bones [of a dead crazy coyote]" can also cause craziness. "She would stamp her feet, and her eyes would flare up . . . like a deer in the forest when it was frightened. Her mother was probably frightened by a wild animal, a deer or something, when she was pregnant with her." Other prenatal causes include seeing "a person doing hand trembling. Her child grew up to nine or ten years old and then goes crazy and starts to tremble like that . . . my mother was pregnant with me, and she went to a sing and saw sand paintings and that is why I had the fainting." It seems fairly clear that what can cause people trouble if viewed or done can cause similar difficulty for the unborn baby if its mother is the viewer or participant.

The most potent causes of mental illness, however, are those connected with witchcraft. In most cases of emotional disturbance, witchcraft or ghostly influence is suspected. We have already commented on the general mechanism presumed to be operative. A few examples will further illustrate these beliefs: "Some of these witch people, he can put plant pollen, some of these poison pollen, put it in smoke and let you smoke that when he hates you"; "Somebody steal her hair or some piece of turquoise or her skirt or shirt or spit. He done something with it, tied it to a tree. So when the wind blows on that . . . and [it] begins to move, she begins to jump around like that. When the wind doesn't blow, just keeps still, then she's all right"; "If you beat a witch in a game, he makes you crazy. They use loco weeds"; "If a girl repulsed a man who wished to have intercourse with her he might get revenge in the following manner. He went to the place where the girl lived and watched until he could get some of her saliva or dust from the bottom of her moccasins. He took either the dust or the saliva to a jimson weed and while singing tied it to the plant. Then he sang some more songs. The girl would go crazy right away. She would take off her dress and run around naked and everyone would laugh." "They say that a witch can see a pretty girl and if she won't go with him, he can make her crazy." "Coyote men keep their victims on the edge of their nerves, irritable and upset. They stop eating and get thin."

§ The Main Patterns of Psychopathology

Four distinct patterns of psychopathology are distinguishable in the more than 600 cases described in our field materials. One of these patterns is clearly schizophrenia. Although there are many interesting questions relating to the cultural patterning of the symptoms of schizophrenia, in the interests of confining our discussion to patterns that have specific cultural etiologies or meanings, we shall omit this group of cases from discussion. The three patterns that involve distinctly Navaho illnesses are *iich'aa* or moth craziness, ghost sickness, and crazy violence. Only the first of these has a Navaho name, but the other two are known to all Navahos.

IICH'AA (MOTH CRAZINESS)

In some respects, the main type of Navaho mental illness and the kind most clearly treated in Navaho mythology is *iich'aa* or moth craziness. While the symptoms described by Navahos clearly indicate epilepsy, most other forms of mental illness are related to it in some way or other and are described in similar or related terms. Mental illness in general is believed to come in fits during which the person is "not himself." It seems correct to say that *iich'aa* and the *iich'aa* legend have shaped Navaho thinking about all mental illness. Reichard[3] describes *iich'aa* or moth craziness as possession of so little control over oneself that one becomes rash and so out of his mind that he may jump into the fire. While this term seems to be reserved at the present time for the "fits" and "spells"

of epilepsy, it seems very likely that the great bulk of cases of mental illness of all kinds includes such related elements as "fits" of violence and
rage or "spells" of being out of control, of craziness, or of nervousness. It
seems fair to say that Navahos are not clear where *iich'aa* leaves off and
that there is at least a suspicion that it is involved in many illnesses that
are not epileptic.

This type of illness is understood to be specifically caused by incest
between brothers and sisters. The legend is that, after the departure of
the *begochidi,* the parents of the children refused to give them in marriage
to outsiders, with the result that brothers and sisters were married to
each other. Having thus violated the prohibition of their elders, they
became insane and plunged themselves into the fire. The legend states,
"They simply trampled over one another from all sides, in a mad rush
to plunge into the fire." The specific causal agent of the crazy behavior
is a moth that is supposed to be crawling inside the head between the
eyes. (In another account, the moths nest inside the stomach and gradually eat up one's insides.) The moths grow bigger and bigger and fly
around more and more violently, and the victims behavior follows suit.
In the end, the victim circles closer and closer to a fire and finally throws
himself in. Many people claim to have seen such cases, and our data
include many reports of people falling into the fire during their fits.

Most relevant to our analysis is that the action of the moth inside
the victim is believed to cause his crazy behavior. While this behavior
does not exactly represent possession in Western terms, it fits very well
the conception that "that which stands within" determines the outward
form or behavior. One Navaho singer says that a demon gets into the
mentally ill and causes them to burn themselves. Part of the cure for this
illness, as for many other Navaho illnesses, is to "vomit everything that
is inside—to throw up what was inside." In the *iich'aa* complex, what is
inside is the moths that are causing the trouble, and when, in the course
of the curing ceremony known as Mothway, the patient vomits, it is
moth wings that come out. That control of the patient depends on what
the moths are doing is indicated by the following quotation: "He says
it seems like there is something crawling around in the head right between the eyes. When it stops he gets consciousness back." Here we
have the idea that the movements of the moth displace momentarily
whatever else has been causing movement and that, when they stop,
the original force takes over again.

In our survey of Navaho psychopathology, we found that seizures
or fits of some kind are among the most prevalent and most important of
symptoms. Since incidence rates in neither Western societies nor the

Navaho group have been ascertained with any certainty, we are not able to assert confidently that the Navahos have an unusually high incidence of this disorder or group of disorders, but our impression is that the prevalence is very high. Although most of these disorders undoubtedly have physical components, it is very likely that they have psychological components as well, which influence the frequency of occurrence. Three factors seem to be present. One is an understanding of illness in general and mental illness in particular as a consequence of a malevolent power or force that enters the body and becomes temporarily or permanently "that which stands within" the body and gives it life or movement. We have suggested that this conception results in a tendency toward illness of a hysterical type. The second factor is that Navaho mythology and folklore contain elaborate and dramatic treatments of craziness—in the form of fits and spells. These treatments imply that such fits and spells are a prominent form of mental illness and a core around which the social patterning of mental illness can form. The third factor is the high prevalence of a variety of seizures or fits. This prevalence is perhaps, at least partly a function of an anticipation that such things can happen and of a willingness that they should or a belief that they cannot be prevented. The three, it may be seen, go together very well, and together they form a social pattern of illness that has an important place in Navaho culture. None can be taken separately from the others, especially the phenomenon of the illness itself and its incidence. A fourth element of this pattern, the curing process, will be treated at greater length later in this paper.

GHOST SICKNESS

A second type of Navaho mental illness, apparently unrelated to the *iich'aa* legend and to the spells and fits, is more closely associated with the influence of evil power and witches. The symptoms are varied and include a great many of the physical illnesses known to Western medicine. They also include weakness, bad dreams, feelings of danger, confusion, feelings of futility, loss of appetite, feelings of suffocation, fainting, dizziness, fear and so forth. Morgan[4] describes the typical illness: "The individual enters a period of anxiety and generalized fear. This fear seems to emanate from a feeling of helplessness and in some cases terror, which precedes and accompanies the involuntary eruption of unconscious impulses where the individual has little or no control over his mind. He may have delusions about sights and sounds in the dark. He may have repetitive nightmares. He may have hallucinations." Wyman, Hill, and Osanai[5] claim that "the chief symptoms of ghost sickness are fainting or

the loss of consciousness, delirium (lost his mind for a while), bad dreams
(falling dreams or dreams you waste away and are dead), or terror
(especially at night)."

In the same class is the weakness of will that results from the love-
magic of witches. An interview with a Navaho singer illustrates the
mechanism of this kind of illness and also of its cure. The case discussed
is the treatment of a girl who was running around too much—she did
not like to stay home. "Old Navahos, they used to have some kind of plant
—put on hand—he see pretty girl—shake hand with her—got into her
—and that's how it start. . . . [How does it work?] Start funnying on your
skin—all over you—pretty soon it get into your head—you know when
somebody burn trash and steal big fire—smell kind of bad—then into
your head. I told_____ where you start doing that—she said I went
to ceremonial at Gallup—big crowd—one old Navaho man touched me
on my shoulder—from there it started. [Did she feel she couldn't help
herself?] Yes—[How did that work?] Her body was funny and her head
was running around—next day it was the same—starts to go around with
boys. [Do people think that the devil gets into her?] Kind of witches—
they use some kind of plant—nobody know—they put on you, then you
start round and round. [Does something come inside you?] Stay inside
you, especially go in your head. [What goes inside?] The plant—smell
bad, breathe it in—goes in your head inside. [Is it a bad wind?] Kind'a
strong wind. [I've heard some winds are bad, some winds are good. Tell
me about that.] The bad wind is no good—pretty soon everything going
to happen—the tobacco give you good wind—[He is referring here to a
mountain tobacco that is used in a special variant of the Blessing Way
sing that is specifically reserved for "cases that are a little bit crazy—mind
not very strong."] breathe tobacco—that bad wind go away and give you
good wind. [When a person is crazy is it always because of a bad wind?]
Cause when you have bad wind in you, you feel—all time your wind is
kind of strong—just like someone is choking you in there—because your
head is funny—just like you're going to get unconscious pretty soon—your
wind is not very good. [Does_____ have bad wind?] Yes, I can tell—it's
getting pretty strong in his head. He likes to fight with somebody. He
don't care—he thinks he's doing the right thing. [Tell more about that?]
See—when you have bad wind you don't like nobody—you don't like to
eat—maybe you go out maybe you breathe strong wind—maybe you fall.
These old witches put different plants on you. They go over where
somebody die—get a little piece of meat maybe [he is referring to human
flesh] and grind it, mix it with four or five different kinds of plants—
especially they go where there's a crowd—get it in their hand. Each plant

have strong wind—mix together it goes inside you—it goes right on top and then you breathe it. . . ."

In discussing another person he had treated with the Mountain Tobacco Blessing Way, he said, "She always have bad dreams, she said she was dreaming that she had been dead and all her children cried—because their mother was dying—so I go to Blessing Way and bad dreams go away. This Blessing Way will kill that. [Why did she have bad dreams?] Because she lost one of her daughters—great big daughter—dead for two years. Daughter's devil or ghost tried to jump on her when she's asleep—that's what give her the bad dreams. She's dreaming about her daughter, the one she lost—she go with her. [How does the ghost make her have bad dreams?] This girl, the one who died, really love her mother, that's why she comes back to her every night—kind'a the devil spirit. [Could it be a good spirit?] No. [How did bad dream get started?] She go fast asleep, bad spirit come on her—then she start dreaming—pretty soon she gets scared and jump out of bed. Come on your breath. Almost choke her then. [Is badness always in the form of a wind?] Yes, the bad wind—and bad spirit come and choke you—the devil choke you. [Is power always a wind?] Yes, nobody sees it. Just like your feelings. [What do you mean?] Catch your breath and go inside—in your head and that's it."

A third case, of a boy who could not sleep for thinking about his good mother who had died [seventeen years before], was treated with mountain tobacco. "[What does the smoke do?] Go inside—all get lonesome go away—sure feel happy like boy—he breathed it in—all the bad stuff all go away. Just like clean his head. Clean his inside so now he's all right."

What is apparently supposed to happen to the victim of witching or a ghost is that the witch's power or the ghost itself comes into the victim and takes over, either causing him to behave in strange ways or to weaken, sicken, or have troubling thoughts. It is a clear case of possession, although this term is not used directly. The proper treatment is in the same vein. A good wind, the smoke of the mountain tobacco, is breathed in, and it drives the bad wind or bad spirit (for they are the same) out. In the curing ceremony, there is often a struggle between the good and evil powers to see which will dominate. The behavior of a man in the middle of an Enemy Way sing prescribed to deal with the effects of the evil ghosts of his enemies was described: "He kind'a got stiff and couldn't hardly breathe. He was crying and it looked like he got all excited. I was thinking that the skeleton [the presumed trouble in this case was that the patient had had contact with a skeleton in an old Pueblo ruin] that was bothering him was trying to beat him instead of that medicine giving him a good spirit. Maybe that skeleton was trying to get ahead. But then the medicine man did something to him. So that skeleton got chased away. [How could the skeleton affect him, how did it work?] I wouldn't know—might make him sick, maybe be bothering his stomach, bothering his head, and all of a sudden he's fainting. Just like you eat an apple and it bother your stomach. Maybe the spirit had some kind of thing to bother it."

Reichard[6] has stated that Navaho ceremonies have two ends: One is the attraction of good powers so that evil can be warded off; the other is purification, the dispelling of evil powers that have already intruded. There appear to be two separate sets of ceremonies, one for each of these functions. In the latter type, the evil is exorcised through a cleansing and purification process. Since evils are believed to enter the body, curing is aimed at getting them out, mainly by emetic and sweating rites, although, as we have seen, smoking may accomplish the same purpose. Reichard's informant states,[7] "You must throw up, because if you don't, bad things will stay in you and make you sick." The process of purification is actually a good deal more complicated than we have described it, and there is a great variety of means that may be utilized. The end, however, is always the same—the exorcism of the evil power that has intruded itself into the body.

As we have suggested, this conception of etiology and of the curing processes has the greatest possible consequences for understanding the nature of the illnesses themselves. Illness is visualized as belonging, not in the realm of behavior or action over which the person has control and for which he accepts responsibility, but rather in an ego-alien realm with which the person does not identify. On the contrary, he regards the illness as an attack on his self, a negation of what he feels himself to be. While this conception probably has considerable justification with respect to physical illness, neurotic disorders involve actions of the patient himself and are composed entirely of his behavior. Avowal of helplessness to control the very actions to which one is devoting energies is a self-deception similar to the one Freud had in mind in his analysis of the process of hysteria. The dominant element here is the maintenance of innocence in the face of contrary facts, a refusal to recognize what one confronts. This refusal to know is the phenomenon that led to Freud's conceptualization of the unconscious.

The Navaho example makes it clear that conceptions of illness and of curing patterns go together and that it is useless to attempt a cure with methods that do not fit the beliefs of the person who is ill. It is not Navaho mental illness alone that is hysterical; Navaho curing practices are also hysterical. But we can see that, for a hysterical illness, a hysterical cure is the most rational possibility.

Wyman, Hill, and Osanai[8] describe a case that illustrates this point. "The next day I thought that it was strange to dream that, so I had someone perform motion-in-hand over me. I wanted to find out why I had that dream. This man told me I must have a sing. He said I must have Navaho Wind Way chant and that if I didn't I would get sore hands and then I would go blind. I didn't believe what this man said so I made more silver. I felt perfectly all right so I didn't have that sing, but later on my hand began to itch, then it got sore on both sides and blistered all over. I wasn't able to sleep. When I put my hand under the blanket it was hot, and it pained. My eyes began to go bad, and I couldn't see things clearly. They got worse and worse until I couldn't see anything. So I called in the same man again to motion-in-the-hand, and he told me the same thing as before. So I had this sing, and the medicine was put on my hand. After the sing was over I felt better. I was able to see what's what. When the sing began I wasn't able to see a thing. But I couldn't see as well as I could before that dream."

CRAZY VIOLENCE

Perhaps the most prevalent type of Navaho psychopathology at the present time is a pattern not directly associated with those we have described so far, but containing some of their elements. This pattern can be called "crazy violence" or "crazy drunken violence," although these terms are not those of the Navahos, who seem to have no specific term for it except "going crazy," or "being drunk." The importance of this phenomena seems to have been missed, partly as a result of its usual association with drunkenness, so that it is regarded as a "natural" consequence of drunkenness rather than as a mental illness, and partly because it is often dismissed as typical Indian drunkenness. While this phenomenon is not unique to the Navahos and many of its aspects are common in other Indian and non-Indian groups as well, the symptoms are so regular and recurrent among the Navahos that there can be little doubt of its special significance for them. It may, of course, have special status in other cultures as well.

This phenomenon first came to our attention when we noticed the extraordinary number of violent assaults mentioned in the records of Navaho psychiatric hospital patients and the high incidence of heavy drinking among Navaho men. Most notable was what people did while drunk. The following case is quite typical of this behavior.

A had been moody and irritable ever since his wife had left him three years previously. He spent most of his time at his family's sheep camp and had little contact with anyone other than his brothers, sister, and mother, who occasionally brought things to him. Shortly before our arrival in the field in 1961, he shot at his mother and brother and then shot himself. His mother described the incident:

> On Saturday evening we were over with A. At six o'clock his brothers came around from working to eat with us. I didn't know anyone had been drinking. The boys decided to take A and me to a Squaw dance. I didn't want to go so I didn't. A was drinking, but I didn't know it. He didn't say anything all this time. At nine o'clock he asked me for the keys to the hogan, and I asked what was wrong. He just said, "What's the matter with you?" He got an axe and tried to knock the door down, and he did. I asked one of my boys, "What's the matter with your brother?" I was shaking blankets behind the wagon—the car was by the wagon—I heard the shot. It went right through the trunk of the car. The girl and I ran off. We heard four more shots. I don't know any reason why he should get mad. He shot himself in the head, and he's in the hospital.

A Navaho woman informant was asked what the old people thought about this drinking. She replied, "They say this alcohol is in the blood, and they don't have their right mind. If there's lots of alcohol in you, you just don't know what you are doing. It just drives you crazy. [Sometimes though alcohol doesn't make you crazy?] I don't know, we think they just look like they're crazy—the way they act and talk. The next time we see this person, they're all right, and that's how it's going, on and off. If they take a little they're all right, but if they take a lot they go crazy. We say, 'Why don't you take just a little like the white man does?' I say they have minds, and they know what they're doing. Maybe some of them have bad winds in them." "Going crazy" here involves a number of different elements. One is that "They don't really know what they are doing." Another is that "He doesn't care what he is doing." "He goes wild" is another. But the symptom implied in all these phrases is violent assaultive behavior.

Is the "crazy violence" pattern another variant of the "hysterical" theme? At first glance, it does not seem to be. It is not primarily a disturbance of awareness, although when the individual returns to normality he often does have a disturbed awareness of his behavior or even amnesia. But this amnesia belongs to the normal state and not to the disturbance itself. The violent behavior seems to occur with complete awareness and consciousness. The individual "wants" to do what he is doing, and he will brook no interference either from others or from his own rational controls. In one sense, his situation is the exact opposite of the hysterical person's situation. He embraces his illness. He knows he is acting "crazy," but he does not care, and he aligns himself with his "worse" side. In hysteria, the victim refuses to acknowledge his illness as his own, attributing it to whatever has invaded him. One of our informants, a white trader, distinguishes this "crazy" pattern from that of illness from witchcraft: "With witchcraft they are really scared, and not trying to prove anything." The implication of this remark is that the drunken berserker *is* trying to prove something by what he is doing.

In the crazy violence pattern there is a "heroic" element of honesty and willingness to take the consequences, an element more than slightly reminiscent of some of Dostoevsky's more violent characters. The person is violent and almost inhuman in his brutality, but he knows what he is doing. He is deliberately reckless, and he acts in spite of the consequences to come. He does not avoid pain, suffering, and trouble for himself any more than for his victim. Although his victim suffers, he is ready to suffer also. Evidence for this readiness can be found in the relatively large number of suicides that terminate these violent outbursts. Perhaps the key to this violent transformation from Navaho normality is the suicidal needs that are part of this pattern. The recklessness expresses a willingness to die and to be hurt. This willingness seems to be the dynamic force that dissipates fear and turns one into a raging superman. Religious thinkers have long recognized the power of fearlessness, and it is fearlessness that makes it possible for the Navaho man to do what he wants.

The psychoanalytic interpretation of this violent behavior is that of "acting out," which may be defined as the direct discharge into action of warded-off instinctual impulses and inner tensions. It is impulsive action associated with weak or absent ego controls. Fenichel[9] has written that most impulsive acts serve the purpose of avoiding depression, a connection that seems to apply in the Navaho case. Fenichel makes the distinction between the impulsive character and the true depressive character according to whether narcissistic gratification is demanded for a real object or narcissism has been discharged to the point where demands for gratification are directed to the subject's own superego.

Our own predilection is to look for something more positive than the weakness or absence of control mechanisms. Such mechanisms are amply demonstrated in the normal routines of these men, and, although it is possible that they are soluble in alcohol, we believe that alcohol is merely an element contributing to their weakening. One possibility is that berserk rage represents an attempt to replace or deny some other state that is felt to be "real." That state among Navaho men is most likely to be one of helplessness or powerlessness. Rage is an attempt to deny these experiences and to assert their opposite. It is squarely in the sphere of the ego and is an attempt to control and master the situation, rather than an evidence of the failure of controls. It is perhaps only in the sense that these rage states are attempts to assert what is not that they are related to hysterical mechanisms.

The crazy-violence pattern seems to stand in a different relation to the Navaho scheme of things than do the other two patterns we have described, and it is impossible to understand the problem of psychotherapy until this relationship is analyzed. In the *iich'aa* illness, the patient is being punished for the social transgression of incest—usually with a clan member. He has been bad or has broken the rules and is in the process of receiving his just punishment. The individual has committed a social wrong and suffers for it. The treatment involves repentance and promises not to transgress again. In general, the illness has the social meaning of a dramatic warning to prospective transgressors and is part of the socialization apparatus of the society.

In the ghost sickness, the patient is a victim of the malevolence of others. He himself is innocent but is weak and powerless to protect himself. We have speculated that, since in fact there is no ghost, the symptoms derive from the patient's own beliefs or attitudes. The social definition of the illness, however, is that of an evil attack on the good. In the curing process, the community ranges itself on the side of the victim and musters its strength for his support. From the patient's point of view, his illness is an opportunity to receive much support that otherwise might not be forthcoming.

In the third pattern, the "crazy violence" pattern, the patient is attacking normal social arrangements. Disregarding for a moment the element of possession by alcohol in drunkenness, we know that the individual completely accepts his role as a deviant and identifies with his illness. In fact, his illness consists completely of his purposeful and intentional behavior. The "cure" in this case is to contain the destructiveness and disruption. We find in these cases that the typical community response is first to restrain the miscreant by tying him if necessary or by taking him to jail. Second, the community elders attempt to persuade the man to "settle down" and give up fighting. He and his family are expected to make restitution for any damages. The social pressures are quite straightforward, and there is ordinarily little mention of the supernatural. One has the impression that the community feels helpless to defend itself and that it does not, at the present time, have any techniques for handling this problem. Ceremonial curing techniques are apparently not utilized—mainly because the curing ceremony is not designed to change the patient but to rid him of the illness of which he is a victim. Its function is to exorcise and counteract malevolence—not to to change the malevolent agent himself. The latter conception, which permeates Western psychiatry, seems not to form a part of the Navaho curing pattern.

§ The Treatment Process

The forms of mental illness that we have described are regarded by the Navaho as disorders of ordinary life, and, like such disruptions as physical illness, drought, and storms, they are dealt with through a highly complex ceremonial system. Navaho ceremonialism is designed above all to set right what has become disordered. The ceremonies themselves have been described many times, and our purpose is not to explore their full significance for the Navaho. Outstanding descriptions of ceremonies are to be found in Matthew, Haile, and Wyman.[10]

Navaho ceremonies or chants or sings, as they are also called, are generally regarded as curing rites for most of them are used in treating illness. Ethnographers have noted that, while the primary concern of the Pueblo is for rain, his Navaho neighbor focuses his ceremonial activities on curing. It is something of an overstatement since the Pueblos also have curing rites and several Navaho ceremonies are aimed at producing rain, protecting flocks of sheep, or assuring good luck. Nevertheless, there can be no doubt that the great part of the Navaho ceremonial system is for curing illness. Nearly all the more than fifty major ceremonials are either exclusively for curing or can be used in connection with curing chants.

There is an intricate mixture of the specific and the general in Navaho curing. A vast number of elements of procedure and apparatus appear in the chant system, and all parts are interrelated by their association in mythology. The parts are occasionally lifted from one ceremony for use in another, and, in treatment, the patient's afflicted body parts usually receive special attention. The singer, touching the arms of a patient, says, "May his feet be well." The ancient principle that "like cures like" requires ceremonies to have many elements of similarity to the illness—for example, Red Ant Way is used to treat diseases caused by swallowing red ants. The related idea, that "the part stands for the whole," also appears repeatedly. Despite this use of parts, however, Navaho man is much more holistically oriented than Western man. According to Kluck-hohn and Leighton, "The whole Navaho system of curing clearly takes it for granted that you cannot treat a man's body without treating his mind and vice versa."[11] Navaho therapy takes into account the patient's physical self, attitude, social-group membership, and the other elements distinguished by Western man—but without as much abstracting and compartmentalizing. This holistic orientation also tends to minimize the distinctions between physical and mental illness. Instead, the Navaho distinguish between "sickness" and "hurts." The latter include broken bones and cuts due to accidents and are treated by a separate class of chants, those of Life Way.

The guiding principle underlying all Navaho curing is that super-natural power may be directed toward removing or overcoming evil or toward restoring order by man's proper use of ceremonies. Reichard discusses this principle at length in her book, *Navaho Religion*.[12] She makes the point that the Navaho do not humble themselves in any way to win the favor of gods. Power is at man's disposal through correct use of procedures given to him by the gods in the form of chants. By properly ("compulsively," according to Reichard) using chant ritual, man forces the supernatural to help him. A significant implication of this view is that the patient does not need to reflect on his behavior or examine his motives, conscience, or reactions in order to be helped. There is no exhaustive analysis of intrapersonal dynamics; he need only place himself within the curing system, which, once set in motion, pro-ceeds almost automatically. Another implication is that, for the Navaho, man stands in a basically co-operative relationship with the supernatural. The gods have supplied him with the clearly stated means for marshalling supernatural power. Man uses these means as his intelligence directs, and, when he follows the procedures correctly, the supernatural, in effect, does its part.

In its simplest form, the ceremony is merely a short excerpt from a longer ceremony tried out to see if it helps the patient. In its most complete, longest form, the ceremony is a complicated event indeed, requiring nine days and nights. It is composed of many elements and exacts the combined efforts of a singer, his assistants, and the family of the patient. Such a ceremony is made up of, to quote Reichard, "ritualistic items such as the medicine bundle with its sacred contents; prayersticks, made of carefully selected wood and feathers, precious stones, tobacco, water collected from sacred places, a tiny piece of cotton string; song, with its lyrical and musical complexities; sandpaintings, with intricate color; prayer, with stress on order and rhythmic unity; plants, with supernatural qualities defined and personified; body and figure painting; sweating and emetic, with purificatory functions; vigil, with emphasis on concentration and summary."[13]

The singer, nearly always male, achieves his position after a lengthy apprenticeship. Our inquiries about who might become a singer revealed only that any man who wanted to trouble himself with learning the ceremonies—they must be learned letter-perfect—and had the intellectual abilities to do it might become a singer. Apparently, moral reputation is not especially relevant, nor could we detect personality differences between singers and other Navaho. The singers do not follow the deviant pattern of shamans in other Indian tribes; they may be deviants, but certainly a fair number is of the solid core of Navaho society. The singers are specialists, and many earn reputations for being able to cure very effectively, but few practice chanting exclusively. Most also have sheep and are otherwise occupied. Singers do not set themselves apart from other members of their community, and they do not form priestly orders, as is the custom of the Pueblo neighbors. Because of the chants' complexity, most singers know only a few, and the repertoire of each singer is well known to members of the community. The singer's reputation depends on his success in treating his patients. The highly successful singer may eventually become a comparatively wealthy man. He must not, however, appear too wealthy, or he will surely be suspected of using his ritual knowledge for the evil purposes of witchcraft. Singers are regarded as the wise men of the community and frequently counsel others, including their patients and families. These talks have no place in the formal ceremonial procedure but undoubtedly do have effects on the patient. The acting-out patient, for example, may be seriously counseled to settle down.

Although the singer is the key agent in the curing process, he does not diagnose the cause of the illness or decide which sing to use. Another specialist performs this very important function. The task of the diagnostician or seer is, very literally, to locate the "trouble within," to determine whether the illness is caused by witchcraft, violation of a taboo, or some other break with Navaho standards. These diagnosticians differ from the singers in several respects. They are not, for example, expected to treat illness; they are simply to designate which sing is necessary for the treatment. Furthermore, the diagnostician achieves his position in another way. He is possessed by supernatural powers that enter him, and, as a diagnostician, he serves simply as the vehicle of these powers. He is expected to carry out his function in the "right way," but he does not undergo a long period of training to acquire special skills. A third difference is that many women are diagnosticians, but women are rarely singers.

The source of trouble is located in any of several ways—stargazing, wind-listening, and hand-trembling. Hand-trembling is apparently the method most frequently used now. Typically, the hand-trembler acquires his power while watching a ceremony. He feels his hands and arms moving, and it is assumed that a power has entered him and is moving his hands. After word gets around, he may be asked to locate the source of trouble in some case; and as he goes into a trance, his hands move over the afflicted person's body until the source of the trouble is located. That this event is supernatural is emphasized by the stricture that the hand-trembler must not talk to the patient or his family about the case. Our informants gave many examples of the accuracy of the hand-trembler's powers in determining the source of trouble, whether it lay in the unfaithfulness of a wife, lost sheep, or some type of mental illness.

The treatment process involves a great many possible courses of action, but all tend to follow a pattern quite closely. A Navaho, on discovering that he does not feel well, for example, feels dizzy, cannot think clearly, is "sick all over," discusses his symptoms with a relative. They may decide to call in a diagnostician to locate the source of this trouble and prescribe the appropriate ceremonial remedy. The relatives rather than the patient contact the diagnostician and arrange the fee and time, exactly as they later will do with the singer. The rite of divination is comparatively brief and involves both the symbolic ritual so typical of Navaho curing and the power residing in the hand-trembler.

The hand-trembler locates the cause of the trouble and may recommend a singer. Usually a family will follow his recommendation if the singer is available and not too expensive. The singer is engaged about four days before the sing, and his bundle of ritual materials is carried back to the patient's home to prepare for the event. These preparations generate an air of excitement as everyone involved cleans the hogan and gathers firewood, food for the family and the many expected guests, herbs, clean sand for sand paintings, and all the other items necessary for the ceremony.

The actual sing is an exceedingly complex event; Kluckhohn and Leighton have compared the singer's task to that of memorizing a Wagnerian opera, including "orchestral score, every vocal part, all details of the settings, stage business, and each requirement of costume."[14] We shall not go into detail in describing the ceremonies. While there are important differences among sings, chiefly in terms of the legends on which they are based, there are enough common features so that this description by Wyman is sufficient:

In a typical Holyway chant, there are ten or twelve more or less standard ceremonies. The *consecration of the hogan* by the singer, who places corn meal and sprigs of hard oak on or above the four cardinal roof beams, opens the ceremonial at sundown. An *unraveling ceremony* follows after sundown, lasting about an hour, in which bundles of herbs, feathers, and so on, tied with a wool string that will unravel and come free when its end is pulled, are applied to the patient's body and unraveled. This symbolizes release from evil. A *short-singing* of an hour or more follows, often accompanied by drumming on an inverted basket. If a sandpainting is to be made, *setting-out* of symbolic bundle prayersticks (stuck upright in a mound of earth outside the hogan door) is performed just before dawn. Thus all beings, human and supernatural, are notified of the procedures within. Just after dawn, a *sweat and emetic ceremony,* for the internal and external purification of the patient and any others who want it, is held only if the chant is of five or nine nights' duration, for this ceremony must be repeated four times and lasts an hour or two. An enormous fire, kindled with a fire drill induces copious sweating, and an emetic extract is used for both drinking and bathing. After the vomiting, the singer sprinkles everyone with a fragrant herb lotion. After breakfast, "jewel" offerings, painted reeds stuffed with wild tobacco ["cigarettes"] and/or prayersticks are prepared for an invocatory *offering ceremony* to attract the Holy People. After a long litany, these are deposited in specified places at some distance from the hogan. In the forenoon of the last day, a *bath ceremony,* with yucca-root suds, provides further purification. The *sandpainting* is then begun, and it is usually completed by early or mid-afternoon. The bundle prayersticks are brought in from the set-out mound and placed around the painting, and corn meal is sprinkled on it. On the last day only, symbolic designs are painted on the patient's body, and a bead token that becomes his property and a head plume for recognition are tied in his hair. The patient then sits on the sandpainting while the singer administers medicine to him and applies sand from the painted figures to corresponding parts of his body. Thus the patient is identified with the supernatural beings represented in the painting, and he becomes strong and dangerous like them. That is why he must observe four days of restricted behavior following the ceremonial, lest others be harmed by contact with him. The sandpainting is erased, and, after the patient has left the hogan, the sand is deposited outside it to the north. An *all-night singing* occupies the final night, and the ceremonial is closed by the *dawn procedures.*

Consecration of the hogan, bath, body painting and token tying, *all night singing,* and the dawn procedures occur only once in any chant. The other ceremonies are repeated four times in a five- or ten-night performance; they are performed only once in a two-night chant, except for the sweat and emetic, which cannot be given at all. In a nine-night chant, the short-singings, setting-out, and sandpainting ceremonies are moved ahead to the fifth, sixth, seventh, and eighth days.[15]

Some ways of controlling supernatural power are apparent in this description. Prayers and songs are used to invoke the deities, while sand paintings capture power and bring it nearer to the patient. Power is concentrated for better handling by drawing it into a small sand painting or a buckskin or by limiting its scope by drawing lines of pollen to create barriers to evil. The purification rituals of emetic, sweating, and continence help to prepare the patient to receive the benefit of the ceremony. The patient remains quite passive throughout, but he is expected to have an attitude of acceptance and to focus his attention on the ceremony. One of our informants said, "When I sit on the sand painting and hear the singer's prayers, I think that all of my friends are close to me."

Our classification of types of disorder is based on behavior. The Navaho, however, base their ceremonial system on etiology. The classification of Navaho ceremonials offered by L. C. Wyman and C. Kluckhohn[16] divide the curing chants into three categories: Holy Way, Life Way, and Evil Way. Only the Holy Way and Evil Way chants have much relevance for mental disorders, as the Life Way chants are for physical hurts. Holy Way chants are used in dealing with disorders arising from contact with lightning, thunder, and such god-related animals as snakes, bears, or deer. The Evil Way group is for trouble from ghosts, either Navaho or alien. In all the ceremonies, there are elements of removing evil and attracting good, but the chief difference between the purpose of the Holy Way chants is that much more attention is given to exorcising evil in the latter group of chants.

The three types of mental disorder described in the first part of this paper are treated by one or the other of these classes of ceremonials. Th *iich'aa* illness, caused by incest, is treated by the Moth Way sing in the Evil Way category, a portion of a larger ceremony called Prostitution Way by Haile and Kluckhohn and Recklessness Way by Reichard. Father Berard has described the major function of this sing as to define the limitations of sexual intercourse; the legend tells of incest among the gods and the tragic outcome. The Moth Way chant is not well known, however, and may be virtually obsolete. Furthermore, it is not clear from Father Berard's account whether or not it is truly a curing ceremony or merely one that mitigates the bad effects of incest. Our informants were similarly divided on this issue. Several informants stated that there was no cure for the *iich'aa* illness.

Most patients with the *iich'aa* (epileptic-like) symptoms were said by some, usually near relatives, to be suffering from something other than *iich'aa*. The case of one young woman is typical. B had had several seizures during the past winter and spring. Her mother-in-law told us that she knew these were symptoms of *iich'aa* and that this girl had had sexual relations with her brother. The mother-in-law was successful in obtaining a divorce for her son and sent B back to her family. B's family, on the other hand, and most of the people we talked with, including the hand-trembler who had diagnosed her illness, blamed the trouble on a fright she had experienced as a child when lightning had struck near her. She was treated for the lightning illness at the expense of her family but without improvement. Than all the people involved were convinced that her case was incurable.

Ghost illness is believed to be due to evil forces, especially witchcraft, and generally calls for an Evil Way ceremonial. We did find that the initial ceremony was quite often a Blessing Way, which is not, strictly speaking, appropriate for exorcising evil but does help to strengthen the afflicted individual and contains some exorcistic elements. The behavior or symptoms of those infected by certain animals or lightning are so similar to those of persons influenced by witchcraft that we have included the two together as "ghost illness." In both cases, the individual's body is invaded by some power. The treatments differ, however, depending on whether the power is essentially evil (usually associated with spirits of dead humans) or related to nonhuman holy beings.

The last category of disorder, that which we have termed "crazy violence," seems to us to be apart from the ordinary illness-cure complex. There are apparently no consistent definitions of etiology for this behavior, and therefore no specific ceremonials can be prescribed. We found that in a number of cases there had been no ceremonial action—the offender had been handled as a criminal in courts or had been turned over to agencies providing psychiatric treatment. In other instances, violence was attributed to a head injury caused by a fall from a horse, for example. In these cases where the injury usually was not readily apparent and the etiology remained in doubt, the Blessing Way was cited as the usual treatment.

Navaho curing techniques are undoubtedly effective in a great many cases. We have little direct evidence of their effectiveness, but our informants were all able to cite instances of favorable response to treatment. It is our impression that, of the three types of behavior disorder, the ghost-illness cases were most likely to improve. *Iich'aa* was regarded as virtually incurable, and many cases of episodic violence of which we learned were regarded as remaining potentially dangerous. One instance of change in a person with ghost illness involved a young man whom we interviewed during our first summer of field work. He had become very disturbed—talking incoherently, running through the woods, threatening violence—and his family attributed his trouble to his violation of taboos during a curing ceremony for his father. A series of chants was held for the young man, and, in our next summer's field work, we found that he had had no further trouble. He had received no modern psychiatric treatment during the year, and his recovery was attributed by those who knew him to the curing ceremonies.

We also found, of course, many cases that either did not improve or actually seemed to become worse despite ceremonial treatment. Usually, the explanation was that either the right chants were not included or the series was not continued long enough. One case, perhaps the only clearly diagnosed case of schizophrenia in one community, was the subject of much disagreement and concern in the community. She was believed to have been afflicted originally with hand-trembler's illness, a disorder caused by misuse of supernatural power. She had not been properly treated with Hand-Trembler Way chant in the Holy Way group because her oldest son had become a Christian and opposed using Navaho religion. She became worse, was hospitalized for several months, and was discharged in partial remission. Years later and still psychotic by both Navaho and white standards, she had become the source of recriminations and discord among members of the family. Many still believe that Navaho treatment would have helped her.

Although biological and chemical treatment is used in ceremonies, it is generally in forms of such low potency that they can have little effect. Mountain tobacco is used in many ceremonies, including Beauty Way (of the Holy Way group), but the smoke has no greater physical effect than ordinary tobacco, and only very small quantities are inhaled. A few powerfully narcotic drugs are known to the Navaho and are used in their ceremonies. The root of jimson weed is one. It is used in Life Way ceremonies to relieve pain and in larger quantities is hallucinogenic. Apparently, however, it is not actually used in ceremonial treatment of mental disorders. The rites of purification—sweat baths and vomiting—may have some beneficial physical effect, but it seems most likely that the effect is again largely psychological. In one sense, all Navaho curing is psychotherapy. Looked at another way, however, none of it is psychotherapy as we know it. In the sense of verbal interaction between patient and therapist, with the goal of changing behavior through increased insight and self-awareness, psychotherapy hardly exists at all.

The effectiveness of Navaho curing ceremonies appears to reside in two processes. One of them is suggestion. The elaborate procedure of purification aims to convince the patient and the community that the "bad stuff" is vanquished and can no longer cause trouble. To the extent that the ceremony is accepted, the patient believes that the causes of his difficulties are gone. Since his difficulties were initially based on a similar process of suggestion or autosuggestion, in that they were organized around the belief that some malevolent agent had attached itself to him or was possessing him, the cure, in an important sense, reverses the process of the illness. The problem in this kind of cure, of course, is that the whole cycle may repeat itself again and again. In fact, there is some evidence that it does.

The second effective agent seems to be reaffirmation of the solidarity of the community and indeed of the whole pantheon of Navaho deities with the patient. The ceremony surrounds him with concern and good will and serves as a kind of reintegration of the social group, with the sick person not only a solid part of it but at its very center. We have seen that this aspect of the ceremony has more to do with the protection of the person than with curing or purging him of already established evil power. But the two aspects undoubtedly reinforce each other psychologically.

We also believe that they tend to support the hypothesis that was our starting point: that the processes of psychotherapy that prevail in any cultural group are integrated with conceptions of the nature of illness and its causes.

Notes

1. C. Kluckhohn and A. K. Romney, "The Rimrock Navaho," Florence Kluckhohn and F. L. Strodtbeck, eds., *Variations in Value Orientations* (New York: Harper & Row, Publishers, 1961); and J. Ladd, *The Structure of a Moral Code* (Cambridge, Mass.: Harvard University Press, 1956).

2. B. Haile, "Soul Concept of the Navaho," *Annali Lateranensi*, VII (1943), 59-94.

3. Gladys A. Reichard, *Navaho Religion* (2 vols; New York: Pantheon Books, Inc., 1950).

4. W. Morgan, *Human Wolves Among the Navaho* (Yale University Publications in Anthropology, No. 11 [New Haven: Yale University Press, 1936], 7).

5. L. Wyman, W. W. Hill, and I. Osanai, "Navaho Eschatology," *University of New Mexico Bulletin* (1942), p. 377.

6. Reichard, *op. cit*, I.

7. *Ibid.*, p. 109.

8. Wyman, Hill, and Osanai, *op. cit.*, p. 3.

9. O. Fenichel, "Neurotic Acting Out," *Psychoanalytic Review*, 32 (1943), 197-206.

10. W. Matthew, *The Mountain Chant* (Report of the Bureau of American Eth-

nology, No. 5 [1887], 385-467; Haile, *Origin Legend of the Navaho Enemy Way* (Yale University Publications in Anthropology, No. 17 [New Haven: Yale University Press, 1938]; and Wyman, ed., *Beautyway: A Navaho Ceremonial* (New York: Bollingen Foundation, 1957).

11. Kluckhohn and Dorothea Leighton, *The Navaho* (Garden City: Anchor Books, 1962), p. 309.

12. Reichard, *op. cit.*, I.

13. *Ibid.* p. xxii.

14. Kluckhohn and Leighton, *op. cit.*, p. 229.

15. Wyman, *op cit.*, pp. 8-9.

16. Kluckhohn and Wyman, *Navaho Classification of Their Song Ceremonials* (Washington, D.C.: Memoirs of the American Anthropological Association, 1938), p. 50.

Victor W. Turner

An Ndembu Doctor in Practice*

THIS CHAPTER consists mainly of an extended case study of an Ndembu *chimbuki* (which I shall translate as "doctor," though "ritual specialist" or "cult-adept" would be equally appropriate) at work. I knew Ihembi well and during a period of six months attended a number of curative rites over which he presided. He was a member of the Ndembu tribe of Mwinilunga District in the extreme Northwest of Northern Rhodesia, among whom I did nearly two and a half years of fieldwork from 1950 to 1954 and about whom I have published a book and several articles.[1] The Ndembu are a relatively conservative people, an amalgam of Lunda invaders from the Katanga and autochthonous Mbwela and Lukolwe. They are matrilineal and virilocal;* have a senior chief and about a dozen subchiefs, four of whom are recognized by the British administration under the Native Authority; and grow cassava as their staple crop along with finger millet, maize, sweet potatoes, and a variety of cucurbits and other relish plants. They have no cattle and only a few sheep and goats (although large areas are free from tsetse-fly infestation). Until recently, hunting was the predominant male pursuit and was accompanied by a richly elaborated ritual system involving beliefs in the punitive and tutelary powers of hunter ancestors or "shades" (as I shall call them henceforward). Ndembu live in small circular villages each of which consists of a nuclear group of matrikin, one of whom is headman, surrounded by a fringe of cognatic and affinal kin.

These facts are relevant to the account that follows, for disease among the Ndembu must be viewed not only in a private or "idiographic" but also in a "public" or social structural framework. All societies have, of course, a functional interest in the minimization of illness, as Parsons has pointed out.[2] But the Ndembu go further in positing a social explanation for illness itself. All persistent or severe sickness is believed to be caused

* A system in which a woman normally resides in her husband's village.

either by the punitive action of ancestral shades or by the secret malevolence of male sorcerers or female witches. The shades punish their
living kin, so the Ndembu declare, for negligence in making offerings at
their village shrines, for breaches of ritual interdictions, or "because kin
are not living well together." My own observations suggest that, whenever
rites to propitiate or exorcise the shades —as distinct from private treatment by herbalists—are performed, there is a factor of social conflict
present. The "ritual of affliction," as I have called it,[3] constitutes, in fact,
a phase in the complex process of corporate life and has a redressive
function in interpersonal or factional disputes, many of which have long
histories. Even when a person's fault has been slight, he may be "caught
by the shades," the Ndembu think, as a scapegoat for his group if it is
full of "grudges" (*yitela*) or "quarreling" (*ndombu*). Therapy then becomes a matter of sealing up the breaches in social relationships simultaneously with ridding the patient (*muyeji*) of his pathological symptoms.
Attributions of disease to sorcery or witchcraft are frequently made in the
context of factional rivalry, especially when the factions support rival
candidates for office during the old age of its incumbent, whether he be
chief or village headman. All deaths are attributed to sorcery or witchcraft, but only those of structurally important individuals are singled out
for special ritual attention. When minor personages die, the identities of
their secret destroyers are left to speculative gossip and rumor, and no
action is taken. But, in the course of lively factional struggle, the death
of even an infant may precipitate accusations and counteraccusations. In
villages that markedly exceed the average size of thirty men, women,
and children, such accusations may precede schism—when a dissident
faction leaves the parent village and builds elsewhere on the pretext that
it is escaping from witchcraft, which is believed to have a limited geographical range of efficacy.

In their treatment of disease, the Ndembu, like ourselves, recognize
symptoms and distinguish between diagnosis and therapy. But there the
resemblance ends. Ndembu do not know of natural causes for diseases
but, as we have seen, believe that either punitive shades or envious
sorcerers produce them. Their diagnosticians are diviners, and their therapists are in effect masters of ceremonies.

§ Divination

Divination is a phase in a social process that begins with a person's
death, illness, reproductive trouble, or misfortune at hunting (for illness
is only one class of misfortune that is mystically caused). It continues

through discussion in the victim's kin-group or village about the steps to be taken next, the most important of which is a journey to consult a diviner (distant diviners are believed to give more reliable diagnoses than local ones). The fourth stage is the actual consultation or séance attended by the victim's kin and often by his neighbors. This séance is followed by remedial action according to the diviner's prescription. Such action may consist of the destruction or expulsion of a sorcerer or witch; the performance of ritual by cult specialists to propitiate or exorcise specific culturally defined manifestations of shades; or the application of herbal and other "medicines" according to the diviner's advice by an herbalist or medicine man.

I have recently published an account of Ndembu leechcraft.[4] It is sufficient to state here that whatever may be the empirical benefits of certain treatments, the herbal medicines employed derive their efficacy, according to the Ndembu, from mystical notions, and native therapy is an intrinsic part of a whole magico-religious system.

The divinatory consultation is the central phase or episode in the total process of coping with misfortune, and it looks both backward to causation and forward to remedial measures. Since death, disease, and misfortune are, as we have noted, usually ascribed to exacerbated tensions in social relations, expressed as personal grudges charged with the mystical power of sorcery or witchcraft or as beliefs in the punitive action of ancestral shades intervening in the lives of their surviving kin, diviners try to elicit from their clients responses that give clues about the patterns of current tensions in their groups of origin. Divination therefore becomes a form of social analysis, in the course of which hidden struggles among individuals and factions are brought to light, so that they may be dealt with by traditional ritual procedures. It is in the light of this "cybernetic" function of divination as a mechanism of social redress that we should consider its symbolism, the social composition of its consultative sessions, and its interrogation procedures.[5]

§ Therapeutic Rites

The curative rites are performed by a number of cult associations, each devoted to a specific manifestation of the ancestral shades. Thus a shade that manifests itself as *nkula* afflicts its living kinswoman with menstrual disorders of various kinds, a shade that "comes out [of the grave] in *isoma*" causes miscarriages, and so forth. The patient in any given cult ritual is a candidate for entry into that cult and, by passing through its rites, becomes a cult-adept. The particular shade that had afflicted him in the first instance, when propitiated, becomes a tutelary who confers on him health and curative powers for that particular mode of affliction. Although the tutelary shade is an adept's kinsman or kinswoman, cult membership cuts across membership of descent groups and territorial groups. Cult members make up associations of those who have suffered the same modes of affliction as the result of having been seized (perhaps "elected" would be a more appropriate term) by deceased members of the cults. Since there are many cults and since the nuclear symbols of each refer to basic values and beliefs shared by all Ndembu, it may be said that the total system of cults of affliction keeps alive, through constant repetition, the sentiment of tribal unity. Ndembu secular society is characterized by the weakness of its political centralization, by the high spatial mobility of its individual members and of its groups (due to shifting areas of cultivation and the emphasis on hunting), and by the tendency of villages to split and reassemble. This secular mobility (and lability) is counteracted to some extent by the embodiment of tribal values of unity in the cults of affliction.

§ The Ihamba Cult

This necessarily truncated account of Ndembu divination and cult therapy must suffice as background to Ihembi's practice. Since this doctor specialized in the Ihamba cult, I shall briefly outline its characteristics. In the first place, the term *ihamba* refers among the Ndembu to an upper central incisor tooth of a deceased hunter. It forms an important element in a complex of beliefs and symbolic objects associated with hunting ritual—especially with ritual associated with those hunters who employ firearms. It is believed that the two upper front incisors of a gun-hunter (*chiyang'a*) contain much of his power to kill animals. If one of these teeth is knocked out or drops out as a result of pyorrhea, the hunter must preserve it. When a gun-hunter dies, these incisors are removed. The left incisor is said to belong to "his mother's side," the right "to his father's." The teeth must be inherited by appropriate relatives who are initiated members of the gun-hunters cult (*Wuyang'a*).

An inherited *ihamba* is carried in a pouch with a long sash of white or colored cloth. The pouch itself (called *mukata*) is made of white cloth. The *ihamba*, concealed beneath a long flap, is embedded in a paste of corn meal mixed with the blood of slaughtered game. Above it are inserted two cowrie shells (*mpashi*), which are known as "the eyes" (*mesu*).

With these *mesu* the hunter's shade is said to "see animals" in the bush and to confer similar powers on their owner. The inheritor takes the *mukata* pouch into the bush with him when he goes hunting. With the carrying sash are folded strips of the dead hunter's clothing. When it is not in use, it is hung up in a shrine consecrated to hunters' shades. Women are forbidden to approach this shrine closely. Should they do so inadvertently, they are believed to develop menstrual disorders or to bleed to death after their next childbirths. This prohibition derives from a basic principle of Ndembu ritual, that "the blood of huntsmanship" (*mashi aWubinda*, from *Wubinda*, which stands for "generic huntsmanship") must not be brought into contact with "the blood of motherhood" (*mashi amama*) or the "blood of procreation" (*mashi alusemu*). For example, when a hunter's wife is about to give birth he must remove all his hunting gear from his hut and its vicinity, lest it lose its efficacy. Behind this principle lies the notion that, for a child to be born, the maternal blood must coagulate around the fetus. Hunters shed blood and cause it to gush and flow. Again, women give life, while hunters take it. The two functions are antithetical.

It is necessary to distinguish between two ritual usages in connection with *mahamba* (the plural of *ihamba*). An *ihamba* may be inherited by a renowned hunter and then be used as a charm or amulet to bring him good fortune in the chase. On the other hand, some *mahamba* are believed to afflict the living by burying themselves in their bodies and causing them severe pains. In such cases the afflicting *mahamba* are believed to be of two kinds: Some are from the corpses of hunters whose incisor teeth were lost before burial; others are "escapees" from *mukata* pouches or from calabash containers in which they had been placed after extraction by Ihamba doctors. The Ihamba cult consists of male adepts, who must be initiated hunters of the gun-hunters' cult, and the purpose of the rites they perform is to extract *mahamba* from the bodies of persons afflicted by hunter-shades. The *mahamba* are said to be the incisors of the afflicting shades. To remove an *ihamba*, the senior adept or "doctor" makes an incision on any part of the patient's body and applies to the cut a cupping horn (usually a goat's horn) from which the tip has been removed. After the horn (*kasumu*) has been sucked, it is plugged with beeswax. The doctor's intention is to "catch" the *ihamba*, which is believed to "wander about" subcutaneously.

What are the symptoms of *ihamba* affliction? Here are some of my informants' comments. Nyamuvwila, the aged wife of a village headman, said that she had been "eaten" (*ku-dya*) in the chest, neck, and shoulders by an *ihamba* that had "fallen" into her body. The *ihamba* came from her uterine brother, a hunter whose *ihamba* tooth had not been removed before burial. After his death, "it wandered about and went after meat." Another woman from the same village had "become sick" (*wakata*) "in the back," because an *ihamba* had "started to bite" her. My best informant on ritual matters, Muchona, in describing to me the circumstances surrounding a particular case of *ihamba* affliction, said, "Chain [the patient] comes from the village of Makumela, his mother's village. That is also where the shade of *ihamba* [*mukishi wehamba*] has come from. His grandfather is the shade, the mother's brother of his mother. He is the one who has fallen on his grandson to obtain blood from him. He has come that he may be known [remembered]. When they have sucked him out [as an *ihamba*], they should offer him the blood of an animal [smear the *ihamba* with the blood of a kill after the hunt], so that they may stay well [live in health, mutual accord, and prosperity], and that the patient, who was sick, may also stay well. They pray to him that they may put him in a pouch of cloth and sing and dance with drums for him [at a gun hunters' rite]." According to other informants, an *ihamba* can be seen moving about under the patient's skin (muscular spasms, perhaps) "like the movements of an insect (*nyisesa yakabubu*)." It is said to "catch him with its teeth," the plural form *mazewu*, "teeth," being sometimes used for the single tooth that has been extracted. It "flies in the air" to reach its victim, whose blood it demands.

Its attributes suggest that the *ihamba* epitomizes the aggressive power of the hunter. It also represents the harshness of internalized norms, since an *ihamba* only "bites" when there has been transgression of moral or customary rules. At the unconscious level of meaning, behavior associated with *ihamba*—"eating," "biting," "going after meat"—and its removal by "sucking" and anointing with blood suggests that *ihamba* beliefs may be connected with the orally aggressive stage of infantile development.

An interesting feature of the Ihamba cult is its comparatively recent introduction into Ndembu territory. It has been grafted onto the rites of the long-established hunters' cult and shares much of its symbolism. But this cult, with many tribal variations, has a wide geographical range among the West Central and Central Bantu peoples. Certain linguistic features indicate that Ihamba was borrowed by Ndembu from the Luvale and Chokwe peoples in Angola. It has certainly spread rapidly in the postwar period. One major difference from the hunters' cult proper is that, while the *ihamba* is almost invariably a manifestation of a male shade, its victims include at least as many women as men, although women may not become Ihamba doctors since membership in the curative cult is restricted to initiated hunters.

Two further features of Ihamba should be noted. The cult has spread precisely where hunting has been on the decline because of the increasing scarcity of game and the increase of population. Apparently, by frequently performing Ihamba, the Ndembu maintain in fantasy the values, symbols, and trappings of a highly ritualized activity that is rapidly losing its economic importance. The penetration of the modern cash economy into the pores of Ndembu social organization, together with an accelerating rate of labor migration to the industrial towns of the Northern Rhodesian Copperbelt, have created new economic needs and new tensions in traditional social relationships, while new relationships based on trade and contract are insidiously undermining corporate bonds. Ihamba may, therefore, be seen as part of a rearguard action that Ndembu culture is fighting against change. In the projective systems of modern villagers, the shades of hunters may well represent, at one level of social experience, the guilts and anxieties of those who are compelled by changing conditions to act in contravention of traditional standards.

Another sign that Ihamba is a response to cultural change is reflected in the fact that the rite contains its own built-in phase of divination. The traditional diviner, it is true, may well diagnose a person's illness as due to an *ihamba* affliction, but it is not strictly necessary. It is enough for someone to dream of a hunter-shade when he is ill and then to consult an Ihamba doctor to have the rite performed for him. Furthermore, when the rite begins, the doctor divines by peering into medicated water in an old meal mortar, in which he claims to be able to see the "shadow-soul" (*mwevulu*) of the afflicting hunter. By asking questions of the patient and his kin, he declares, he can then identify the particular relative who has "come out in *ihamba*" (*wunedikili mwihamba*). He may also claim to detect sorcerers and witches who have seized the opportunity of the patient's *ihamba*-caused debility to attack him. As we shall see, part of the process of removing the *ihamba* consists in the doctor's summoning kin of the patient to come before the improvised hunters' shrine (identical with that used in the hunters' cult) and inducing them to confess any grudges (*yitela*) and hard feelings they may nourish against the patient. The tooth will "not allow itself to be caught," he will assert, until every ill-wisher in the village or kin-group has "made his liver white" (or, as we would say, purified his intentions) toward the patient. The patient, too, must acknowledge his own grudges against his fellow villagers if he is to be rid of the "bite" of *ihamba*. It is curious how the symbolism of oral aggression pervades our own speech-ways in the context of small-group behavior: "envy's poisonous tooth," "the bite of malice," "the mordant utterance," "back-biting," "the sting of jealousy," "being eaten up with jealousy," and so forth. There is a parallel here, too, between the Ndembu notion of the hunters' tooth preying on the living and our saying that someone is "hounded by guilt" or "a prey to remorse."

Ihamba (as well as other Ndembu rites that involve the sucking of objects, including bones, graveyard-soil, and stones, from the bodies of patients) is a variation on that widespread theme of primitive medicine that Erwin Ackerknecht has called "the stone of the medicine man."[6] He quotes im Thurn that, for the Indians of Guiana at least, the foreign substance "is often if not always regarded not as simply a natural body but as the materialized form of a hostile spirit." Given this premise, im Thurn goes on to argue, "the procedure is perfectly sincere and in its way rational. An invisible force is dealt with visibly by means that are meant and understood to be symbolic." Nevertheless, I can confirm that the Ndembu—except for the doctors—do believe that the *ihamba* tooth of a specific hunter relative is actually extracted from the patient's body. The doctor confines skepticism to the issue of whether the tooth is that of a human being or of an animal (like a monkey or a pig). He leaves untouched the question that sleight of hand may have been used in making the "extraction." The doctors must themselves be aware of their own trickery, although I never managed to persuade one to admit that he had used deception. My own guess is that doctors sincerely believe that their therapy—which includes the use of washing and drinking medicines ("lotions" and "potions") and of cupping techniques—has a positive efficacy and may also believe that in some mystical fashion they actually do withdraw an influence inimical to the patient's welfare from his person. At any rate, they are well aware of the benefits of their procedures for group relationships, and they go to endless trouble to make sure that they have brought into the open the main sources of latent hostility in group life.

§ Therapeutic Procedure

Before getting down to specific cases I shall briefly describe the manipulative techniques of an Ihamba doctor. We must consider, for example, whether or not there may be certain unintended or inadvertent benign consequences for health from Ndembu practices that are overtly determined by magico-religious ideas without empirical foundation. It seems possible that the bloodletting that accompanies the doctor's efforts to "capture" the elusive tooth may have beneficial effects on some patients. There may also be in the procedure something analogous to modern shock treatment—treatment that, as Lessa and Vogt have suggested, "stimulates an internal reaction capable of returning the organism to health."[7]

It is more difficult to establish whether or not the use of "medicines" confers any physical benefit. The medicines employed are the leaves, bark scrapings, and roots of forest trees and bushes. The principles underlying their use are not derived from experiment but form part of a magical system, as is clear from a listing of the properties attributed to them by informants. I have collected a considerable body of this kind of exegetical material not only about Ihamba medicines but also about many other kinds of rite, and in almost every case notions of sympathetic or contagious magic control the selection of vegetable or animal medicines.

LIST OF IHAMBA MEDICINES

NDEMBU TERM	BOTANICAL NAME	INDIGENOUS EXPLANATION FOR USE
1. *Musoli*	*Vangueriopsis lanciflora*	a. It comes from *ku-solola*, "to make visible" or "reveal." b. It has fruit that are eaten by *duiker* and other woodland game during the early rains. Ndembu say that the name is connected with the power of the tree to draw forth animals from their hiding places in the bush and make them visible to the hunter. What is made visible is good, what is concealed is often bad. *Musoli* medicine is given to barren women "to make children visible." c. It is the senior (*mukulumpi*) medicine of Ihamba, the first to be collected. The doctor addresses the *musoli* tree and says: "You *musoli* tree of animals (of huntsmanship), come quickly, may this *ihamba* come out quickly, so that the patient may get well soon." He then guesses where the tap root lies and hoes up the ground. If he finds it at once, it augurs well that the tooth will be found quickly. d. *Musoli* means "to speak openly or publicly." It refers to the confession of grudges described earlier.

LIST OF IHAMBA MEDICINES (*Continued*)

NDEMBU TERM	BOTANICAL NAME	INDIGENOUS EXPLANATION FOR USE
2. *Museng'u*	*Ochna pulchra*	a. The name comes from *ku-seng'uka,* "to multiply." b. It has many small black fruits—it stands for "many animals" or "many children."
3. *Mututam-bululu*	*Xylopia adoratissima*	The name comes from *ambululu,* a small bee that makes nests in the ground or in old termite mounds. Such bees come in swarms to the *mututambululu* tree to gather its nectar. In the same way, many people will come to the drum (rite) at which it is used, and many animals will come near a hunter who has been washed with its medicine.
4. *Mufung'u*	*Anisophyllea boehmii*	From *ku-fung'a,* "to gather together a herd of animals."
5. *Mutata*	*Securidaca longipeduncu-lata*	This word means "to heat huntsmanship" (*Ku-tatisha Wubinda*).
6. *Muneku*	*Randia kuhniana*	It comes from *ku-nekama,* "to sink down" —which means that a *mufu* or "zombie" raised by a sorcerer's curse must "change its mind" (*ku-nekuka*) about afflicting the patient and sink down into the grave again. It will be recalled that the grudges of the living must be confessed during Ihamba because the Ndembu believe that protracted grudges animate the mystical powers of sorcery and witchcraft if not brought into the open. In any case, sorcerers and witches and their familiars are always likely to be present in large assemblies of people or so the Ndembu think.

§ Commentary

Other medicines employed in Ihamba have similar characteristics. They represent aspects of huntsmanship or protect the patient and the congregation from sorcery and witchcraft. Many of the medicines are borrowed directly from the hunters' cult rites and appear to represent *inter alia* the afflicting hunters' shades. At any rate, in other rites of affliction, the pieces of medicine leaves adhering to the patient's skin after he or she has been splashed by a leaf-broom are said to "stand for the shade," in that each represents a cluster of values associated with the cult of hunters' shades, and, in a sense, to identify the patient with that shade. Other antisorcery medicines in Ihamba include a root dug up from under a path leading into the village. This root is used because Ndembu believe that sorcerers conceal destructive medicines beside or beneath paths to injure or slay their personal enemies. The root-medicine "makes known" the sorcery and renders it innocuous. The doctor thus signifies that he has exposed the hidden sorcerers and can if necessary counter their malignant magic.

The main point to note in connection with these medicines (which are pounded by the doctor and his assistants in an old meal-mortar, soaked in water, and then both splashed on the patient's body and given to him to drink) is that they are ostensibly used because, through analogy, they confer on the patient certain powers and qualities conducive to strength, good luck, and health. The semantic links of analogy may derive from the name of the object used (by a species of serious "punning") from its natural properties, as they are conceived by the Ndembu, or from both. But it is doubtful that the medicines have any pharmaceutical value at all; it is sufficient that they are not toxic.

§ Ihembi, the Ihamba Doctor

This brief account of the cultural structure of Ihamba suggests that whatever efficacy the rite possesses—and it does have ameliorative effects on patients, as I can testify after witnessing more than a dozen performances, some of them in villages I knew really well—resides in the degree of skill wielded by the doctor in each instance of its performance. It is hardly likely to be attributable to the bloodletting and the application of medicines. We must therefore examine the form that Ihamba ritual takes in the light of what Radcliffe-Brown has called "the actually existing network of social relations." I propose therefore to say a few words about the personality of one Ihamba doctor, Ihembi, and then to describe his practice of his craft in two concrete situations.

Ihembi was a man about seventy years old, white-haired, dignified, but with a smile of singular sweetness and charm. He had the throaty voice characteristic of the Ndembu hunter, but he put it to lucid and eloquent use. I first met him at the court of a "progressive" subchief, Ikelenge, when I was collecting from the chief and his councilors the official history of his chiefdom and the royal genealogy. There was a full muster of elders from the chief's area present, and they were encouraged to contribute to the discussion. Among the most vociferous was Ihembi, who tended to raise objections to the chief's narrative at crucial points. I found out afterward that Ihembi belonged to a branch of the royal lineage that had formerly supplied chiefs to the realm but had been permanently excluded from the succession several generations before after a bitter and unsuccessful dispute with another branch over the incumbency of the chieftainship. In compensation, the victors had given the defeated branch, that of Matembu, a ritual office. The members of Matembu resided in a single large village, several miles from the capital, and their headman performed important ritual functions in the installation of each new Ikelenge chief, at chiefs' funerals, and in periodically purifying the royal insignia. Ihembi thus belonged to a social group with ritual status that had nevertheless a permanently "marginal" or "outsider" quality in political terms. Within the Matembu matrilineage, Ihembi had further "dispossessed" characteristics. Although he came from a senior branch of that lineage and was chronologically senior to its headman, he did not hold political office—probably because in his youth he had migrated to another Lunda subtribe, that of Shinde in Balovale District, many miles to the South of Mwinilunga District, where he had married and raised a family. There he had also practiced as a diviner. More important for this analysis, he had become initiated into the hunters' cult and had later learned the medicines and techniques of Ihamba, allegedly from the Luvale people who live intermingled with the Lunda in Balovale District. At a comparatively old age he had returned to the Ikelenge chiefdom, where he found the headmanship of Matembu already occupied. He did not fall into apathy but applied himself vigorously to his practice as an Ihamba doctor and earned quite a substantial income, for people were prepared to pay ten shillings or even a pound for an "extraction." Chief Ikelenge, who paid careful heed to the views of the Christian missionaries in his area, on more than one occasion fined Ihembi for fraudulently exploiting the people. Nevertheless, Ihembi managed to carry on his practice and enjoyed a wide reputation. In many ways, he was typical of Ndembu doctors: capable, charismatic, authoritative, but excluded from secular office for a variety of reasons, some structural, some personal. He was the typical "outsider" who achieves status in the ritual realm in compensation for his exclusion from authority in the political realm.

It was not long before Ihembi and I were on terms of friendship
that soon developed into the "joking relationship" between "grandfather
and grandson." This friendship enabled us to speak very frankly to one
another and to perform mutual services. I gave him gifts from time
to time, and he allowed me to attend his Ihamba rites and explained
much of their symbolism for my benefit. In this short paper, I can do no
more than discuss briefly two performances. They were held for the
same patient and formed part of a series of seven rites performed for
him, of which I was fortunate to observe three in close detail. Three of
the seven were Ihamba rites, two belonged to the hunters' generic cult
of Wubinda (since the patient, though not a gunhunter, trapped and
snared antelope), one was the antisorcery rite called *Kaneng'a* and one
was a recently introduced rite called Tukuka in which the patient is
believed to be possessed by the spirits of live Europeans or of alien
tribesmen. The large number of these rites, all performed within a few
months, indicates that the patient was seriously disturbed. Furthermore,
as I have argued, it indicates that there was serious disturbance in his
network of social relations.

§ Ihembi and the Case of Kamahasanyi

It is at this point unavoidable that I should deploy the divinatory
apparatus of the social anthropologist: the genealogy, the hut plan, the
village census data, and the condensed life history. For the events I shall
discuss fall within a social field with many dimensions, several of which
must be exhibited and scrutinized if we are to make any sense at all of
the observed behavior and the monologues (the prayers and invocations)
and dialogues of the participants. I may say, too that, in an intuitive or
pragmatic fashion, the information and even analysis I shall submit
were fully mastered by Ihembi, whose business it was to study social
relationships in order to diagnose the incidence and pattern of tensions
and to attempt to reduce them in his handling of the rites. We have
noted earlier how Ihamba contains its own built-in system of divination.
What I have written elsewhere of the divinatory process among the
Ndembu holds true, therefore, *a fortiori* for the Ihamba doctor in his
divining capacity. I wrote[8] that "the diviner clearly knows that he is
investigating within a social context of a particular type. He first estab-
lishes his clients' locale—the Senior Chief's area, then the subchief's, then
the vicinage (the cluster of neighboring villages), and finally the village

of the victim. Each of these political units has its special characteristics:
its factional divisions, its inter-village rivalries, its dominant personalities,
its nucleated and dispersed groups of kin, all of them possessing a history
of settlement or migration. An experienced diviner will have already
familiarized himself with the contemporary state of these political sub-
systems from previous consultations and from the voluminous gossip of
travelers. Next he ascertains the relationships between the victim and
those who have come to consult him. He is assisted in this task by his
knowledge of the categories of persons who typically compose a village:
the victim's matrilineal kin, his patrilateral kin, his affines, cognates and
unrelated persons. He finds out the type and nature of the victim's
relationship to the headman, then focuses his attention on the headman's
matrilineage and discovers into how many sub-lineages it may be segmented. By the time he has finished his interrogation, he has a complete
picture of the contemporaneous structure of the village, and of the
position in its relational network occupied by the victim."

These remarks refer to diviners who are consulted by clients from
distant regions and who operate by the manipulation of symbolic objects,
as well as by the exhaustive interrogation that accompanies it. The clients
try to trip up the diviner by feeding him false information, and it is the
mark of a "true diviner" if he avoids this pitfall. But the Ihamba doctor
is in the more fortunate position of operating in a village not far from
his own, whose inhabitants and their interpersonal relations are known
to him, and of having had full access to the patient's dreams (which
induced him and his kin to call in the Ihamba doctor in the first place)
and to the gossip and opinions of the patient's neighbors and relatives.
Nevertheless, he builds up his picture of the social field and its tensions
in much the same way as the specialist diviner does and acts on this
knowledge in his therapeutic practice. By tactful cross-examination of
the participants and by keeping his eyes and ears open, he discovers the
likes and dislikes of the patient, the village headman, the members of
the patient's domestic family and matrilineage, and so forth.

In the case of Kamahasanyi, which I shall describe shortly, Ihembi
already knew the principal participants, and his two assistants, Mundoyi
and Mukeyi, had distant patrilateral ties with the patient. What is more,
before the second performance of Ihemba he spent a day and night in
the patient's village, where he was able to size up the situation.

My own acquaintance with Kamahasanyi's village had been long and
close, for my first camp had been in the neighborhood, and my wife and
I had attended a girl's puberty ritual there. Furthermore, I had collected

census and budgetary information not only in this village of Nswanamundong'u but also in many other villages of the Mukang'ala chiefdom,
of which it formed a part. It was while I had been visiting Nswanamundong'u that I first became aware of Kamahasanyi's troubles. His snares
had failed to catch *duiker* antelope for many weeks, and he had had the
hunting rite Mukala performed to placate the angry shade. This shade
was that of his maternal grandfather, the late chief Mukang'ala, he told
me, and the same shade had "come out in Ihamba" to afflict him "with
pains in his whole body." An Ihamba rite was to be performed for him
the day after my arrival by a Luvale doctor temporarily residing in the
neighborhood. I mentioned to the villagers that I knew Ihembi well, and
they immediately besought me to bring the great doctor and his assistants (who helped him with the collection of medicines and with various
ritual tasks) from the Ikelenge area in my car. He could "help" the
Luvale, they said, who was "only a little doctor"—they even hinted that
he might tactfully take over control of the rite. They also asked me to
bring to the performance a man called Samuwinu, whom they described
as "the real headman" of the village. He had fled from the chiefdom at
the accession of the present chief Mukang'ala Kambung'u, fearing the
latter's sorcery. For Samuwinu had been a candidate for the chiefly
"chair," and, indeed, the male members of the nuclear matrilineage of
Nswanamundong'u belonged to a branch of the royal matrilineage of
Mukang'ala chiefdom. Their village was a "royal village." The villagers
told me that the shade afflicting Kamahasanyi "in Mukala" and "in
Ihamba" was doing so because it was angry that a "younger man" had
become headman while a member of its own generation (genealogical
generation) remained alive. A member of the junior adjacent generation
to Samuwinu had been appointed as headman by the villagers. The shade
was incensed too, they said, because it had been slain by the sorcery of
the present chief, a slaying that had been unavenged for several years.
Its wrath had been manifested in other ways. Once there had been a
whirlwind that had ripped the thatch from the hut of the new headman
Kachimba, and people claimed that they had seen flames leaping above it.
Villagers said that they had dreamed that the late chief's shade had
come to reproach them. Not only was it aggrieved that it had been
ensorcelled, they alleged, but also because the British authorities had a
few years previously withdrawn recognition from the Mukang'ala chieftainship, which had been merged with that of Senior Chief Kanongesha.
The shade, that of Mundong'u Kabong'u, blamed the people of the
chiefdom and in particular those of his own village for allowing this
merger to happen.

The persecution of Kamahasanyi by the late chief's shade was therefore not so much aimed at him personally as in his representative capacity.
When I asked one informant why Mundong'u had not afflicted Kachimba,
the acting headman, he replied that the shade "wanted to shame" everyone by "catching" one of the villagers. It was not Kachimba but the village
folk (enimukala) as a whole who had behaved irresponsibly. They should
have made Samuwinu headman, and the latter should have remained in
the area to represent his matrilineage fittingly. Indeed, it was Kachimba
himself who begged me earnestly to bring Samuwinu to the Ihamba
performance so that Samuwinu could invoke the shade on Kamahasanyi's
behalf. The shade, he said, would listen to Samuwinu, who was his
uterine brother, as well as "real headman" but might well reject his own
intercession. I learned later that several villagers secretly despised
Samuwinu for running away and indeed for not pressing his claim for
the chieftainship with vigor while he could. As we shall see, this whole
case history is pervaded by the theme of failure to undertake responsibility
and failure to live up to expectation. Part of the work of a doctor is to
encourage people to discharge the obligations of their status well and
not seek escape from them.

But, while the villagers were sure that Mundong'u Kabong'u's shade
was afflicting Kamahasanyi and that other misfortunes assailing them
collectively at that time (like loss of crops because of wild pigs, quarrels
between village sections, bad luck in hunting) could be laid at his door,
it was thought highly probable that other mystical agencies were also at
work. Some thought that Kamahasanyi was being bewitched by someone
in the village, a line of inquiry that soon engaged Ihembi's attention and
that he discussed with me. Others thought that the spirits of living
Europeans were "troubling" him. Kamahasanyi himself had recently gone
to Angola to consult a diviner there and had been told that his own
father's shade, as well as that of Kabong'u Mundong'u, had "caught" him
in Ihamba. This diagnosis, supported by the fact that Kamahasanyi had
frequently dreamed of his father's shade, opens the way for an investigation of Kamahasanyi's life history and an analysis of his character and
temperament that must be postponed until our sociological analysis has
been made. The point I want to make here is that, when misfortune is
attributed to mystical causes in Ndembu society, it is common for *many*
sets of disturbed social relations to be scrutinized by the interested
parties. The vagueness of the mystical beliefs enables them to be
manipulated in relation to a great diversity of social situations. Eventually the crucial tension is isolated and dealt with.

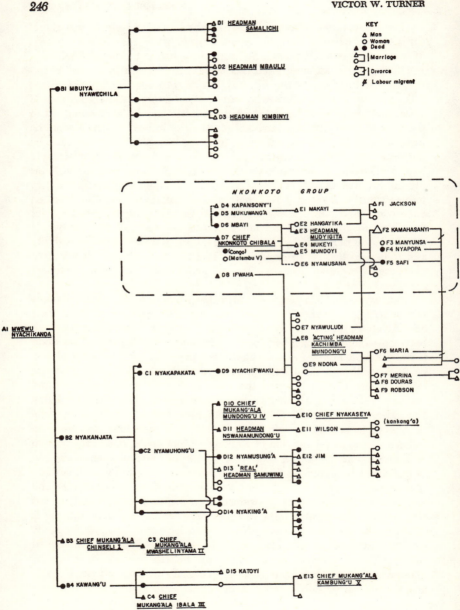

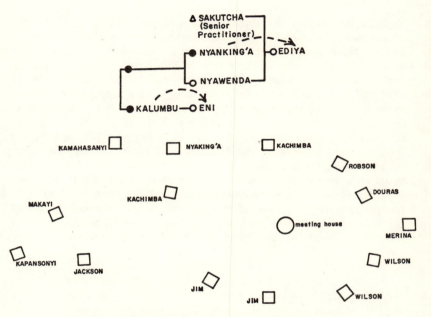

FIGURE 2. Hut Plan of Nswanamundong'u. Village.

FIGURE 1 (*Opposite*). Genealogy of Nswanamundong'u Village.

§ The Structural Context of the Case
of Kamahasanyi

In order to give the reader a clear understanding of the social
factors that Ihembi had to take into account in his handling of the two
Ihamba performances he conducted for Kamahasanyi (in the first of
which he removed what he claimed to be Mundong'u Kabong'u's *ihamba*
and in the second of which he removed that of Kamahasanyi's father
Mudyigita), I shall have to use a genealogy and a hut plan of Nswanamundong'u. Since the nuclear matrilineage of that village belonged to
the royal matrilineage of the Mukang'ala chiefdom, I have included in
the genealogy other branches of the royal lineage, for they are part of
the total field influencing the behavior and ideas we are examining.

To simplify the analysis I shall subdivide the social field of Nswanamundong'u into its component social entities—various kinds of group,
subgroup, category, and relationship—and exhibit them in a series of
interpenetrating dimensions of relationships. These relationships consist
of white-black relations; political relations between branches of the
Mukang'ala royal lineage; intravillage relations; intrafamilial relations.

WHITE-BLACK RELATIONS

For the present analysis, this set of relations constitutes a set of
perduring conditions full of chronic tension and conflict. The chieftainship of Mukang'ala had been abolished about four years before my
arrival in the area. The area was in a state of seedy decrepitude. The
court house at the capital village was falling into disrepair, as was the
Mission Out-School, closed down after the abolition of the chief's chair.
Those who had occupied paid positions under the Native Authority had
returned to their villages of origin and reverted to the lives of peasants
and hunters. Indeed, the "primitive" appearance of Mukang'ala's chiefdom was the result of regression and of "dedifferentiation," of the breakdown of the modern political structure of Native Court and Treasury
with their paid officials. It was not due to isolation from modern trends
of change for the chiefdom extended almost to the British Administration
Headquarters. Local sources of cash income had dried up with the death
of the local government. Men had either to go to the Northern Rhodesian
railway 300 miles away to find paid work or to cultivate their cassava
gardens and hunt in the bush—mainly with traps, snares, bows, and
spears, since they had not the cash to buy guns nor the command of

European and chiefly patronage to obtain licenses to purchase am-
munition.

Among those who had regressed to "bush" life was Kachimba, the
acting headman of Nswanamundong'u. His smattering of literacy had
been enough to obtain him the post of court clerk in the days of the
chiefdom's official recognition. Now he had become a shy figure who
normally evaded a headman's duty of supplying hospitality to wayfarers
and, as often as not, was away in the bush when people called. His
villagers and many others in the former chiefdom used to blame him
for the loss of his authority. He had been brusque and unco-operative
toward European officials, it was said, and many stated that he had been
considered "dirty" and "unhygienic" in the way he ran his capital village.

RELATIONS AMONG BRANCHES OF
THE MUKANG'ALA LINEAGE

The abolition of black authority by white power had repercussions
along several dimensions of social relations in the black sector. Among
branches of the royal matrilineage, it led to widespread emigration of
important men from the chiefdom. Several went to Chief Ikelenge's
area to the North. This area was highly prosperous in terms of modern
cash economy. Several European traders and farmers held land there
and offered opportunities for paid employment. Its chief was young,
progressive, literate, and in favor with the government, in contrast to
Mukang'ala. The dissident Mukang'ala royals, notably Samalichi (D1),
Mbaulu (D2), and Kimbinyi (D3) all prospered and became headmen
under Chief Ikelenge. Kimbinyi became, in addition, a wealthy trader.
Samuwinu (D13), the "real headman" of Nswanamundong'u, who had
fled to Ikelenge's area before the abolition, had not prospered, but he
was reckoned to be a man of weak character, who had failed to meet
the crisis of his life with courage.

The defection of these royals left the Mukang'ala lineage divided
into two branches: one descended from Nyakanjata (B2), the other from
Kawang'u (B4). I shall call them the Nyakanjata and Kawang'u lineages.
The incumbency of the chieftainship had alternated between these two
lineages since Mukang'ala II—there had been earlier chiefs than those
shown, but their genealogical connections are irrelevant to the present
account. This alternation was never institutionalized but was the result
of power struggles. Mukang'ala III, Ibala, who had fought against the
British when they first came, had been slain, it is said, by the sorcery of
Mundong'u Kabong'u (whose shade was believed to be afflicting Kama-

hasanyi). He was believed to have been ensorcelled in turn by Mukang'ala
V, Ibala's sister's daughter's son, of Kawang'u lineage.

It is probably because Nyakanjata lineage, most of whose members
resided in Nswanamundong'u, had in the past provided so many chiefs
that its members did not emigrate but continued to stay in Mukang'ala's
chiefdom. I do know that they cherished hopes that the chieftainship
would be restored to official favor and recognition. Among those who
hoped was Jim (E15), an intelligent, enterprising young man who had
worked as a labor migrant in Southern Rhodesia. He was widely recognized as the likely heir of the present incumbent. In Nswanamundong'u,
where he lived, it was Jim rather than Kachimba who took the lead in
village matters and who offered hospitality to strangers. The biggest
feather in his cap came when he sponsored a circumcision ceremony—a
role normally performed by the chief in such a small chiefdom—at which
three of his own sons were initiated. Jim's political strategy was twofold:
to support the present incumbent in his frequent appeals to government
for renewed recognition and to try to build up a following for himself
from Nyakanjata lineage and from anyone else who could be induced
to support his future claim for office. He had, therefore, a strong interest
in preventing internecine strife in Nswanamundong'u and in maintaining
friendly relations between it and other villages. It is hardly surprising
therefore that he was among the foremost in asking for Ihembi to perform
the Ihamba rite to propitiate his mother's brother's shade, a rite that was
known to have beneficial effects on village relationships. It is also interesting that he performed the task at each ceremony of sucking the cupping
horns of Kamahasanyi's body.

INTRAVILLAGE RELATIONS

Jim's concern that Nswanamundong'u should remain united sprang
from a real fear that it would split. A comparison of the hut plan with
the genealogy shows that, although the village is small, it is divided into
two distinct sections. One is inhabited by Headman Kachimba (E8),
his wife, and his adult children, Merina (F7), Douras (F8), and Robson
(F9); by Jim (E12), his two wives, and his junior children; and by
Wilson (E11), son of the late headman, and his two wives and junior
children. The other is occupied by what I have called "the Nkonkoto
Group," consisting of a solitary old man, Kapansonyi (D4), his classificatory sister's son Makayi (E1) and his wife, and their adult son
Jackson (F1). Between these sections are the two huts of Kamahasanyi
(F2) and Nyakinga (D14), Kachimba's mother's mother's sister's
daughter (whom he calls "mother"). These siting arrangements reflect

social structure. It seems that about thirty-five to forty years before the events I record, many members of the Mukang'ala lineage fled to Chief Nkonkoto's Ndembu chieftainship in what was then the Belgian Congo, probably to escape from the forces of the British South Africa Company, which Chief Mukang'ala Ibala (C4) had opposed. There they inter-married with some Nkonkoto villagers and made friends with others. Eventually they returned and, in the course of time Mundong'u Kabong'u (D10), the senior man in Nyankanjata lineage succeeded to the chief-tainship. Some Nkonkoto people tried to exploit their ties of affinity and friendship with Nyakanjata-lineage members to obtain paid employment under the Native Authority. They sought Mundong'u's patronage to get work in the Public Works Department or the Native Court. Makayi, one of this group, sent his son Jackson to the Mission Out-School at the capital village. They built their huts beside those of Nyakanjata people. For a time, all went well, but when I knew them the Nkonkoto group, reduced in number to those I have mentioned, were a pretty disgruntled bunch. They seemed to hold their fellow villagers from the Nyakanjata lineage, especially Kachimba, responsible for the decline in fortune of the chiefdom. And they had no good word to say of Samuwinu (D13), who had defected. Relations were particularly tense between Makayi and Kachimba. Neither would sit in a group when the other was present, although both were on good terms with Jim (E12), who made it his business to be friendly with everyone.

It was into this situation of strain between the Nyakanjata lineage and the Nkonkoto Group that Kamahasanyi arrived, a short time before my own first visit to the village. He, too, had come from Nkonkoto chief-dom, where his father Mudyigita (E3) had been a great headman and a famous hunter. Furthermore, Mudyigita was the son of a former Chief Nkonkoto (D7). Since Kamahasanyi's mother, as we have seen, belonged to the Mukang'ala royal lineage, he was certainly well connected on both sides. There are several peculiarities about Kamahasanyi's life history that made it most unfortunate for him that he had plunged into a situation that exacerbated conflicts between maternal and paternal loyalties. For it was as though his endopsychic conflict had been objectivized and given social form. Through his paternal link with the Nkonkoto group, Kamahasanyi was exposed to the grievances ventilated by Makayi and his people. As a member of Nyankanjata matrilineage, he heard the counteraccusations of his maternal kin. As can be seen from the hut plan, Kamahasanyi built his hut between those two groups, indicating his dual allegiance. A stronger character might have acted as a mediator between his matrilineal and patrilateral kin. Indeed, I have recorded several instances of men who played this very role. But Kamahasanyi "retreated from the field" into what I can only think was neurotic illness. The key to an explanation of this illness may be found, I suggest, in the circumstances of his life and in his temperament.

§ Kamahasanyi's Life History

Kamahasanyi was exceptional in Ndembu society for the great length of time he had resided in the village of his father's nuclear matrilineage. When he finally came to settle with his mother's kin, he was past his fortieth year, and his father had been dead for several years. It not infrequently happens that sons reside with their fathers for some years after their own marriages, especially, as in Kamahasanyi's case, when the father is a headman and can extend to his son certain privileges and assistance in economic matters. But it is rare for a man in advanced middle life to do so, unless his mother is his father's slave (*ndung'u*). There was no evidence that Kamahasanyi's mother had been a slave, though it may well have been hushed up. If his mother had been a slave, Kamahasanyi, by matrilineal descent, would have inherited her status and would himself have been inherited by his father's matrilineal heir, unless his relatives had redeemed him by a substantial payment. Since they were too poor to have done so and since Kamahasanyi claimed to have made large payments of bridewealth for two of his wives in the Belgian Congo, he must have been a man of independent means. At all events, he seems, in his youth, to have been his father's favorite and to have received from him considerable assistance in accumulating bridewealth.

Members of the Nkonkoto group told me that Mudyigita, Kamahasanyi's father, was a man of great force of character. In this respect, he presented a sharp contrast to his son. Kamahasanyi was effeminate in manner and was reckoned to be "womanish" (*neyi mumbanda*) by his fellow villagers. He plaited his hair in a feminine style known as *lumba*, and he spent much of his time gossiping with women in their kitchens. Furthermore, although he had been married four times, he had failed to beget children. An interesting feature of these marriages is that three of them were with cross-cousins. Two of the three were with patrilateral cross-cousins, that is, with members of his father's matrilineage. Such marriages are one means, in Ndembu society, of forging closer links with one's father, since one's children thus belong to one's father's matrilineage and will inherit and succeed within it. One will then live uxorilocally in one's father's village and not move to the village of one's maternal kin. Ndembu generally consider that men of mature years who live uxorilocally or patrilocally (with their father's kin), are men who evade their responsibilities, for the major sphere of a man's struggles for status and power is the village of his primary matrilineal kin. Here it is that a man may hope to become a headman or, if he is royal, to become a chief. Here it is, also, that a man is expected to help his matrikin in legal and ritual matters and to share his economic surplus. Kamahasanyi had shirked these duties and had obviously been dominated by his successful father. After Mudyigita's death, according to my informants (Ihembi's assistants, Mukeyi and Mundoyi, who were Mudyigita's seminal brothers), Kamahasanyi's continued residence in his village aroused irritation and resentment. He had never really pulled his weight in corporate matters, and he was urged to return to "his own people," to Mukang'ala's chiefdom. He paid several visits there, and on one visit married Kachimba's daughter Maria (F6), his first matrilateral cross-cousin. It is quite clear that unconscious incestuous drives influenced Kamahasanyi in his choice of mates. Cross-cousins are, it is true, preferred marital partners, but few Ndembu marry as many as three in a lifetime. They are the easiest partners to obtain, which would have been in accord with Kamahasanyi's tendency to take the line of least resistance. It is probable that his father and later his mother's brother had arranged these cross-cousin marriages for him. Like his father, his fourth wife Maria was a dominant personality who, both before and after her marriage to Kamahasanyi, took lovers when she felt like it. For a time she lived with her husband in Mudyigita's village, where she made large cassava gardens. The Belgian authorities paid relatively high prices for cassava meal, which went to feed the copper miners in the Katanga Union Minière belt so that Maria, and through her Kamahasanyi, prospered for a while. But when Kamahasanyi's senior wife, his patrilateral cross-cousin Safi (F5) died, his patrilateral village kin demanded a large "death payment" (*mpepi*) from him and from his matrilineal kin. The custom of paying *mpepi*, apparently introduced from the Luvale tribe, is a financially crippling one. It is connected with the notion that the matrilineal kin of the deceased have the duty of consulting a diviner about the cause of death (to ascertain whose witchcraft or sorcery was responsible for it). Diviners charge high fees, and the surviving spouse and his kin are required to hand over a large payment in cash or kind to cover diviners' fees, as well as to compensate for the loss of the deceased's services. It is unusual, however, for *mpepi* to be demanded in the case of cross-cousin marriage, for the partners are considered kin as well as affines. But as

Kamahasanyi had had to pay high bridewealth for his cross-cousin wives —again an unusual circumstance—so he was asked to pay a high *mpepi.* These facts indicate, I think, the villagers' dislike of the man. Kamahasanyi was dilatory in paying *mpepi,* and it was then alleged by his patrilateral kin that his wife Maria, with his connivance, had bewitched Safi to death, as cowives are often believed to do. The result was that Kamahasanyi and Maria were virtually forced to leave Nkonkoto chiefdom and return to Maria's village in Northern Rhodesia, although not before Maria had sold her cassava gardens at a profit, making Kamahasanyi more dependent upon her than ever.

Kamahasanyi had, therefore, returned at last to his own matrikin. But the fact that he was known to have been forced to do so and his reputation as a "difficult" person to have around made his welcome a rather cool one. Again, as I have said, he was confronted in Nswanamundong'u with an external duplication of his own inner conflicts, for his new village was neatly divided into groups consisting respectively of his maternal and paternal kin. The Nkonkoto group not only felt grievances against the Nyakanjata lineage as a result of the "putting down" of the chieftaincy as described, but they also shared the hostility of their Congolese kinfolk toward Kamahasanyi.

A further complication arose. Before her marriage to Kamahasanyi, Maria had taken as her lover one of the Nkonkoto group, Makayi's son Jackson, an educated young man who had hopes of employment as a clerk in a European enterprise. On her return to Nswanamundong'u, Maria took up openly with Jackson again. So brazen was this relationship that several times when he was walking with me Jackson ostentatiously "avoided" Maria's mother Ndona (E8), rushing away from the path when he saw her advancing toward him—as though she were his mother-in-law! Kamahasanyi was said to be impotent, and to all appearances he was complaisant about the liaison. On the other hand, Maria fulfilled many of her wifely duties to Kamahasanyi. She worked beside him in his cassava gardens (indeed she did most of the work!), and she brewed finger-millet beer for his guests. She even accompanied him to Angola to consult a diviner about his health and fortune. This devotion may have been tendered because Kamahasanyi occupied a structural position of some importance in the village. As may be seen by consulting the genealogy, Kamahasanyi was a full member of Nyakanjata lineage and was therefore, according to Ndembu rules, a possible candidate both for the chieftainship of Mukang'ala and the village headmanship. In view of Jim's (E12) strong claims, by virtue of blood and intelligence, to become chief in the future, it was unlikely that Kamahasanyi would succeed to the chair. But, on the other hand, since Jim, if he became a chief, would set up a capital village of his own, it was possible that Kamahasanyi would "continue the name" of Nswanamundong'u by succeeding to its headmanship and scraping up a modest following of matrikin, cognates, affines, and anyone else he might persuade to reside with him. At least, Maria, with her strong will and energy, might do these things with her husband as nominal headman.

Despite his disadvantages, Kamahasanyi had a strong sense of his own importance. Even in a society whose members like to stress their connections with chiefs, Kamahasanyi was more snobbish than most. For example, when I discussed the history of the Mukang'ala chiefdom with senior men like Kachimba, Jim, and Wilson (E11), he would brush aside or interrupt their accounts and tell me "what really happened." He was the only one who could tell me the full, sonorous clan formula of the Saluseki clan to which the Mukang'ala royal lineage belonged—the clan (munyachi) has ceased to have any political and has retained little social importance. He was also proud of his paternal link with the Nkonkoto chieftainship. He was, as I have said, conceited about his appearance, braiding his hair and oiling his body. He had brought with him from the Belgian Congo several dilapidated books in French, which he could not read but which he clearly considered to be status symbols. His attitude toward me was that we were both civilized men among barbarians, whom he despised and who could not understand him.

The symptoms of his illness consisted of rapid palpitations of the heart; severe pains in the back, limbs, and chest; and fatigue after short spells of work. He felt that "people were always speaking things against" him—though he excepted Jim from blame—and finally he withdrew from all village affairs and shut himself up in his hut for long periods. He complained to me and to Ihembi that the villagers ignored his sufferings to the extent that no one had bothered to consult a diviner to find out what was wrong with him. In the end, ill though he was, he had had to travel many miles to Angola to consult a diviner himself. I cannot say with clinical certainty whether Kamahasanyi's symptoms were real or imaginary. My own feeling is that they were mainly neurotic. At any rate, when the ritual sequence was over, Kamahasanyi was perfectly able to cultivate his gardens, to set traps for game in the forest, and to travel considerable distances to visit kin and friends. And to all outward appearances there was nothing much the matter with him; he talked animatedly and at length to anyone whom, like Ihembi and myself, he considered sympathetic. It is probable that most of his symptoms were psychosomatic—with a few rheumatic pains, a common Ndembu ailment, in addition—and were an unconscious way of obtaining the attention of his fellow villagers.

§ The Performances of Ihamba

The material I have presented—and much more—was known to Ihembi, who discussed it with me and with his assistants Mundoyi and Mukeyi, who were themselves patrilaterally connected with Kamahasanyi and had grown up in the same part of the Belgian Congo. All of it was taken into account and put to therapeutic use by Ihembi, not only in the formalized situation of ritual performances, but also in the informal talks he held during his stay in Nswanamundong'u with Kamahasanyi, Maria, Jim, Kachimba, Makayi, and other interested parties. I would like, first of all, to present some of Ihembi's diagnoses of the causes of Kamahasanyi's illness and misfortune and then to consider his conduct of the Ihamba performances. Ihembi, like other Ndembu believed that these causes were all of a mystical type. He was not at all like a Western psychiatrist working with the concept of mental illness.

After the first performance of Ihamba, in which he had, as anticipated, tactfully taken control of the proceedings from his Luvale colleague (with great delicacy he had first asked his permission to do so and later gave him a half-share of his ten-shilling fee), Ihembi told me that, while it was true that Kamahasanyi had been "bitten" by the *ihamba* of his "grandfather" Mundong'u Kabong'u, other entities had also been at work. He had himself removed the late chief's incisor, and he had been correct, he said, in his view that the shade was angry because a proper headman had not been installed in Nswanamundong'u. He knew that he was correct, he went on, because the shade had caused the patient to "tremble"° (*ku-zakuka*) after Ihembi had "addressed" (*kwinka nyikunyi*) the proper questions to it. But later he had divined by gazing into a meal mortar full of pounded medicines and sprinkled with powdered red clay (with the generic sense of "blood") and white clay (which may mean "innocence," "health," "strength," certain manifestations of ancestral shades, and so forth). There he had "seen" another *ihamba*, probably that of the patient's father. Kamahasanyi, it may be recalled, had dreamed of his father's shade. Ihembi said that Mudyigita was angry with his son for having quarreled with his (Mudyigita's) matrikin.

° A sort of rhythmic shuddering, indicative of possession, which begins in time with the drum rhythm and afterwards may become uncontrollable.

Since Kamahasanyi had dreamed on successive nights that the shade had stood between the forked branches of a hunters' shrine set up in front of his dwelling hut, Ihembi resolved to perform Ihamba at that very place.

But in addition to *mahamba*, said Ihembi, sorcery and witchcraft were partly to blame for Kamahasanyi's troubles. When he first divined, he thought he saw in the medicated water the "reflection" or "shadow-soul" (*mwevulu*) of Wilson. He "saw" further that Wilson had "raised a *musalu*," a kind of malignant ghost, by means of a curse, after quarreling with Kamahasanyi. I can confirm from my own information that Wilson strongly disliked Kamahasanyi and resented his coming to the village. Since he was not a matrilineal kinsman, Wilson was less constrained about expressing his hostility, for matrikin must in public maintain the fiction of amity in their relations. But, on going more deeply into the matter, Ihembi learned, since he was a great diviner and not easily deceived, that the "reflection" of Wilson had been "put in his *ng'ombu*" (his divining apparatus) by the "real witches." These witches were Kamahasanyi's wife Maria and her mother Ndona (E9), Kachimba's wife. They wanted to "kill Kamahasanyi for his meat," since Ndembu witches are thought to be necrophagous. They had sent their familiars (malignant little beings known as *tuyebela*, who take the forms of small domestic animals or tiny men with inverted feet) to "beat" Kamahasanyi with hoe-handles. This behavior accounted for some of his symptoms. Beside, Ndona preferred Jackson to Kamahasanyi as a son-in-law and wanted the latter done away with.

He told me that he had informed the villagers that, before he could "make another Ihamba," he would have to perform a rite known as Kaneng'a or Lukupu ("splashing with medicine"), to make the witches realize that in a general way "they were known." Lukupu also had the effect of driving off witches' familiars. He would not mention any names openly, since "there was enough trouble in the village," but the performance of Lukupu would act as a sharp warning to the witches to call off their familiars, for otherwise he would expose them publicly and take drastic ritual remedial action. To perform Lukupu was also, in my opinion, Ihembi's way of sharply jolting the quarrelsome villagers into reconciling their differences and behaving better toward their kinsman Kamahasanyi. For to imply so bluntly that witchcraft was at work in the village was the sharpest rebuke Ihembi could make and played on the Ndembu villagers' deepest fears.

Ihembi told me that it was in his mind to advise Kamahasanyi to divorce Maria and to go to reside in Chief Ikelenge's area, where his widowed mother was now living with Kamahasanyi's younger brother—

not far from the "real headman" Samuwinu's hut (D13). He might thus hope to escape a horrible death. In the end, however, he decided against this course and worked to make "the livers of the Nswanamundong'u people white towards one another," to remove the state of mutual ill-feeling. This removal would "please the shade," which would stop afflicting Kamahasanyi.

In this projective guise, Ihembi was really dealing with the undercurrents of personal animosity and sectional rivalry in the village. He was also clearly trying to emancipate Kamahasanyi from the guilts and anxieties attendant upon his belated removal from his late father's sphere of influence. Kamahasanyi had to be made over, as it were, to the matrilineal sphere, which was also the arena of adult responsibility.

I shall pass over the events of the Lukupu rite, which I observed, except to note that Ihembi made Kachimba (E8) throw, on behalf of the whole village, a portion of white clay (*mpemba*) into the medicines with which Kamahasanyi was washed to betoken that all had "good feelings" toward him. Makayi, too, attended the rite, which was held in the bush far away from the village.

§ The Second Ihamba Performance

I shall not give a "blow by blow" account of the rite here but shall confine myself to its social implications. It is necessary to know, however, that, after certain ritual preliminaries, including the collecting of medicines in a prescribed formal manner, an Ihamba rite proceeds in a series of stops and starts. The "stops" occur when the cupping horns (*tusunu*) are attached to the patient's body; then follows a phase of drumming and singing, in which all present join, and the patient goes into a trembling fit. If he shakes off a horn or two in his convulsions, the doctor bids the drummers stop playing, removes the horns, and investigates them. If he finds nothing in them, he makes a statement to the congregation about why the *ihamba* has not "come out"—which usually entails a fairly detailed account of the patient's life story and of the group's interrelations—then he invokes the shade, urging it to "come quickly" and finally invites village members to come, in order of sex and seniority, to the improvised hunters' shrine set up for the shade and confess any secret ill-feeling they may have toward the patient. The patient himself may be invited as well. Then cupping horns are affixed once more, drumming and singing commence again, and the "big doctor" passes the time until the next round of verbal behavior in dancing, purifying the village by ritually sweeping out huts and paths, or going out into the bush to bring back some new medicine plant.

Ihembi's greatest skill was in managing this stop-start routine so that, after several hours of it, the congregation felt nothing but a unanimous craving for the removal of the *ihamba* from the patient's body. The intense excitement whipped up by the drums; the patient's trembling; mass participation in the sad-sweet or rousing hunters' cult songs, which are sung to "please *ihamba*," followed by the spate of confessions and the airing of grievances, the reverent or hortatory prayers addressed not only by the doctor but also by village elders to the shade to "make our kinsman strong," the sight and smell of blood, which often pours in gouts from the horns: All these elements make a dialectical and dialogical pattern of activity that generates strong sentiments of corporateness, reduces skepticism, and maximizes sympathy for the patient.

Ihembi was also skilled in allocating appropriate ritual tasks to the patient's kin. For example, he asked Nyaking'a (D14) to bring in a calabash of water to be consecrated to the making of Ihamba medicines. Nyaking'a had been a friend of Kamahasanyi's mother while both were married out in the Belgian Congo. She was Kamahasanyi's classificatory "grandmother," and she had been ritual instructress to Maria some years earlier at her puberty rite. Because of its importance at life crises, Ndembu regard water as an "elder" (*mukulumpi*) or most venerable "thing," and Nyaking'a's friendly relationship with the disturbed marital pair was thus recognized.

Jim (E12), the tactful aspirant to the chief's chair, helped in the sucking of horns, thus demonstrating that he wanted to rid the patient (and his village) of troubles. Samuwinu was asked to invoke the shade before others did, since he was "the real headman."

Wilson was asked by Ihembi to put a piece of white clay on the fork of a hunters' shrine-tree in token of his friendly and pure intentions toward Kamahasanyi, of which, as we have seen, there had been some doubt. Ihembi made the faithless Maria go into the bush to bring leaves from a *mudyi* tree (*Diplorrhyncus condylocarpon*). This tree, as I have shown elsewhere,[9] stands for "motherhood," "matriliny," and "womanhood" (its white latex secretions are likened to mother's milk). It also stands for "auspiciousness." Maria chewed the leaves and spat the juice on her husband's temples, feet, and hands, centers of thought and activity, and tapped him smartly on the back and head with a small hand rattle—"to give him strength." By these acts, she reaffirmed her wifely duties toward the patient and her good will—the reverse of witchery.

Others too numerous to mention were assigned minor parts in this ritual drama by that old impresario Ihembi, who sought, as I have seen him do again and again in ritual contexts, to get everyone working together, despite the issues that divided them in secular life, "to please the shade," and thus to cure the patient. Once when the women attenders did not sing loudly enough, Ihembi made them come closer to the compact men's group and exhorted them to sing up. "It is very important," he said, "that you should give your power to help Kamahasanyi." For, in Ndembu belief, singing is not merely a pastime or aesthetic activity but a way of generating "power"—which can be used by a doctor for healing purposes.

After·a number of people had admitted to ill feeling or negligence toward Kamahasanyi, the patient himself spoke out. He complained vehemently that his matrilineal kin (*akumama*) had not moved a finger to help him when he was ill. He had been forced to go to a diviner himself, although he was unwell. It was fortunate, he said, that Maria, his wife, had gone with him. But, he added, now that he had told his grudge to everyone, he thought that all would be well. His hard thoughts had kept back his cure. It was also lucky that Mundoyi and Mukeyi, Ihembi's assistants (who had performed many ritual tasks) were present, for they were Kamahasanyi's (classificatory) "fathers" (see genealogy), and it was his father who had been troubling him.

I should like to conclude my account of the performance with an extract from my field notes, written up shortly after I observed it in 1951, to convey something of its atmosphere and flavor:

Mundoyi now took the *duiker* horn out of Kamahasanyi's hair over the brow, washed it, filled it with medicine, and replaced it at the back of his head. He did the same with the blue *duiker* horn at the back, replacing it at the front. He blew his whistle twice. Kamahasanyi started to quiver again violently, and the cupping horn on the left of his neck fell off, unpleasantly spilling what looked like a small chunk of flesh. Next the horn on his temple fell off. Ihembi sat very quietly, not registering any emotion at all. I felt strongly that what was being drawn out of this man Kamahasanyi was, in reality, the hidden animosities of the village. To all appearances, Kamahasanyi was in a state of complete dissociation.

Now Ihembi fitted a long thin *duiker* horn on the little finger of his right hand, took a mongoose-skin purse in his left hand, and pointed the horn at one of the cupping horns, wiping the patient's skin just above it as he did so. The whole congregation rose to their feet as one man, and Ihembi fastened on the twitching Kamahasanyi, who fell on his side, writhing convulsively. Kamahasanyi cried out and sobbed when Ihembi removed the blood-dripping horn in a large skin-purse. Mundoyi and Kachilewa (an Ihamba adept from a neighboring village) threw large quantities of medicine over the patient. Ihembi rushed to the small calabash (containing medicine and blood from other cuppings) and threw the cupping horn now concealed by the purse into it. He then spat powdered white clay on the really ugly bulge on Kamahasanyi's neck where the horn had been, "to cool and purify it." Kachilewa now held his hand poised over the leaf-concealed calabash while all of us waited intently. He removed the leaves and dredged with his hand in the bloody mixture. After a while he shook his head and said "Mwosi" ("Nothing in here"). We were all disappointed. But Ihembi with a gentle smile took over. He plunged his fingers into the gruesome liquid and when he brought them up I saw a flash of white. Then he rushed with what was in his fingers out of the avid circle of onlookers. From the edge of the village, he beckoned to the elders and to me. Led by Samuwinu and Kachimba, we went one by one to Ihembi. It was indeed a human tooth, we had to say. It was no bush-pig's tooth, nor a monkey's. Jubilantly we told the women, who all trilled with joy. Men and women who had been on cool terms with one another until recently, shook hands warmly and beamed with happiness. Kachimba even smiled at Makayi, who smiled back. Several hours later a mood of quiet satisfaction still seemed to emanate from the villagers.

These events took place toward the end of my first field trip. More than a year later, when I visited the village again during my second tour, I found that several changes had occurred in its composition. Of the Nkonkoto group none remained in Nswanamundong'u. Old Kapansonyi had died, and Makayi had emigrated to Chief Ikelenge's area, while Maria's lover Jackson had gone as a labor migrant to the Copperbelt mining town of Chingola (where I met him by chance in the street one day—he said he was never going back to village life). Kachimba's sons Douras and Robson had built new huts elsewhere in Mukang'ala Chiefdom. But Kamahasanyi was still in residence, Maria was still his wife, and indeed he had added to his personal following by persuading his younger brother and sister to reside in Nswanamundong'u. Furthermore, he had increased his prestige by becoming an adept in some of the cults into which he had been initiated through suffering—though not in Ihamba, for he was not a gun-hunter. In terms of social morphology, therefore, Nswanamundong'u had shed its patrilateral attachments and was reduced to its matrilineal nucleus, although it had increased in size. Kamahasanyi gave me the impression that he was enjoying life, was accepted by his fellow villagers, and was liked by his wife. He showed me with pride his new cassava gardens and told me that he was now successfully snaring game. It looked as though Ihembi's "therapy" had "worked," if only for a time!

§ Conclusion

It seems that the Ndembu "doctor" sees his task less as curing an individual patient than as remedying the ills of a corporate group. The sickness of a patient is mainly a sign that "something is rotten" in the corporate body. The patient will not get better until all the tensions and aggressions in the group's interrelations have been brought to light and exposed to ritual treatment. I have shown how complex these interrelations can be and how conflicts in one social dimension may reverberate through others. The doctor's task is to tap the various streams of affect associated with these conflicts and with the social and interpersonal disputes in which they are manifested—and to channel them in a socially positive direction. The raw energies of conflict are thus domesticated in the service of the traditional social order. Once the various causes of ill feeling against Kamahasanyi and of his ill feeling against others had been "made visible" (to use the Ndembu idiom), the doctor Ihembi was able, through the cultural mechanism of Ihamba, with its bloodlettings, confessions, purifications, prayers to the traditional dead, tooth-drawings, and build-up of expectations, to transform the ill feeling into well wishing. Emotion is roused and then stripped of its illicit and antisocial quality, but nothing of its intensity, its quantitative aspect, has been lost in the transformation. Ndembu social norms and values, expressed in symbolic objects and actions, are saturated with this generalized emotion, which itself becomes ennobled through contact with these norms and values. The sick individual, exposed to this process, is reintegrated into his group as, step by step, its members are reconciled with one another in emotionally charged circumstances.

Yet there is room within this communal and corporate process for the doctor to take fully into account the nuances and delicate distinctions of interpersonal relationships. Ihembi, for example, dealt with the idiosyncratic relationships between a father and a son, a husband and a wife, an uncle and a nephew. But his main endeavor was to see that individuals were capable of playing their social roles successfully in a traditional structure of social position. Illness was for him a mark of undue deviation from the norm. The shades punish such deviation. In this time of rapid change, the shades of old hunters are particularly likely to be sensitive to breaches of traditional norms, since hunting is for Ndembu the activity around which has formed the basic constellation of tribal values. It is therefore appropriate that hunters' shades should "bite" those who are most exposed to modern changes.

Stripped of its supernatural guise, Ndembu therapy may well offer lessons for Western clinical practice. For relief might be given to many sufferers from neurotic illness if all those involved in their social networks could meet together and publicly confess their ill will toward the patient and endure in turn the recital of his grudges against them. But it is likely that nothing less than ritual sanctions for such behavior and belief in the doctor's mystical powers could bring about such humility and compel people to display charity toward their suffering "neighbor"!

Notes

1. V. W. Turner, *Schism and Continuity in an African Society* (Manchester: Manchester University Press, 1957); Turner, *Ndembu Divination: Its Symbolism and Techniques* (Rhodes-Livingstone Paper Number Thirty-One [Manchester: Manchester University Press, 1961]); and Turner, *Lunda Medicine and the Treatment of Disease* (Rhodes-Livingstone Museum Paper Number Fifteen [Lusaka: Government Printing Office, 1963]).

2. T. Parsons, *The Social System* (New York: The Free Press of Glencoe, 1951), p. 430.

3. Turner, *Schism*, p. 292.

4. Turner, *Ndembu Medicines.*

5. Turner, *Ndembu Divination*, p. 18.

6. Erwin Ackerknecht, "Problems of Primitive Medicine," *Bulletin of the History of Medicine*, 11 (1942), 503-21.

7. W. A. Lessa and E. Z. Vogt, eds., *Reader in Comparative Religion* (New York: Harper & Row, Publishers, 1958), p. 343.

8. Turner, *Ndembu Divination*, p. 18.

9. Turner, *Ndembu Medicines*, pp. 131-7.

Catherine H. Berndt

The Role of Native Doctors
in Aboriginal Australia

THE INDIGENOUS CULTURE of the Australian continent was much more complex than is sometimes supposed and much more diverse. But there were also pervasive similarities, not least in the cluster of beliefs and practices centering about native doctors—or, as earlier writers called them, medicine men. These similarities mean that, ideally, no one area should be considered in isolation from others. Conversely, to look only at the over-all scene is to minimize the importance of local context in relation to actual cases. This paper attempts to keep a balance between the general and the particular. The first section deals with the broader Australian perspective; the second concentrates on a specific region— western Arnhem Land, in the extreme North of the continent.

The Australian Aborigines were traditionally hunters and food-collectors, with no fixed settlements and relatively few material goods. For all practical purposes, their social units were small. Face-to-face relations predominated, both actually and potentially through extension of the classificatory system of kin terminology to include everyone within each person's social world. Seminomadic though these people were, their attachment to their own land was strong. It provided a personal anchorage, in an emotional and spiritual sense, and a firm basis for social continuity in the shape of social units built around either or both of two criteria: genealogical or quasi-genealogical descent and territorial affiliation. The land was a visible and tangible symbol of the mythical beings who had created it, peopled it, provided vegetable foods and natural species in their proper places, and, above all, set in train the rules that all living things were expected to follow. These beings, in spirit form, were be-

believed to be still accessible. People could get in touch with them by means of the appropriate ritual and so ensure that, through their influence, the "right" way of life would continue undisturbed. In other words, Aboriginal societies were tradition-oriented and permeated by religion. Religion, the ultimate source of all the most important sanctions, served also to underwrite a host of minor ones and to legitimize the hard core of the authority structure.

Nevertheless, despite the relative conservatism of these societies when compared with a number of others, there was some room for individual variation. What was more, causation was not defined simply in "ultimate" terms. Misfortunes and troubles were not ascribed simply to the will or caprice of a deity or to the working-out of some inscrutable providence or fate. More often, answers were sought at the level of human affairs themselves—in the realm of black magic, or sorcery. Not all cases of illness and death were so classified—particularly those of the very young and the very old, who were viewed as being extremely close to the supernatural or extranatural dimension anyway. But in the great majority, even when the immediate cause was observable or readily inferred (snake bite, for example, or attack by a crocodile or shark, a spear wound, a severe fall), the "real" responsibility was held to lie with another human being.

In a fashion typical of any sorcery-complex, social relations, and especially interpersonal relations, were accorded pre-eminent importance. The part played by the human will in manipulating the lives of others was overemphasized; physical, or rather physiological, factors were subordinated to "psychical" or "psychological" factors. The human organism was believed to be vulnerable to influences directed by persons operating at a distance from it, with no direct physical contact necessary for achieving the desired ends, but the ill effects brought about in this way could often be countered or reduced by prompt measures of a comparable kind. Up to a point, both types of action (designed to injure or to heal) were open to any adult to master and to use. But knowledge and skill varied, and, before a man could be regarded as a specialist or expert, he was usually obliged not only to learn the relevant techniques but also to undergo a preliminary experience—a dream or other "revelation" or a ritual initiation[1] that would provide him with the necessary formal status.

This status rested, then, on something more than individual human ability. It involved the intervention of some supernatural force, which endowed the practitioner with magical power. In a few areas, this power was believed to be inherited.[2] But it was not necessarily irrevocable. For example, in certain Northern Territory tribes it could be weakened or even lost through some action on the part of its possessor: eating "too much fat," letting a large ant bite him, drinking "anything hot,"[3] or misbehaving. Spencer and Gillen[4] report that they "saw a man lose his power simply because, during a fight, he had struck a tribal father, who was a doctor much older than himself, with a boomerang."[5] There is provision here for explanation of failure to achieve the desired results; these and other plausible excuses can represent "an honourable way out."[6] In other instances, neglect of special prohibitions and rules relating to eating and drinking was said to lead to illness and possible death.[7]

All Aboriginal languages appear to have had special terms for persons equipped with such power. Most were men, a few women; rarely, the recipient is said to have been singled out through a dream experience in childhood, although active practice did not follow until later.[8]

In areas like East Kimberley[9] the healing, protective, and life-sustaining aspects of such activities were separated from the destructive or death-dealing aspects. For practical purposes, the overlap between them was ignored in order to clarify the issue of "who is responsible," distinguishing "good" from "bad." In other areas, like northwest central Queensland[10] and among the Narrinyeri of the lower River Murray in South Australia,[11] the distinction was blurred to the extent that the complete range was seen as the province of one all-round specialist, probably on the assumption that sorcery could be combated most effectively by someone who was himself an expert in that field as well. There was identification between "sorcerer" and "healer," at least to the extent that the same person was believed to be equally competent in both spheres: to engage in both types of activity. In other areas again, the two roles were vaguely distinguished, although it was acknowledged that they might be performed by one and the same person; a "native doctor" ("clever man," "powerful man," or "medicine man") in one situation might be a "sorcerer" in another.

A native doctor was not merely someone believed to be capable of curing minor cases of illness or upset, which at an elementary level were mostly handled by people themselves without specialist attention. Plant and other substances were used freely as simple medicaments. He could expect to be called upon to help in a variety of circumstances. Predominantly, he was a mediator or buffer between humanity in general and the supernatural, the contingent, helping men to cope with the unforeseen and dangerous emergencies of life. He could, it was said, see and control ghosts and other potentially harmful spirits and beings, including manifestations of the Rainbow Snake; through divination, identify the "murderer" or sorcerer after a death; interpret dreams; advise on ritual precautions to avert possible misfortune or point out what ritual precautions had been overlooked or inadequately observed; "find" new ceremonies or new versions of old ones; assist in cases of difficult childbirth; and play a major part in fighting and revenge expeditions, safeguarding the well-being of the participants and ensuring a successful outcome. He was expected also to identify the "sorcerer" who had been responsible for the illness of his client[12] or even to identify a "potential evil-doer."[13] And not only did his initiation involve, in many cases, the insertion or absorption of some material substance—pearl shells, *maban*, in the Western and Great Victoria deserts; "flints" in Queensland;[14] "stones and other objects" in parts of the Northern Territory.[15] An important feature of the curing process itself consisted of removing from the patient's body the illness or infection itself or a symbol of it in material form—a stone, stick, bone, frog, and so forth.

Both the "power" on which the doctor draws, then, and the "evil" that he combats in his treatment of illness are conceptualized as both visible and tangible. In the first case, the manifestations are visible to him but merely inferred by others. In the second, the important thing is that they *should* be seen by others, including above all the patient himself (or herself): They provide clear "proof" that what was causing the distress has now been removed. As Elkin says such performances represent "the outward expression and means of the doctor's personal victory over one or both of two factors: first, the malevolent activities of some person practising sorcery on the sick man or woman; and second, the patient's willingness to remain ill or even to die. The latter must be counteracted, and the will to be healthy and live be restored."[16]

§ Western Arnhem Land

European contact was earlier and more intensive in the West of Arnhem Land than in the East. The people of the coast and off-shore islands, in particular, apart from their long term association with "Macassan" (Indonesian) traders and later with Japanese pearlers, had a small European military settlement established (but subsequently abandoned) in their territory in the early years of the nineteenth century, at Port Essington. Farther inland, the drift toward the main Darwin-Alice Springs road was supplemented by eastward influences from that direction. One consequence has been that the people who traditionally inhabited the "buffalo country" between Darwin and the East Alligator River are today almost extinct.

This river now marks the western boundary of the Arnhem Land Reserve. A Church Missionary Society station has been centered there for some years at Oenpelli, the site of a former buffalo-shooting and later government station; the Methodists have a "half-caste" settlement at Croker Island not far from Port Essington, although changes are imminent there, and a "full-blood" station farther east at South Goulburn Island. Gunwinggu speakers, moving westward, now represent the dominant population in the Alligator River region and a fairly high proportion of that at Goulburn Island, originally Maung territory. Maung and Gunwinggu territories traditionally overlapped near the coast; the Maung recognized even closer cultural ties with the Jiwadja (Yiwadja), originally located around Port Essington but now, with the virtual disappearance of the Marlgu and other "tribes" from the Croker Island area, extending into the islands as well. Gunwinggu, Maung, and Jiwadja meet at both the Oenpelli and Goulburn Island Mission stations, together with members of other "tribes" from farther east, south, and southwest; there is some movement between the two, as well as a gradual but continuing drift to the West and Southwest.

These larger "tribal" or language names are used for convenience both by the people themselves and by outsiders. The more basic identification, however, rests on membership in a named, not coresident, territorial unit of patrilineal descent and on moiety, phratry, and subsection affiliation of matrilineal and indirect matrilineal descent.[17] Clearly, the tribal labels oversimplify the position, both traditionally and in respect to actual persons. And this observation applies to the region with which we are primarily concerned here: the mixed population, mobile in varying degrees, centered around the East Alligator River, with special reference to the period between 1947 and 1950. (I revisited the area briefly in 1958 and again in 1961. Early in 1964, I revisited South Goulburn Island, working with Gunwinggu speakers there.) Its complexity should be borne in mind, although to avoid confusion the major reference is to the Gunwinggu, and only Gunwinggu terms are indicated.

THE TRADITIONAL PICTURE

The Gunwinggu and their immediate neighbors have separate terms for native doctor and for expert or "professional" sorcerer; although some kinds of sorcery are said to be available to everyone, "professionals" are always men. The native doctor is, in Gunwinggu, a *margidbu* (or *margid*), a word very much like the eastern Arnhem Land *marnggid*[18]—from *marnggi,* meaning "know." And in local opinion he is, in fact, a knowledgeable man, a person of more than ordinary intelligence and enterprise. But here too his ability is not a result of individual effort. It must come to him from without. He cannot, merely by wishing or by personal endeavor, achieve this status.

In several accounts, the initiation he must undergo resembles in part the more elaborate types reported from other areas (for example, the Great Victoria Desert and western New South Wales).[19] Briefly, the postulant is swallowed by the Rainbow Snake, vomited in the shape of a newly born infant, and ritually restored to adult stature as a *margidbu.*[20]

In other reports, the procedure is simpler and much more informal. Typically, the experience is unsought. A man going along by himself encounters unexpectedly a spirit or ghost, especially the ghost of a close relative like his father or his father's father—even a mother's brother, although there is more emphasis on transmission of power from father to son. The man falls to the ground as if dead. The ghost proceeds to insert into his head a length of very thin bamboo, *gunrong,* sometimes identified with a spirit snake. (People say that this *gunrong* can be heard at times rattling in a *margidbu's* head: that when he bites anything they can hear a loud and unnatural noise.) Then he blows into the man's ears (according to other accounts, into all the other body apertures as well), giving him "breath" (*gunngole*), equivalent in this case to "spirit" or "power." The man, reviving, stands up. He is a *margidbu* now, a "powerful man," and, no matter what happens, this power cannot be dissipated or taken from him. There are, however, degrees of power. Some men have more than others, and this fact is inferred from the effectiveness of their endeavors over a period. Their claims are more often substantiated; their reputations extend over a wider region; the patients they agree to treat are more likely to recover.

A "powerful man," like his counterparts in other regions, is credited with ability to perform marvelous feats. He can, it is claimed, climb into the sky; render himself invisible; collect from about himself the small flies that, in this semitropical environment, hover around ordinary people and draw attention to their presence even when they try to escape notice; see ghosts and spirits invisible to ordinary persons and follow them unobserved; report a death long before the news comes by ordinary messenger; come into contact, through dreams, with people at a distance; interpret strange events; perceive the threat of danger unsuspected by others; find out what is frightening an unborn baby, so that it refuses to emerge from its mother at the appropriate time, and kill the offender—for example, a goanna or blanket lizard. With the help of his familiar(s), he may "compose" songs and dances; a shrewd observer of what is going on around him, he can refer in his songs to incidents or to sweetheart relationships that the people concerned thought were unknown to anyone but themselves.

If a child, as it grows, is perceived to be "deaf," apparently unable to take in what is said to it or respond intelligently to the questions or demands of people around it, a *margidbu* may be asked for advice or at least for an explanation. The child may not be able to speak in a "normal" way; perhaps only its mother can understand and interpret its words. It may refuse ordinary food and show a preference for mud or pebbles. The *margidbu's* diagnosis is likely to be that a malignant spirit or ghost has taken the child's spirit or soul and has made the child's tongue "soft" so that human speech is impossible.[21] He may attempt, or so he claims, to recover the child's spirit and thus restore him to normality; but if he reports failure, he is usually in a position to indicate other difficulties that have militated against success—for example, one of the parents may have broken a taboo, or the trouble may be of such long standing that he can do nothing to remedy it. Occasionally, it is said, a *margidbu* may abuse his power by injuring or killing someone who has offended him, by sending his spirit snake to "bite a person's head" or a spirit hawk to "eat a person's heart." In myths, *margidbu* are reported to be able to send the Rainbow Snake (Ngaljod), a flood and storm and also a "bad mother"[22] symbol, to "swallow" (drown) whole camps with all their inhabitants because of a grudge against one of them. And if confronted by the Rainbow, approached by swirling flood waters, *margidbu* can hold disaster at bay at least for a time.

Pre-eminently, however, a *margidbu* is a man to whom people turn for help in times of trouble or personal crisis. They are armed to some extent against minor accidents or misfortunes; to a degree, they can cope with everyday difficulties. But in cases of illness, anxiety, or death or when conflicting rumors are rife on a topic that concerns them deeply, the *margidbu* is expected to provide positive support, particularly emotional support.

This support is not always forthcoming. A western Arnhem Land "powerful man" is no more ready than native doctors elsewhere to sacrifice his reputation for a lost cause, and there are conventionally accepted provisos that safeguard him here. A *margidbu,* summoned to a patient's side, may scrutinize him carefully first before agreeing to treat him. For example, he may tug lightly at a lock of the patient's hair. If it comes away in his hand, the case is clearly hopeless, and he refuses to handle it: "He will die: You have called me too late." On other occasions, the patient or his relatives may not want him to proceed, on the grounds that he asks too much in the way of recompense, but this attitude is not customary, if only because an offended *margidbu* is regarded as a bad enemy. Again, a *margidbu* may accept a case and diagnose what is wrong, but he may warn the patient's relatives that he cannot answer for the consequences unless they follow his instructions exactly. He may tell them, for instance, that the patient is certainly ill but that with treatment "he may get up in three days, if you don't cry. I'll make him better—but remember, if you cry you'll injure him, he'll get worse. Sit quietly, let your tears flow silently if you must; but if you cry noisily, he is sure to die."

If there are no setbacks of this sort, people say, if a *margidbu* is called in promptly and his orders are obeyed to the last detail, he can heal the most difficult patients, suiting his treatment to the case in hand. In this region, there is less emphasis on sucking, massaging, and removal of objects than elsewhere—in eastern Arnhem Land, for instance. Here there is rather more stress on the simple use of "power," the "laying on of hands," so to speak, accompanied by exhortations and the use of simple medicaments. But one feature that is widespread in all areas where native doctors are involved in healing and reassuring "ordinary" people is of major importance in western Arnhem Land: the need for faith and confidence on the part of the *margidbu's* patients, or clients.

Claims about the superhuman exploits of "powerful men" are not locally regarded as fantastic or unreal, nor are they merely embellishments, unessential additions to the main body of information relating to the activities of such people in ideal as well as in actual terms. Realistic and down-to-earth as the Gunwinggu and their neighbors are in many respects, they do not see their own territory as merely an impersonal setting for themselves. The land is rich in sacred and semisacred sites; the bonds between human and other living things, including plants, are well established in current mythology. But in local belief there are other inhabitants, too: spirits of various kinds, including ghosts—since it is said that, while one part or one manifestation of a person's spirit goes to the land of the dead, another part may remain behind in the country it knew in life. These spirits or ghosts are capricious, and "new" ghosts especially are described not only as erratic but also as resentful of the living.

In popular belief, a *margidbu* can deal effectively with beings of this kind, or at least can provide some protection from them. From that point of view, he is providing a practical service. But over and above this service, his association with the supernatural and marvelous imbues him with an aura of special privilege and knowledge. It suggests that his actions in this respect have supernatural backing, that he can draw on a resource of power that is not available to other people. This power is the basis of his reputation, which his personal record as a practitioner may enhance or diminish. It is a vital aspect of his equipment, underwriting his claims and supplying a "reason" for satisfying the fundamental requirement of the *margidbu's* profession: The patient or client must have faith. The point is illustrated succinctly in a popular local story, one variant of a common myth that accounts for the origin of death.

In this Gunwinggu version, Moon and Spotted Cat, travelling together, were taken seriously ill. Unable to move about or to eat, they were barely alive. Finally, Moon managed to revive himself. He rose up, making himself alive again. Before he went into the sky, he tried to revive Spotted Cat; but he could not do so *"because Spotted Cat didn't trust him."* In consequence, Spotted Cat died, and that is why now people die forever. If only Spotted Cat had trusted Moon, nobody would have died. "We look up at Moon and say, 'He's a truly powerful *margidbu.*' He appears to die, but he always returns after three days. And we human beings could have done the same . . ."

THE CONTEMPORARY PICTURE

For some years, the mission station at Oenpelli was small and understaffed. Its work was carried on almost entirely in English, without concern for the local languages and with emphasis on the formal Anglican service modified scarcely at all for local participants. English biblical names were substituted for personal names among quasi-permanent residents. Numbers of children were taken into the mission dormitories, and traditional betrothal and marriage arrangements for them were discouraged or forbidden in favor of partners chosen by the mission.[23]

But outside this immediate core of activity, the mission station did not make a strong impact on the local population, except in regard to material needs. Even then, since the country was fairly well supplied with native foods and the mission only sporadically banned the issue and use of tobacco, which these people had learned to treat as an indispensable item of diet, they were less dependent on the station for satisfying such needs than were Aborigines in harsher regions of the continent. The mission was not a center of active proselytizing, and, although its few staff members showed much concern with Christian rites and beliefs on the station itself and less tolerance of Aboriginal rites and beliefs than their Methodist neighbors on the coast, their lack of direct interest in such rites and beliefs meant that, in practice, a great deal of traditional life could continue in the immediate proximity of the station without more than occasional interference.

There was a small two-bed hospital under the charge of a missionary sister, who also ran an out-patients' clinic; but for a long time most women were reluctant to bear their children there, preferring the familiar environs of the camp. For a long time, too, until the recent improvement in medical services, people who suspected (or whose relatives suspected) that they might be suffering from leprosy would "go bush" at any suggestion that a flying doctor plane might be on its way to the station, which had a small airstrip. Others, especially younger people with minor sicknesses or injuries (from camp quarrels, for example) who liked the prospect of a trip to Darwin, welcomed the possibility. But even among the young, belief in the powers of local *margidbu* seemed to be as strong as belief in the efficacy of European medical treatment. The aura of power that surrounded Europeans was not taken wholly for granted. Their failures were remembered even more vividly than their successes. A death in Darwin hospital, far from home, was (as usual in such cases) counted as a mark against the hospital, despite the familiarity to local ears of the plea that the patient had not been made available for treatment until "too late."

This outline, sketchy as it is, suggests a number of pertinent considerations. Alien contact, mediated in this case largely through the mission as one culminating influence in a long series, had led to some reorientation in local living without completely eradicating either the traditional values or the modes of behavior through which they were expressed. The presence or availability of new agents for healing physical illness and injury (nursing sisters, flying doctors, hospitals) and of agents for spiritual "healing" or help, did not mean that these agents were readily accepted by the local people. In neither case was serious effort made to integrate the newer patterns of action and belief with what was already there. Despite the use that was made of both services, there was considerable uncertainty about their "real" relevance. Physical cures were more quickly and more fully appreciated; they supplied clearer "proof" that the new measures were in some degree effective. On the religious side, however, particularly in view of the relatively formal way in which a great deal of the teaching was presented in a largely unfamiliar language, there was more room for doubt.

In this situation, then, new needs were being established and "old" ways being upset; but the agencies that were concerned simultaneously with implementing changes and with attending to physical and spiritual welfare were not organized in such a way that they could successfully achieve either goal. Many opportunities were therefore open to *margidbu*. They were asked for advice or help frequently, sometimes by people who were attempting at the same time to draw upon European sources, sometimes as sole consultants or temporary ones (for example, in a night emergency or when there was a suggestion that Europeans would not be in a position to diagnose or to "understand," or to help).

This behavior was the more likely because one *margidbu*, Wilambilam, a man of predominantly Jiwadja affiliations, although his two wives were predominantly Gunwinggu, had been selected as local "headman" by the mission and was allowed a fair amount of latitude in mediating between the missionaries and the camp in general. His status in this respect reinforced his status as a *margidbu*, but one of his close brothers, Namadbara, was also a *margidbu* in his own right. Both were rather quiet and reserved men who took their reputations as "powerful men" quite seriously. Both had considerable influence, although it would have been greater had they been more outstanding and more deeply involved as leaders in the sphere of men's sacred ritual; the fact that they were not in their own paternal territory militated against them in this respect.

Four short examples will suffice to show the kinds of problems with which they were most often asked to deal.

The first is a simple case of injury and healing. A woman of the Wadaman tribe in the Katherine area had married a Maiali-Gunwinggu man. In the wet season of 1949-50, he was visiting relatives at Oenpelli, but although she came with him she was lonely and unhappy, jealous of his local associates and anxious to return to the main north-south road. She nagged at him continually and finally one evening struck him with a tin billy can. He responded by hitting her forcibly a couple of times on the back of the head with a heavy firestick. She fell to the ground, with blood flowing from the wound, a trickle from her mouth, and bloodshot protruding eyes. People nearby, afraid that she was dead, sent urgently for Wilambilam: "It's not good that she should die here, she's not one of our countrymen. The police will get us!" Wilambilam came hurrying, his wife beside him carrying a kerosene lamp. He did not touch her at first but stood looking at her from a little distance away. Then, satisfied, he came near and felt her, examining the wound. "It's all right," he said at last. "She won't die. It's only that the 'string' at the back of her neck was hit, and that's why her eyes are coming out." He felt her pulse, and he "made her well," he gave her strength—some of his own "spirit" or "power." Then he said, "Let her drink water now." She opened her eyes, drank, spoke, and then slept. Two days later, she had recovered; her husband took her back to her own country as Wilambilam suggested and as she herself wanted.

The second "healing" incident involved Namadbara and Wilambilam and a third close brother as a subsidiary figure. A young man took ill one cold season in the late 1940s and instead of recovering became gradually worse. He lost weight, his cheeks became hollow and his body like a skeleton: Presently he could not walk at all but lay semiconscious in his camp. His pulse was so weak that people were sure his spirit had already almost left him. His relatives gathered around him, wailing and gashing themselves in mourning "because he was so young"; but some of them were already beginning to make trouble for his wife, accusing her of not taking care of his belongings and so leaving him vulnerable to sorcery. One of them, however, sent for old Namadbara and his brothers, who came with their wives. They built up the fire, covered him with a blanket, and got water for him. Old Namadbara moved the women and children aside: "Give me room!" They moved quickly. He came close to the patient and touched him, while Wilambilam touched his feet. They "felt" him all over. Then they told the women, "Get hot water, and bathe him now and then. Don't use cold water, and don't keep on bathing him, or he'll become worse. Bathe him now, and then when the sun is just rising bathe him again. We'll come back soon and 'heal' him again. After that he will be well. It will take three days." They "felt" him again and repeated, "Don't cry, he'll be all right, in maybe three days." The patient slept quietly, for a long time, while Namadbara and his brothers "watched over" his spirit, guarding it, putting it back into his body. After a time he woke and asked, "Who were those two men touching me?" His relatives gave him food and told him. "I saw two men in my dream," he said, "washing my body with very cold water, making me feel well again. I don't know where we were: somewhere up in the sky perhaps. I don't know that place, it was a different place altogether, where those powerful men always go." From that point he grew stronger, and, in a few weeks, he was quite well again.

The third case centered mainly on the after-effects of a death. A young woman died, leaving a baby daughter who fretted for her. The dead girl's mother, Wurgamara, and sister, Melinggir, mourned for her too. Their grief was accentuated by the child's continuous crying—which they themselves were unwittingly encouraging by their own behavior. They were involved also in another crisis just then. Melinggir, endeavoring to leave her elderly husband for a younger sweetheart, had already eloped and been brought back; and the episode was causing a series of upsets in the camp. It was fairly clear that the first man would relinquish her, but in

the meantime she (and, indirectly, her mother) was the focus of recriminations from his immediate kin, and the affair had led to some bad feeling
between her and her mother. Wurgamara showed signs of emotional
strain, far more so than Melinggir. She accused a number of people of responsibility for the death, through working sorcery or merely through
neglecting the dead girl. Especially, she would start noisy arguments with
her husband late at night when people were trying to sleep, reproaching
him with running after other women, abandoning her and the dead girl.
Finally she would break down in tears to wail for the girl and the "motherless" baby. This behavior continued for several nights. Her husband tried
to soothe her. "Why are you always seizing on that corpse [with words]?"
he used to ask. "Talking won't bring her back. That's how it has been from
the very beginning. By talking about those who are dead we can't revive
them, make them alive again. We are not *margidbu*, to go up into the
sky and below the ground, or whatever it is that they do. . . ." At last
he called in old Namadbara and Wilambilam to help. When the two men
came, they stood "listening" attentively for a time, without speaking, then
moved around, still "listening." Presently they reported the reason for
the child's crying: Her dead mother was crying too, wandering about the
camp in search of her, trying to take her away to the land of the dead.
"Her ghost is here with you," they told Wurgamara and Melinggir. "She
wants her child. Take the child, build up a big fire of ironwood leaves,
with plenty of smoke. Hold the child close beside it, don't leave her
away from the fire. Then her mother won't be able to seize her for fear
of burning her hands. And you two women, don't cry. Let her ghost go
quietly away. Look after the child. You are her own mother's mother
and her "mother." Care for her, so that the ghost can depart leaving the
child behind with you, in your charge. . . ." They underlined the dependence of the child, its need for affection and care, and the two
women's joint responsibility for its welfare now that its mother, their
own daughter and sister, had left it in their keeping. In this way, they
tried to draw attention away from the actual death and to heal the partial
breach between Wurgamara and Melinggir by reminding them of the
closeness of the bond between them and by giving them a positive interest in common. This advice did not immediately resolve the trouble.
But it came at a strategic point, at the peak of the crisis; after it, Wurgamara gradually became more "settled," quieter, and more reconciled to
her daughter's new marriage.

    The fourth case is a little different. It comes from a period of uncer-
tainty when people were eagerly awaiting the arrival of wet-season stores
for the mission and also for supplies for my husband and myself, supplies

in which they knew they would share. Stormy weather and repairs to the barge concerned had several times delayed its departure from Darwin, and rumors were rife about when it could be expected. European foods (flour, tea, and sugar), which the Aborigines liked, were almost finished. What was more, they were "starving" for tobacco, which the mission had refused to distribute at that time but which they knew was expected among our stores. In addition, the low-lying ground around the Oenpelli billabong had been flooding after heavy rains, and the water level underneath the "dry" ground had been rising so that some of the new tin huts in the camp had toppled aslant. In this time of speculation and crisis, Namadbara and Wilambilam called people together for a series of ceremonies. Wilambilam had seen in a dream, he said, his spirit familiars, which had told him to summon everyone so that their friend, the "frog that died," could come to life again. He was speaking about a spirit familiar or spirit child of Namadbara, sometimes identified with a sacred-secret object, believed to be buried under the ground. "This frog is a *margidbu,* he wants to live again. Come and share in his end-of-mourning feast, let us 'work' together in this rite. . . ." People assembled at the ceremonial ground or "ring place." In the course of the ceremony, a dream-message was conveyed to them from the two spirit familiars— who were invisible to everyone but the *margidbu* brothers. "Don't worry," was the gist of this message. "Everything will be all right. We didn't let those houses fall over for nothing. [It was a sign.] The boat with the stores couldn't come before, because of the frog that died. We buried him, and now we have revived him through this ceremony, and all will be well. Don't be anxious, the boat will come soon. Perhaps the day after tomorrow you will hear word of it. It is on its way and everything will be all right. . . ." For the time being, people appeared to be relieved. "We believe those two *margidbu,*" several of them said. "They always know, those spirits tell them in dreams. . . ." It so happened that several days after the last ceremony word came that the barge had in fact left Darwin at last. Although it was no more than could reasonably have been expected after a delay of some weeks, earlier conjectures based on spirit pronouncements reported by Namadbara and his brother were forgotten, and this one was acclaimed as another example of accurate forecasting. (Later, it so happened that the stores met with misfortune. The barge had unloaded them at the mouth of the East Alligator River on to a small boat that made its way upstream until it grounded on a mudbank and all the goods had to be abandoned. They could be recovered in time only with great difficulty. No reference was made, however, to the fact that no dream-prediction had suggested this possibility. It was taken simply as a combination of inept European seamanship and the well known hazards of the flooding wet-season river.)

In these four examples, no "extra" techniques or physical skills were employed—nothing that people other than *margidbu* could not have attended to themselves. There was no prolonged massaging or manipulation or removal of objects, and from that point of view the treatments and responses were not "typical" of native doctors' healing procedures in general. Use of smoke from ironwood leaves and wood is a conventional means of discouraging ghosts and other unwelcome spirits. The suggestion here is merely that the mourners were so distraught that somehow nobody thought of it. But in all these cases the emphasis is on providing reassurance, on restoring confidence, and on doing so in a familiar and therefore comforting way. The approach of Namadbara and Wilambilam, in this respect, is characteristic of that expected of *margidbu* throughout this region. What they lack in medical skill they make up, to some extent, in knowledge both of the local situation and of traditionally effective means of dealing with crises.

There is no need here for detailed inquiry into a patient's background and early experience. Traditionally, and even today, much of ordinary living takes place in public, and little secrecy is associated with it—as Wurgamara's case implies. People have personal experiences, of course, but they are rarely private in the sense of being concealed from others. Even when a *margidbu* comes from a different area, called in perhaps because of his superior skill or reputation, there are plenty of people to supply the information he needs about personal case histories and about social relations in that *milieu*. Even in sorcery cases, which have not been included here because of the extra discussion they would entail, the *margidbu's* identification of "who did it" rests heavily on his knowledge of local relationships; this knowledge influences, for example, decisions concerning such matters as on whom it would be politic to cast blame and when to do so (usually after the first shock of anger and grief has died down after a death, when people are in a position to look at the matter more calmly).

Ideally, *margidbu* are men who are not so preoccupied with religious or sacred affairs that they pay little attention to the empirical world about them. On the contrary, it is their interest in that world, their curiosity and concern with what goes on in it, that supplies them not only with "case material" but also with the experience on which to build up their own generalizations—applied, in turn, to the new cases that confront them. Their attention is directed, not simply to specific individuals, but to individuals in context—an orientation that is not conspicuous in the treatment of minor illness but emerges most obviously in crises of a more clearly "social" kind. This observation holds in the contemporary situation of change no less than before, especially since now different Aboriginal traditions are impinging on one another, as a minor part of the more far-reaching clash between different ways of living exemplified in Aboriginal-European contact. While points of strain between introduced and traditional ways continue to exist, it is likely that the demand for this intermediate category of quasi-psychological treatment will continue too. The contact situation is perceived by many Aborigines as fraught with perils and difficulties, not only from such agents of the alien society as police (whose reputation in the past has not always been favorable), but also from welfare agents, whose aims are couched in terms of helping, protecting, and healing.

The position in western Arnhem Land today, as elsewhere in Aboriginal Australia, has improved immensely in recent years. But as official policies of assimilation have gathered momentum and as measures designed to bring about Europeanization in all but a physical sense have been accelerated, the strain on formerly tradition-oriented Aborigines has increased. True, it is no longer fashionable to sneer at native doctors as "impostors" and "charlatans," as so many early observers did. There is much greater appreciation today of the part such men have played in their own societies; in part because psychosomatic aspects, or the role of emotional factors in producing or exacerbating functional disturbances, are much more widely recognized than they were even a few decades ago. Also, far more material is available on the traditional construct patterns of what native doctors (and sorcerers) do: how they become initiated, what rites they must undergo, what myths are drawn upon to validate both initiation and practice, and so forth. But little detailed research has been carried out in the "actual" situation, from the point of view of the doctors reporting their own cases and from that of the patients or relatives, skeptics as well as believers. The best account on this score, even after a lapse of almost thirty years from the date of its publication (nearly forty from the period of the field work on which it was based), remains Warner's classic study of the north central Arnhem Landers.[24] Nor has much been written, apart from this work, except in a general way or in passing references, on the range of types that the label of "native doctor" can cover. The "profession" offers opportunities for the brightest and most alert men (occasionally women) in a society to exercise initiative and imagination, albeit within a traditional framework. But it can also provide a refuge for persons more interested in dreams and trances and in communicating with spirits than in the people around them—or for "misfits"—just as it allows scope to charlatans or to those with an eye to the personal benefits they may be able to derive from it.

The techniques evolved in Aboriginal Australia for coping with such disturbances are, or were, less elaborate and less systematic than in a number of other regions. Native doctors were not equipped to cope with serious injuries or illness, and the view that such illness, like magical power, came from a source external to the organism itself was a handicap to any extension of their healing powers to include more "realistic" explanations of disease. Notwithstanding these limitations, their role as amateur psychiatrists or amateur psychotherapists has not been accorded the attention it deserves. This absence of attention may be explained perhaps by their attempt to combine two kinds of healing, physical and "psychological," drawing on magical or supernatural claims—whereas attempts to heal the "whole man" or the "whole person" have only in relatively recent times been fully accepted by practitioners working within the western European tradition. In any event, even when they have identified in part with alien authority (and Wilambilam and Namadbara, for instance, are now back on the coast,[25] living in partial independence of Europeans, emotionally if not materially), there have been hints of rivalry and competition, even of open conflict. This rivalry is even more noticeable when the native doctor has taken the stand of representing traditional ways and expresses antagonism to the new era—including "new style" doctoring.[26]

Training in "human relations," unfortunately, has not often been a feature of preparation for administrative, missionary, educational, and "welfare" work in Aboriginal Australia. Where it has been, it has rarely been combined with anthropological training to provide the essential cross-cultural perspective. Similarly, anthropological study, both of the traditional situation and of the changing scene today, even when accompanied by an interest in welfare problems, has usually stopped short of this particular aspect—and in any event, such research is not designed to achieve clinical or therapeutic ends. The contribution that native doctors could have made, especially in this transition period, has rarely been acknowledged. Furthermore, where belief in their powers has been deliberately undermined, a process made easier by the obvious defects of some of their techniques (notably the removal of "foreign" objects from their patients) and by their lack of medical knowledge, this loss of faith in itself has affected their results. At the same time, there has been a decline in opportunities for and sponsorship of initiation rites for the "making" of such doctors.

The passing of native doctors from most parts of the Australian continent is symptomatic of the passing of Aboriginal traditional culture itself, but it points also to the passing of a force that could have been turned to advantage in assisting the Aborigines in their contacts with Europeans and in the changes that were inevitably entailed.

Notes

1. Some quite detailed accounts of such initiatory rites are available in the literature. For summaries, see A. P. Elkin, *Aboriginal Men of High Degree* (The John Murtagh Macrossan Memorial Lecture for 1944, University of Queensland [Sydney: Australasian Pub. Co., Ltd., 1945]); Elkin, *The Australian Aborigines. How to Understand Them* (3rd ed.; Sydney: Angus & Robertson, Ltd., 1954); and R. M. Berndt and T. Vogelsang, "The Initiation of Native Doctors, Dieri Tribe, South Australia," *Records of the South Australian Museum,* VI (1941), No. 4.
2. B. Spencer and F. J. Gillen, *The Northern Tribes of Central Australia* (London: Macmillan & Co., Ltd., 1904), p. 448.
3. *Ibid.,* pp. 481, 485.
4. *Ibid.,* p. 484.
5. H. Basedow, *The Australian Aboriginal* (Adelaide: F. W. Preece, Ltd., 1925), p. 180; and W. L. Warner, *A Black Civilization* (Rev. ed.; New York: Harper & Row, Publishers, 1958), pp. 217-8.
6. Elkin, *Aboriginal Men,* p. 17.
7. Spencer and Gillen, *op. cit.,* p. 485.
8. See, for example, S. Gason, "The Manners and Customs of the Dieyerie Tribe," J. D. Woods, ed., *The Native Tribes of South Australia* (Adelaide: Wigg, 1879), p. 283.
9. See P. Kaberry, *Aboriginal Woman, Sacred and Profane* (London: Routledge & Kegan Paul, Ltd., 1939), pp. 212, 251-2.
10. See W. E. Roth, *Ethnological Studies among the North-West-Central Queensland Aborigines* (Brisbane: Government Printer, 1897), Sections 89, 90.
11. G. Taplin, "The Narrinyeri," Woods, *op. cit.,* p. 134.
12. Roth, *op. cit.,* Section 263.
13. *Ibid.,* Section 199.
14. *Ibid.,* Section 260.
15. Spencer and Gillen, *op. cit.,* p. 479.
16. Elkin, *Aboriginal Men,* p. 16.
17. See Elkin, Berndt, and C. H. Berndt, "The Social Organization of Arnhem Land, I:Western Arnhem Land," *Oceania,* XXXI (1951), No. 4.
18. Warner, *op. cit., passim.*
19. See Berndt and Berndt, "Preliminary Report of Fieldwork in the Oldea Region, Western South Australia, *Oceania,* bound offprint, 1942-5; and R. M. Berndt, "Wuradjeri Magic and Clever Men," *Oceania,* XVII (1947), No. 4, and XVIII (1947), No. 1.
20. See Berndt and Berndt, *Sexual Behaviour in Western Arnhem Land* (Viking Fund Publications in Anthropology, No. 16 [New York, 1951]), pp. 167-8.
21. For a brief outline, see Berndt and Berndt, "The Concept of Abnormality in an Australian Aboriginal Society," *Psychoanalysis and Culture* (New York: International Universities Press, 1951), pp. 75-89.
22. Among the Gunwinggu, the Rainbow is occasionally identified as male, more often as female. She is "our mother," but she is usually represented as a threatening

figure, against whom certain ritual precautions are necessary, particularly at such times of crisis as menstruation and childbirth. In secret-sacred rituals in this region, several of the principal mythical characters are also referred to as "our mother," whether or not they are viewed as differing manifestations of the same figure; but then they are usually viewed as good and beneficent, associated with fertility and with the continuation rather than the destruction of life. The associated myths do not draw this distinction sharply, however, but infer that both aspects may be present in any or all of the characters concerned.

23. See Berndt and Berndt, "An Oenpelli Monologue—Culture Contact," *Oceania*, XXII (1951), No. 1.

24. See Warner, *op. cit.*, Chapters 7 and 8 *et passim*.

25. Early in 1964, I learned that Wilambilam had died suddenly a few weeks before.

26. An interesting example of this antagonism in west central Arnhem Land is given by an Aboriginal trained as a medical assistant, as reported by a Darwin journalist. See D. Lockwood, *I, the Aboriginal* (Adelaide: Rigby, Ltd., 1962), pp. 230-5.

Michael G. Whisson

Some Aspects of Functional Disorders Among the Kenya Luo*

THE KENYA LUO are the most southerly group of the Nilotic tribes of East Africa and live along the shores and hinterlands of the eastern side of Lake Victoria. Traditionally a pastoral people, the tribesmen are now sedentary cultivators but retain many of the values of pastoralists. During the period of effective British rule, from about 1900, the population has probably more than doubled, and in parts of the tribal area there is considerable pressure on the land, as the population density is more than 300 per square mile, the soil poor, and techniques very simple. The main economic activity is subsistence farming, most of the work being done by the married women. Most of the men who are able to obtain jobs outside the tribal area go out to work, leaving their wives and families at home to work their land. The men return in middle age or when unable to obtain employment, to work their land and herd their cattle.

There are two forms of social organization and two ways of categorizing the universe for the Luo today. There is the traditional system of social organization, religion, values, and ideas, and there is the system that has been imposed by the British administrators and missionaries. Behavior in any situation is conditioned by compromise between these two systems and can usually be understood only by reference to both. In the two cases examined in detail here, the interaction of the two systems and the conflict of values involved are illustrated. In each case, the patient suffered a minor physical disorder, which developed into a

* This paper was produced under the auspices of the East African Institute of Social Research, Makerere University College, with the aid of grants from the Christian Council of Kenya, the Anthony Wilkins Scholarship Fund of Cambridge University, and the Goldsmiths' Company of London.

serious functional disorder. The division between organic and functional disorders is one that is not clearly made in Luo categories of thought, and, in order to explain the cases described, these categories and beliefs must be clarified.

§ The Traditional Approach to Disease

The Luo tribe believes itself descended from a single ancestor, and all the social groups within the tribe think of themselves as the descendants in the male line of one ancestor or ancestress. The tribe is divided into about twenty subtribes, most of which have one dominant group and a number of smaller groups, which live with the dominant group for mutual support. Marriage within the group is forbidden but may take place between different groups within the subtribe and between members of different subtribes. At marriage, a girl traditionally went to live in her husband's homestead, often several miles from her own home.

Homesteads belonging to one group were usually grouped close together along a ridge or round a hill. Members of the group might invite friends, in-laws, or refugees from intersubtribal wars to join them, however, and in some places, homesteads belonging to different groups might be mixed. The group that first occupied the ridge was considered to be the owner of the land, and those who came later were its tenants. Tenants could be ordered to leave their homesteads at any time, but numbers were an advantage for the defense of the ridge.

The homestead was the most important unit of the whole social organization. The owner lived with his wives, his sons, their wives and children, and his own unmarried daughters. A man would build his own home only when he had adult sons who would be able to help him to defend it. A man might also have other relations in his homestead— a mother, brother, or in-law—or a tenant. Within the homestead, the owner had complete authority, although each woman had rights over some of the cattle, which formed the major part of the wealth of the homestead. The owner distributed the land attached to the homestead to the women for their use, and the sons of each woman would inherit from their mother. Each woman had her own house in the homestead, which formed the focal point of the group made up of herself and her children. She had her own granaries, and all the produce from her plots of land was hers alone. The wives of the owner were considered to be in competition for his favors and for the patrimony over which he had final rights of disposal. Full brothers were considered to be united in all that they did and opposed as a group to the sons of other women in the homestead. When a group divided and its parts fought, the quarrel was frequently described in terms of conflict between the descendants of cowives.

Disputes within the group on the ridge would be settled by the owners of the homesteads concerned and the senior man of the group. In a dispute demanding the detection of an offender—suspicion of theft or witchcraft—a diviner (*ajuoga*) would be called in to assist. Disputes between groups within the subtribe might be mediated or arbitrated by a respected leader who usually came from a large group and who usually possessed magical power to support his decisions. Disputes between subtribes were resolved by fighting unless influential men on both sides could arrange an agreement. Such men would have wives from the families of influential men in the opposing subtribes. Magical power and political power tended to go together, and an influential man was believed to have supernatural power to influence people and to attack those who crossed him. An "attack" of this sort would take the form of disease, and the disease could only be cured by neutralizing the magical cause.

The complex of ideas concerning religion and magic was bound up with that concerning the causation of disease. There were several forms that supernatural power might take. The powers were not clearly ranked, with one supreme and the others gaining their force through delegation. With respect to disease, they may best be understood as a set of tools for doing a number of jobs. Some powers were regularly associated with certain manifestations of sickness, but any might, in the last resort, be the cause of any sickness. Religious ideas were not invoked to defend a theological position but in order to explain a situation and to indicate the correct course of action to remedy it.

God, the creator of the world (*nyasaye*) also created the other powers but did not control them. Widespread epidemics, famines, and droughts were associated with His power. He might be propitiated by prayer and sacrifice but was not subject to the influence of individuals in the way in which the other powers might be influenced. If all means had failed in an attempt to cure a patient, the diviner and the elders would suggest that the illness was the work of God and must be accepted. If the patient were violent, he might be restrained with ropes, but he would be fed and treated as kindly as possible. It was feared that, if he died, his spirit would return to possess any one who had ill-treated him and cause them to suffer in the same way.

Some men claimed to be able to cure violent lunatics (*joneko*). The victim would be tied up for several weeks, and the practitioner would produce worms, which he claimed to have extracted from the head of the patient through his nose. The patient would be given various herbs and roots and often severely beaten. Some, suffering from cerebral malaria, would recover and thus enhance the reputation of the practitioner. It was not thought possible to cure a violent lunatic permanently, however, although some men, using the described method or that for the treatment of spirit possession, claimed to be able to do so. If a man was obviously mad but not violent, various causes and treatments to be described later would be suggested and tried, and if he did not respond, God was named as the cause of the madness. The patient would then be left to roam about. He would be treated kindly, fed, and given work to do if he could do it.

The ancestral spirits might also bring disease to their descendants. The diviner might ascribe disease to the spirits' anger at the patient's breaking a taboo or neglecting a ritual or merely to their desire for attention in the form of a sacrifice. Any condition caused by ritual impurity was called *chira*. If a child was born feet first, deformed, or albino he was *chira*—caused by ritual impurity. If a man lost weight rapidly and became too weak to move, his condition might be ascribed to his failure to bury a relation properly, thus bringing about *chira*. Such diseases might take any form from tuberculosis to hallucinations—the term used described the supernatural cause, not the signs or symptoms. The cure could only be completed if the supernatural cause was divined and dealt with. The organic condition might be treated with roots or herbs or might cure itself, but the cure would be ascribed to the intervention of the ancestral spirits and the removal of the ritual impurity that had brought about the disease. Ancestral spirits were often thought to hover around the homesteads of their descendants, appearing in dreams to ask favors of the living or to warn them of danger. Disease was the sanction to force the living to maintain proper relations with the dead.

While the intervention of the ancestors might be capricious, the diseases ascribed to them or to God were usually felt to be punishments for the sins of the patients or their families. A man who broke a tribal rule might expect to be punished for it by the ancestors or by God in the form of disease. Any man attacked by disease therefore would feel obliged to examine himself and his relationships with the ancestors. A very minor organic disorder—like several days of constipation—might create a considerable overlay of fear or guilt and reduce the patient to

helplessness until the rituals were performed and the ancestors propitiated according to the traditions of the society and the directions of
the diviner.

The Luo also believed in a class of spirits that were not ancestral
but that sprang directly from God. These spirits (*juogi*) were not subject
to God, however. They were free to roam the world, although they were
usually associated with natural phenomena of some sort. One group was
associated with the islands in Lake Victoria, one with a species of euphor-
bia tree, another with the lakes and rivers other than Lake Victoria,
another with the sun, another with a mythical water snake, and another
with a tribe that was very fierce in war. For each group of spirits, there
was a special group of practitioners who would be able to cure all those
attacked by spirits in that particular group. A practitioner was always
supposed to be able to tell if a patient was suffering from the same
spirits as possessed him, but if he failed to cure the patient, then he
could claim that two spirits were present, only one of which was subject
to his influence.

The disease of spirit possession (*juogi*) came into a category quite
separate from that of *chira* or those ascribed to witchcraft and sorcery.
The patient usually had a feeling of general ill-being rather than specific
pains and had failed to respond to other forms of treatment. The practitioner could only deal with the spirits if he had been possessed by them
himself and had himself been cured previously. After attending a large
number of cases with the practitioner who cured him, the former patient
might find that he himself had the power to cure others. As long as a
practitioner lived, the people whom he cured, whether they were practitioners themselves or not, would maintain close relationships of friendship
and dependence with him. A former patient would describe the man who
cured him as "the father of my spirits."

The patient might go to the practitioner by himself—guided by the
spirits, according to the beliefs related to his problems. There he would
stay for a number of months for treatment and return to his home when
cured and when sufficient payment had been made by his homestead
to satisfy the practitioner. The practitioner might also be called to the
homestead of the patient, where he would recognize "his" spirits and
take the patient away. The case of Ann, to be described later, is typical.

The attacks of the spirits of possession are said to be entirely capricious, but as the case analysis illustrates, such is far from being true. Social
causes of primarily functional disorders are recognized by the practitioners and made explicit in terms that the members of the homesteads

can understand. The organic origins of a disorder, if any, are not recognized explicitly by the practitioner; responsibility for the disorder is laid upon the spirits, and the cure is effected by their being brought under control. They are not expelled but remain with the patient forever.

Disease might also be caused by sorcery and witchcraft. Minor ailments like stomach ache after a heavy meal might be ascribed to a woman with an evil eye who had looked at the patient while he was eating. The diviner might designate the person who had made the patient sick. The accused would deny knowledge of having attacked the patient and declare that, if he was indeed responsible, then all evil would be removed from the patient. If he did not wish the patient well, and the patient did not recover quickly, he might be blamed more seriously and counteraction with magic taken against him. The diviner would also make small cuts on the body at the point paining the patient, place a horn over the cuts, suck and produce some half-digested food from his mouth, which, he would claim, he had sucked from the body of the patient.

Witchcraft accusations of this sort were frequently made within the homestead between cowives and particularly against those who had no children. It was believed that a witch would not give birth unless she were married to a witch. Witchcraft was also said to be inherited. Since marriage took a woman into the homestead of her husband's family and no man would ever admit responsibility for a union being sterile or that he was a witch, blame was almost invariably attached to the woman.

More serious disease might be caused by magic or sorcery. Over a number of years, a man might build up a reputation for having bought or otherwise acquired the power to kill his enemies by magic (*bilo*). He might also be spirit-possessed (*jajuogi*), but the two forms of power were not necessarily associated. He was able both to cure and to cause disease, and he might trade openly in medicine and clandestinely in magical or real poisons.

The accusation of sorcery and attribution of a disease to sorcery were made by the diviner, but factors other than chance might lead him to this particular diagnosis. The sudden collapse of a patient, be it physical or mental, would be ascribed to magical or real poison. If the patient was known to have aroused the enmity of a well known sorcerer or a person known to consort with sorcerers, the obvious conclusion would be drawn. If the patient or members of his household had seen offensive and strange objects about the place shortly before the patient became sick, the cause of the disease would then be known, and counter-measures could be taken even if the identity of the person causing the attack was uncertain. An offensive object could be located by a skilled practitioner and sent back to its original owner. Until the cause was ascertained, however, the patient could not recover, and experiments might be tried to locate the supernatural source of the trouble before it killed the patient.

Those who lived by sorcery were expected to die by sorcery, although the strongest practitioners would claim that they could only be killed by poison and not by man-directed supernatural forces. Their craft, despite the work of healing that they did, was considered to be generally evil.

These elements then were the possible causes of disease, whether mental or physical. Hallucinations were attributed to spirits of possession or, more often, to spirits of the dead who came in various guises to attack those who had caused their deaths or neglected ritual duties. Depression was considered to be the work of spirits of possession, as were hysteria and cerebral malaria. There were some categorizations according to signs or symptoms, as has been indicated, but for the most part the categorization of disease was in terms of the causal agency.

In contrast to common belief in the West, organic disorders were considered to have supernatural or mental origins. The Luo sought the motive and social causes of all disorders, rather than the organic causes for which their scientific knowledge ill equipped them. As a consequence, their appreciation of social causation and their ability to cope with functional disease was probably well developed. Within a simple society, the number of possible social causes of functional disease are low, compared with those in a complex Western society. A man experienced in his simple society and intelligent enough to observe or learn certain correlations between social disorders and individual complaints of sickness could well predict a course of events and so gain a reputation for supernatural knowledge and power.

§ The Impact of Western Medicine

This system of ideas has been in close contact with Western ideas, as represented by missionaries and British administrators, for most of the present century. The missionaries, through their preaching and their schools, have attempted to demolish the old system of ideas and to replace it with Western theories of causation. Few, if any, of the tribe have escaped these theories completely, although most still maintain faith in some of the traditional practices, especially those relating to spirit possession. An experienced missionary doctor observed, "There are some things which they know we cannot cure." The organic disorder may be diagnosed and treated, but the patient does not feel well until he has passed through the costly course of treatment described in the cases later in this paper.

With conflicting systems of ideas have come organizational changes that have encouraged acceptance of new ideas. The tribal wars and free movements of individuals and groups have been stopped, and a man may be forced to live close to an unpleasant neighbor because he cannot get land elsewhere. Large numbers of active men have been forced out of the tribal area to obtain work to pay for taxes, clothes, and school fees. Hospitals and dispensaries form a thin network over the entire area, providing medical treatment at small cost to the people. Outside the two hospitals, there is only one doctor for about 600,000 people, however, and subordinate staff rarely have more than eight years of formal education and three or four years of training. There is no psychiatrist with intimate knowledge of tribal ideas of disease causation and contributory social factors.

The members of the tribe have tended to accept the medical services as an addition to their resources for coping with all forms of disease, rather than as a substitute for the old methods. When a person is sick, a number of factors determines the course of action to be followed in his behalf. The distance from his homestead to the nearest shop that sells patent medicine, the dispensary, or the local expert in native herbs will be considered. The cost of each is a consideration—in cash for the first two and possibly also in kind for the last. The seriousness of the complaint will be considered and also the opinions of the patient and those in the homestead as to which of the agencies is likely to be most successful. Dispensaries are known to be successful with cuts, ulcerated wounds, malaria, constipation, and diarrhea under most circumstances. Vague but sustained feelings of sickness cannot be cured by them, however, and the diviner or spirit-possessed practitioner may then be called in.

In a case in which the patient suffers for a long period, a number of agencies may be tried. The local herbal cure may be tried, followed by a patent pill from the shop. The dispensary or hospital may also be visited, and finally the patient may be handed over to the spirit-possessed, who, under such circumstances, are said to fail very rarely and thus prove themselves better than the dispensary.

§ The Cases of William and Ann

In the two cases that follow, the Luo categories place the patients quite separately. William was suffering from sorcery carried through objects that had been cursed and placed in his home by human enemies. Ann was suffering from attacks by spirits. According to Western categories, both patients were suffering from mental overlay from organic ills —although in Ann's case it might have been argued that she was suffering only from a mental disturbance following her miscarriage.

The cases illustrate the manner in which various agencies are brought to bear to cure disease that is clearly partly of physical and partly of mental origin. They also illustrate the social background that may be used by the patient and the diviner to establish the reasons for the attack and the identity of the powers or persons involved.

William was born about 1928 and, after receiving his early schooling near his home, spent three years in a mission boarding school. He returned to his home in 1947, where he taught for one year as an untrained teacher before returning to his studies in a mission teacher-training college, where he spent two years. He then returned to his home area to teach once more, but because of his high qualifications, compared with those of the people around him, he received a much higher income than they. He felt that during his years at school and college, he had outgrown all superstitious fancies like belief in magical power and that he was a Christian. He had, however, spent his early years sleeping in his grandmother's house and knew from her teaching all about the Luo supernatural powers. He had also, in his early life, seen many troubles ascribed to them, especially in relation to the highly complicated situation in which he now found himself.

He lived close to the boundary of his subtribal area at a place where there are several groups living together and a shortage of land. Four groups were relevant to the situation. "A" is the largest group in the area and claims to be the original settler, so that all land belongs to it. "B," another large group is linked to "A" through a woman many generations back. "A" and "B" may marry members of one another. "C," to which William belongs, is a small group linked to "A" by the marriage of its founder to a girl from "A." "A" 's members consider "C" 's members to be their tenants, although both groups arrived in the area at the same time. Because of its slow growth and migrations from the area due to the dispute to be described, "C" has the greatest area of land per head of its members. "D" is very small and new to the area but has as its leader a most powerful magician, whose trade has brought him great wealth in women and stock, for which he requires land. He and his group have very little land.

In 1935, William's sister married Fred, the magician from "D," and Fred had been lent some land on the border of his land and that of "C." Land was not scarce at that time, and custom demanded that Fred's request should not be refused. Later the woman left Fred and married elsewhere, but Fred kept the land, as he claimed that the brideprice had not been repaid. Although it was against custom, he defeated William in a court case and kept the land. In other land disputes between "C" and "D," Fred was said to have killed two men from "C" with magic in 1935 and 1942. In 1945 there was a serious fight between Fred and five men (three from "C" and two from "A") in which Fred was badly hurt. He hired a lawyer. When the case was heard, three of the men were imprisoned for five years each and two for two years each, and several men from "C," fearing Fred's power in all directions, left the area with their families, leaving the land to William and two of his cousins, who thus gained large pieces.

William had done well at school and college, despite having a very volatile temperament, and had settled down to become a popular teacher. At that time no member of "A," on whose land the school was built, was doing particularly well academically, and the headmaster belonged to "B." Oscar, the son of Henry, who had founded the school, was an untrained teacher on the staff. Henry had retired as he was overtaken in educational attainments by most of his former pupils.

William had started to pay cattle for a close cousin of his headmaster when a dispute broke out between the headmaster and Oscar. According to kinship relationships, William should have supported "A" against "B," but instead he supported his headmaster and "B." There was a great deal of ill feeling on both sides.

While he was paying for his wife, William also began to build a large house, for she was well educated by the standards at that time and very beautiful to a Luo. One of his cousins, who had been released from prison shortly before, also wanted to marry. He had a difference of opinion with William as to how the cattle received for two girls of their group who had recently married should be shared between them. William neither smoked nor drank and lived at home and was therefore in a good position to save. As the people believed that the school fees went straight into the teachers' pockets, however, some resented his obvious prosperity, apparently at their expense.

Early in 1952 when all these tensions existed for him, he found some birds' wings in his home and later a dirty piece of cloth with something wrapped inside it. He did not open it as he was afraid of what it might contain. When his new house was ready, he went to sleep in it, but after a few weeks he became sick. The only sign was a swelling under the right big toe, which became an abscess. This type of abscess is known as *tong juok* in the vernacular—the witch's egg. It was treated by one of the women married into his homestead, who beat some leaves to pulp and spread them with a cobweb over the sore place. The swelling did not respond to the treatment, and he began to ache all over so that he could not sleep.

After five days, he was taken to the hospital attached to his old mission school more than thirty miles away, where he was admitted. Being a relatively wealthy man, he ignored the local dispensary. After a day, the abscess was incised and pus removed. The following day, his joints were aching, and he still had a high temperature. On the sixth day, his temperature was normal, and, on the eighth day, he was discharged. The hospital noted that his general condition took longer than usual to improve, although the abscess cleared quickly, and that in his subsequent history there was a large overlay of fear and almost terror of spirit possession.

The official records do not include all that appears to have happened in the hospital, however. He felt no improvement after the incision had been made, and, after a few days during which he claims to have become too weak to sit up or to eat, his uncle and a notorious magician, who was a grandson of a close female cousin of his, came to see him. They brought him some medicine, which they gave him—*manyasi*, for purification from evil. A quarter of an hour later, he felt as if everything were spinning round in the room, and, when it stopped, he felt much better and was able to eat. Two days later, he was allowed to leave the hospital, and his sister took him home to his own house again. It may be noted that, at the time when he claims to have been at his lowest ebb, the physical disorder had been completely cleared up.

The morning after he reached home, he felt very sick again, and the magician was called. He was taken to his grandmother's hut. The magician crushed some leaves and boiled them in a pot. William was put under a blanket and the covered pot put under it with him. The top was removed, and the steam rose into the blanket. He began to sweat freely and felt as if coils of rope were being unwound from his body and limbs. The magician gave him medicine to drink and sprinkled the house with more medicine to destroy any remaining magic. Cuts were then made on his hands and feet, and *bilo* (magical powder, the main constituent of which is usually leaf ash, which contains much salt) was rubbed into the cuts, which made them sting.

The magician stated that Henry, the founder of the school, had been responsible for the magic in the home and warned William to be very kind and tactful in his future dealings with him. He said that the magic used was so strong that it would have killed a bad man who tried to use magical protection, but, since William's blood was completely innocent, it could not kill him. Black magic will not destroy a man whose heart is completely pure.

The treatment was repeated on several further occasions, in the mornings and evenings, according to the prescription of the magician. William was able to return to his house but felt afraid, so a cousin and his sister stayed with him for a week. He did not know exactly what might happen but thought that the man who had originally brought the magic might return.

When he had left the hospital, he had been given a certificate by the doctor to enable him to rest and regain the weight that he had lost, and he remained at home for some time before returning to the same school to teach until the end of the academic year. He had been in the hospital from June 18 to 25 and completed the year to December. He was then transferred, at his own request, to a school some miles away, on the grounds that he wished to have more time to study, which he could only get by being away from home.

Since then, he has not taken any native medicine and states that magic cannot harm him now. He has fought and lost a land case against Fred against the advice of his group, who feared that they might all be attacked again. He has fought and won a land case against a man in "A." He married the girl from "B," and she lives with their five children in the house that he built in 1952.

In this case, it may be noted, the social situation was ripe for someone to claim to be attacked by magic—if he fell sick. The history was full of group tensions and accusations of witchcraft or magical poisoning, and William had gained for himself a position of wealth and influence for which his age alone did not qualify him. All the teaching that he had had at the mission proved to be no defense in the moment when he was forced to choose between the natural and the supernatural explanations of his condition. The costs of the hospital were probably no more than $7 for his entire stay there; the old lady who treated him originally probably received no more than the equivalent of a quarter. The magician was given cattle and cash to the value of $70, which was the equivalent of three months' salary for William at that time.

The treatment that the magician provided for William included all the different things that could be done for him. He was given solids to eat, liquids to drink, a steam bath, and medicine through the skin, and his house was sprinkled. Nothing was left to chance; every known method of treatment was used. The prevalence of this attitude toward treatment is illustrated by the many people who go to the dispensaries and demand an injection, in the belief that without one, all that is possible has not been done for them.

The second case to be described here is fairly typical of one of the most common forms of Luo mental disturbance, especially among women, today. It appears as a form of hysteria and is very largely conditioned by social factors. A woman marries away from her own home and, in her husband's home, finds herself in opposition socially and economically to the other women there. In the present situation of land hunger in some places, it may be a real sacrifice for her mother-in-law to give her land to cultivate, as by custom she must. If she produces a son quickly, she will be accepted into the home and will probably have few problems. If she has trouble in childbirth or does not bear a son for several years, she will be considered more of a liability than an asset, and the tensions inherent in the situation may increase until they are unbearable. The situation may be ameliorated by her husband, who can help to smooth relations between his wife and the wives of his father and brothers. Many young men do not remain at home during this period, however, but go to work in the towns outside the tribal area, returning home for only a short time each year. Through employment in the towns, a situation may arise in which one man may earn far more than his brothers. One may earn the equivalent of $140 a month, another about $23, and another no more than he can get from his few acres of exhausted land. Their wives, in adjacent huts in one homestead, may therefore be living at very different standards, even allowing for the help given by the richer brother to the poorer ones for taxes and school fees.

The women are also responsible for the maintenance of the family in a way that the men are not. No matter what natural disasters of flood, drought, pests, or sickness may afflict the lands and the family, the woman is expected to produce enough food for her family, while her husband looks after himself in the town and sends home what he considers necessary for clothes, school fees, and other *ad hoc* expenses that the wife may incur. If he loses his job, his wife is expected to keep him in food as well, with but a small contribution from him to the labor of the home in many cases. Escapes from the endless round of work are few for her. Some drink locally distilled spirits as soon as they can afford to buy or make them. Some turn to the churches, which provide release in the form of possession-dancing. Some join churches that lay great stress upon open confession and, in their weekly testimonies, tell their stories of hardship and tension to the others in the church. The fellow-ship of the churches provides a new common-interest group, within which the members are not usually in competition. Such activities maintain the majority of women in good mental health.

Those who do not join in such activities and who fail to conform to the ideal of producing children find themselves surrounded by tensions that may become too much for them. They may also suffer from inability to produce enough food to maintain themselves in good physical con-dition.

When she falls sick, a woman expects to recover completely within a certain period of time—as most people recover from malaria and other common disorders. If she fails to respond to treatment, doubts im-mediately arise about the true cause of her complaint. The categories that she uses in her thinking are not those of different organic disorders but of classes of supernatural causation. Natural causation may be ac-cepted but only for short periods for many women—and then only as an addition to the possible causes rather than as a substitute for super-natural causes. A mental breakdown may follow if she has no strong religious forces from her church to sustain her. As in cases where magic is blamed for man's inability to cope with his situation, there is nearly always a history of physical disorder before mental disorder in a case of a person said to be possessed by the spirits.

We may now consider a case of spirit possession (*juogi*). Ann was married in February, 1960, and went almost at once to stay with her husband, who was a male nurse in a coast town 550 miles from her home and about 4000 feet below the altitude at which she had been reared. In June, she began to suffer from pains in the head, chest, and stomach and thought that she had malaria. She was taken to the hospital for a short time and then discharged as, she claimed, they were unable to find anything wrong with her and told her she was malingering. At about this time, she had a miscarriage. (William had claimed that the hospital could find nothing wrong with him, but the records showed that he had, in fact, been diagnosed, treated, and physically cured). The pains continued until she was unable to move. The members of her church came and prayed for her, and she felt a little better but after a few days began to have shouting fits and to run wildly in the streets. Her husband said that the Pentecostalists had prayed for her—some of the groups in that area lay great stress upon spiritual healing. She believed that they were from her own Episcopalian church.

In July, her husband, unable to keep constant watch over her, sent her to his home. She could remember nothing of the journey except that she had consumed only one cup of tea on the three-day train journey from Mombasa to Kisumu. When she reached her husband's home, her parents-in-law immediately sent for an expert in dealing with spirits (*juogi*) who lived about eight miles away. The expert diagnosed the trouble at once and took Ann to her home. She could remember nothing about how she was able to walk those eight miles.

The family said that the divination was performed with the aid of a speaking gourd. The gourd is partly filled with small seeds, and the expert sits with her back to the person consulting it. The expert shakes the gourd and asks it questions, to which it replies in a gruff voice. The gourd is also used as a rhythm instrument to stimulate dancing until the dancers begin to shake at the shoulders in spasms, speak "in tongues" (gibber) and become "possessed by the spirits." While the gourd was being consulted, Ann began to perform in this way, which proved that her spirits were in sympathy with that in the gourd, and her parents-in-law paid a small amount to the expert.

Only Ann went to the expert's home, and she remembers only danc-ing a little there but no more. The following day she felt better and two days later felt completely restored. She remained there, however, until November 24, when she was brought back to her husband's home by the expert and some other possessed people. The other people had been treated by the expert in the past and had their spirits under control. She said that, while she had been with the expert, she had been treated kindly, given medicine, and washed daily in water treated with medicine. She said that she could have been brought home earlier, but her husband was in Mombasa, and the cost of the treatment had to be met before she was brought home. After two goats (value about $7), one heifer (about $23), and about $22 in cash had been paid to the expert, she was brought back. She was dressed in a plain dress, over which she wore large shells and iron bells. A creeping plant with strong fertility associations was tied round her. Her face was painted white in the manner of mourners at a funeral. She carried a paddle in her

hand—in memory of a celebrated healer of the possessed who was said
to have used a paddle when he rode round Lake Victoria on the back
of a water snake.

When the returning party reached the entrance of the home, about
50 cents and a chicken (value about 60 cents) had to be given to the
expert before she would allow Ann to enter. Before she could enter the
hut of her mother-in-law, another 50 cents were paid. After still another
50 cents were paid, they began to dance to the rattles and a drum. The
form of dancing was one common to many Luo situations. Dancing at
weddings and funerals, by the supporters of the winning side at football
matches, and by certain of the independent churches during their services is of this type. The body is very relaxed, swinging gently in time
with the rhythmic shuffling of the feet. The dancing was interrupted
occasionally either by the expert's or by Ann's becoming possessed, shaking violently at the shoulders, leaping with the body stiffened, and
shouting as if deliberately exaggerating a belch. This performance continued, with breaks for meals and certain ceremonies, from about
five P.M. on the 24th until about noon on the 26th. They did not sleep
at all on the night of the 24th but took about seven hours rest on the
night of the 25th.

In the morning of the 25th, all the women changed their clothes, and
Ann was dressed with a new creeper and banana leaves. After a little
more dancing, a goat was brought in and held still until it passed water
and a few droppings, after which it was kicked and butted by Ann to
"get the devils out of it." It was then made to walk three times round
Ann as she sat on the floor of the hut (three has a fertility symbolism
for females in Luo rituals). It was then held down and killed with a
knife. Parallel cuts were made on either side of the windpipe, and the
jugular pierced. The blood was caught in a bowl. A strip of skin was
then removed from the beard to the testes—the need for which was
given as the reason for the unusual way of slaughtering the goat—and
this skin was placed over Ann's head. Throughout the whole day, there
were continual arguments about money, and the expert and her friends
demanded more beer at every opportunity, explaining that it was needed
to keep away the devils or declaring that they had had nothing to eat
or drink for a very long time.

The meat of the goat was divided. The right foreleg was placed at
the back of the hut for the devils—and the people of the home ate it
after the devils were judged to have had their share. The left foreleg
and the better half of the meat were put with the best of the entrails

for the expert and her possessed friends. Before they were divided, the entrails were read by a possessed man, who explained that Ann had been suffering from constipation; that the Revivalists in the home quarreled with the other people there and they misunderstood each other; and that a young girl had been buried in the homestead.

Constipation is probably the most common Luo ailment, as the flour used for food is often not boiled sufficiently for it to be broken down into digestible starch. The Revivalists try to minimize their dealings with non-Revivalists and refuse to follow customary rituals for the prevention of misfortune; they are therefore usually in a state of tension with the heathen members of the home. A nubile girl should not be buried in the home of her father. If she has not married, special rituals should be performed and her body buried just outside the homestead to prevent her spirit from bringing sterility to the other girls in the homestead. This rule was of importance in Ann's case, which had really begun with her miscarriage.

After a meal of the meat of the goat, the expert inflated its rectum and treated the ends with magic powder. She tied it round Ann's neck with the words, "May you swell up like the rectum of this goat"—meaning that she should become pregnant. Ann then ate some of the medicine, and the expert spat some over her.

They then left the hut and started dancing outside. Ann next had her head shaved. This ritual cuts people off from their pasts—it is performed at the end of a funeral, and after it the wives of the dead man may be inherited. Money was demanded for this work, and the family was told that, if it was not paid, Ann would not be able to stand up. Later she said that, although she did not know what was holding her down, she was unable to get up until the money had been accepted by the expert.

Ann and her husband then had to beat each other—he first beat her and then ran away while she chased him to beat him. This ceremony was to ensure that she would not run away if he beat her in the future and is also performed in the marriage ceremonies. Much of the ritual performed came from the marriage ceremonies, with the expert taking the part of Ann's parents—who receive large gifts at the marriage of their daughter.

These events occupied about four hours between ten A.M. and two P.M. on the 25th. The group then began to eat again, feeding Ann as if she were a small child. Despite her lack of sleep, she now appeared to be happier and more relaxed than she had been when she first arrived in the homestead. After their meal, they all ran into the nearby gardens "to show her where they are" and then returned to dance. More food was brought for them, and they complained that they were being given very little, although in fact they ate a great deal, until their stomachs swelled visibly.

Ann was then taught how to do all the duties of the home—in the form of a charade. She was shown how to dig, pick vegetables, gather wood, fetch water, grind, and cook. If she were not taught how to do these things by the expert, it was said, the spirits would not allow her to do them in the future. A price was demanded for all the lessons. She was then told to clean out her husband's house, which she did. The party then moved into that hut, and medicine was placed there to ensure that Ann would not be troubled while she was there. Some more visitors arrived, swelling the number of the possessed to about twelve. The number varied between six and twelve throughout the ceremonies. Two men and three women, including the expert, remained there all the time.

They continued to eat and dance, with a break to tell of the spirit that possessed Ann. It was Sumba, which comes from the islands in Lake Victoria inhabited by Bantu fishing folk, who are supposed to have magical power to resist the malaria and sleeping sickness that are endemic there. The party broke up about midnight.

On the morning of the 26th, the group assembled for food in Ann's house, where a fire was lit in a pot and some millet stems burned in it over her head. Ann was then told by the expert that she must always obey her husband, be respectful and obedient to the older people in the home, and obey the rules of *juogi*—her spirits. These rules include certain food taboos, dress taboos, and rules of behavior. She was given medicine to keep evil spirits away from her house. The instructions were given added weight by the expert's cuffing Ann about the head with her fingerless hands (she was a leper from her youth) for entering a house without permission. In this context, the entering of a house had double significance. If a woman enters the house of her mother-in-law without permission—especially the sleeping side—the older woman will not bear again. If Ann broke the rule, she would be attacked by the spirits again.

Small cuts were then made on her body, between her breasts, behind her neck, and on her shoulders, hands, and feet. Medicine was rubbed into the cuts, and the expert chanted, "We worship the spirits because God gave them to us." A white hen was put on Ann's head and told to leave the house—which it did. The chicks that it produced would have the spirits that had troubled Ann. They all danced while the expert sang a song telling how the spirits had come from the lake and how she had cured twenty people. She then demanded that she should be given small amounts of every kind of food that was eaten in the home to take away with her. All members of the home were ordered to dance, as they should be happy when the spirit-possessed leave them, and more food was demanded to help the latter on their journey. While they ate, they argued about how much more money was due to the expert, and Ann was warned to wear the articles that she was given for the rest of her life. They were goatskin finger stools, shells, and a bracelet of cowrie shells. She was also given a list of things that she should not do without the expert's permission and told to come for more medicine to the home of the expert—for which she would have to pay. She had to have permission to eat new crops, to take her child out of the house when it was born (customarily on the third day after the birth of a girl and on the fourth day for a boy), to travel on any vehicle, and to go more than a short distance from the home.

They then left the home, taking with them all that had been used by them or for them during their stay in the home—pots, a broom, cups, plates, and spoons. While the items were being collected, Ann began to shake and gibber again, and everything had to stop once more, while all the people in the home danced—until the expert got annoyed and told Ann to stop, which she did after a few more moments. According to her husband, the total cost in cash and kind amounted to between $125 and $140. According to Ann, the value of all the items was about $105.

On December 15, we went to talk to Ann in her home. She was happy, relaxed, and quite prepared to talk about what had happened. She was able to recount what had been done with remarkable accuracy, and her powers of memory and perception had obviously not been affected by the ordeals through which she had gone. She said that she had not been unhappy in Mombasa but had found life rather lonely there, as there were few women who could converse with her in her own language. The obvious cause of the trouble in the first instance had been her miscarriage. Her mother's mother and her mother's sister had both been attacked by *juogi* in the past, which meant that she knew all the behavior expected of her. About six months later, she returned to Mombasa and seemed to be in good health and spirits.

The pattern followed by most treatments conforms to this one, and the case histories obtained have had several similarities. Stomach pains are usually the first indication that there will be an attack. These pains may be caused by constipation, by difficulties related to childbirth, or by general nervousness, which frequently shows itself in stomach pains and feelings of ill-being. Malaria is endemic in the area and can produce a feeling of general debility. The one serious case of depression that I observed was treated as one of spirit-possession, the parents of the affected girl refusing to allow her to be taken to the hospital. She was taken to two experts over a period of two years, but neither was successful in her efforts. The popular diagnosis was that the spirits were too strong for the experts, and the girl died. No medical examination was possible, and the patient would not speak. The case was considered very unusual by the people around her.

The experts in *juogi* are only called in as a last resort, for their fees are high—up to about $187 for a treatment that may not effect a permanent cure. They also remove the patient from her home and thus deprive it of her labor, while demanding that the home should provide her food while she is being treated. The time that the patient spends in the home of the expert varies, but in the cases studied in detail they have remained for periods of up to a year. The reason given for this long stay is that the price of the cure has to be raised by the family, and the patient does not come home until a large part of this price has been paid. During the time that she is in the home of the expert, the patient is cut off from the social situation that may have caused the disorder, and a long stay may be beneficial to her. With the expert, the patient is given rest and good treatment and allowed to work in the gardens as she likes—instead of being responsible for a family or possibly for in-laws who seek to take advantage of her efforts to prove herself a good wife and asset to the home.

The experts themselves are obviously key people in the system and, in dealing with the patients, have the advantage of having suffered from the same trouble themselves and brought it under control. The expert has a bond of sympathy with the patient, which is expressed by the terms for parent and child used between them and in their shared experiences. When the patient begins to gibber and shake, the expert may do so too. The two remain friends for the rest of their lives, and the expert will teach the promising patient how to treat others.

The treatment itself also has real therapeutic value. When she first enters the expert's home, the patient may be forced to dance to the point of exhaustion, at which point she may become highly suggestible. Later, the taboos, the dress, and the need to keep in contact with the expert help to build a supernatural wall around the patient and make the other women in her home a little wary of her. She has something that others, possibly better adapted to the homestead in which she lives, have not. The repeated warnings to the patient and to the members of her home that they must maintain good and harmonious relations by behaving in a correct and charitable manner underline the importance of social factors in maintaining the mental health of the patient. All this behavior is sanctioned by the threat that another attack may be made by the spirits if the taboos are not observed. The taboos are not arduous, however, serving more to advertise the fact that the patient has been possessed and that she must therefore be well treated.

The rituals that are performed are also important. The patient and the others in the home know from experience that, in other cases in which the rituals have been followed, the patient has recovered, and their performance is appreciated as being necessary if the patient is going to recover. They form an important part of her expectations for recovery. In one observed case, the people of the home reminded the expert that he had forgotten some parts of the ritual.

In the rituals, nothing is left to chance. Every method of treatment that can be used on the patient is used. Even if there is some doubt about what is wrong, if all treatments are tried, the patient must be cured. Ann was washed with treated water at the home of the expert, she was given liquids and solids, she was cut and powder rubbed in, a sacrifice was made, danger was passed from her to the chicken, and her head was shaved. This behavior conforms to the categories used in the Luo analysis of disease. The original specific cause of concern to the patient —her miscarriage and doubts about her fertility—was also ritually exposed and dealt with in the ceremony with the rectum of the goat.

The patient continues to shake, gibber, and drum or rattle for the rest of her life. This behavior reminds the people around her of her condition and provides her with an exhilarating escape from the endless round of work that is her lot as a married woman. She is also ritually joined to the group of the possessed, sharing in the feasts and the dancing that accompany the return of a patient to her home. She may gain the status of an expert to compensate her for her failure to make a satisfactory adjustment to her home and to give her confidence in herself.

There is some indication that heredity plays a part in the condition of the spirit-possessed—most cases studied have had close relatives who have been attacked, but this factor may be primarily environmental, as the patient grows up to fear and possibly to expect an attack. A nephew of one expert dreamed that he would be attacked one day and so become

a healer as famous as his uncle—and subsequently exhibited signs of
mental instability.

A most important factor in the healing process is that the treatment
is given in clearly explicable terms. The healer, in his role as a psychiatrist, explains the cause of the trouble in animistic terms that are readily
understood by a patient who has grown up in a world peopled by such
spirits. The psychiatrist working within a frame of reference that excludes spirits would have great difficulty in curing any patient who
believed himself attacked. This problem lies at the root of many that
doctors have faced in dealing with such conditions in the tribal situation,
particularly those doctors who have strong religious views. Those who
become practitioners vary considerably, but all have the confidence of
the majority of people in their powers to heal. Where sorcery is diagnosed,
the practitioners are usually old men with strong personalities, often
with reputations for having killed others with their magic in the past.
Some can hypnotize their patients and possibly their victims; many more
can instill a great deal of fear into their enemies or into people who
believe them to be their enemies. The experts in spirit-possession may
be of either sex and any age, although most are now women of middle
age or older. The craft of both classes of practitioner is treated with
amused scorn by the better educated, but when trouble strikes, even
those who boast of their Christian convictions and their progress beyond
primitive ways find themselves drawn inexorably back into acceptance
of the powers that form the basis of the society's traditional beliefs—
and into the hands of those who have the confidence to manipulate them.

In this paper, I have taken the two most common forms of functional
disease according to the Luo categories, which are still treated in the
traditional way, and have tried to relate the manner in which they are
diagnosed and treated to the social situations from which they spring.
The categories used by the tribe and their beliefs concerning the relationship between the supernatural and disease play a large part in the success
of treating the various forms of mental disease. They also probably increase the incidence of certain conditions over others, particularly those
that develop out of minor organic disorders.

John Dawson

Urbanization and Mental Health
in a West African Community

AS PART of a multidisciplinary project, carried out by the University of Edinburgh and designed to study the social, psychological, and medical effects of urbanization on the tribal African in Sierra Leone, a program of psychological research was conducted in Sierra Leone from May, 1961, to June, 1962. It was centered on the effects of urbanization, education, and industrial training and employment on the African population employed in the iron-ore mine at Marampa, in the Northern Province of Sierra Leone.

This report deals with those aspects of the research program related to the psychological effects of urbanization and the therapeutic functioning of traditional African psychiatry in both its indigenous role and in the urban situation.

The central hypothesis of this paper is that the cultural background of particular tribal groups determines to a large extent the nature of the adaptive mechanisms evolved by each tribe to overcome the stresses and problems of urbanization. The extent to which adjustment is required is, however, a function of the different sets of problems facing each tribal group in the urban environment. For example, in Lunsar and Marampa, a migrant minority of Mende within an essentially hostile and alien environment face entirely different problems of adjustment to urbanization from those faced by the Temne, who are indigenous to the area. Again, however, Temne from distant chiefdoms must cope with rather different problems from those affecting Temne whose original homes are in the Marampa and Lunsar area.

In order to understand the extent to which social change is affecting the tribal African, we need some historical and cultural perspectives. The first European to mention the Sierra Leone coast was Alvaro Fernandes, a Portuguese who, in 1446, sighted the prominent mountain range of Sierra Leone at the foot of which Freetown now stands. Kup noted in 1961 that the coast was first mapped by another Portuguese sailor, Pedro da Sintra, in 1462.[1] These early European sailors were searching for routes to the rich spice islands of the East. The Portuguese initially held sway over the Sierra Leone coast but were eventually displaced by the French, the Dutch, and finally the English, who arrived in the latter half of the sixteenth century.

In the eighteenth century, British social conscience dictated the formation of a special colony in Sierra Leone to receive those Africans who were in England after their discharge from slavery and also other groups who had been displaced after the American War of Independence. This colony was first settled in 1787 where Freetown now stands, and it was to this port that freed slaves were later brought to settle—the ancestors of the Creoles who live in Freetown today. The Protectorate was proclaimed in 1896.

Various waves of migration had brought different tribal groups to Sierra Leone, usually after major upheavals in one or another of the larger empires to the East. The Limba are believed to have arrived initially in the fourteenth century, and, by 1500, the Susu, Yalunka, Limba, and Loko were living in the North of Sierra Leone, while the Bullom and Temne were in the South. Mende arrived in two waves of migration, the second occurring as late as 1825. There was almost continual warfare in the Protectorate area beginning with the first Mende invasion in the sixteenth century, continued in Islamic *jihads* into the eighteenth century, and culminating in more intertribal warfare and fighting with the British in the nineteenth century. The tribes settled down into their present positions about 1850. Until 1725, tribes in Sierra Leone had been pagan, but in that year a *jihad* was launched by Alpha Bo of Koranko against the Susu and Yalunka, which his successor continued against the Kissi and the Limba. From that time forward, Islam spread through Sierra Leone, particularly influencing the northern and western tribes but not the Mende.

Intertribal warfare between Temne and Mende was almost continuous for a very long period of time, but, with the proclamation of the Protectorate in 1896 followed by the imposition of "Hut Tax" in 1898—by payment of which chiefs thought that they would lose legal rights in their land to the British—Temne and Mende both rose in protest against the British. The rebellion was finally put down, and, apart from minor disturbances, mainly in Temne country, there has been peace ever since.

The tribal groups of the Protectorate area have been divided by Kup into two main language groups.[2] The West Atlantic group, which is thought to be indigenous to the area, includes Limba, Krim, Gola, Sherbro, Temne, and Kissi. The Mende-speaking peoples, the Loko, Susu, Kono, Vai, Yalunka, Mende, and Koranko, are considered part of those tribal groups that have been forced by the expansion and decline of empires from the Western Sudan to the coast.

The Temne-speaking peoples of Sierra Leone occupy an area of 11,000 square miles stretching from the coast on either side of the Rokel River for 110 miles inland. Temne are situated entirely within the Northern Province and the former colony was in Temne country. Farming, fishing, and hunting are the main occupations. The staple crop, as with all tribal groups except Sherbro, is rice, which was first introduced in Sierra Leone in the sixteenth century. The farming economy is based on the growing of subsistence crops on the uplands and in the swamps under the bush-fallowing system, with palm fruit as a cash crop. Men are responsible for brushing the forest and other heavy work, which they do on a communal basis. They also harvest and build and repair houses. Women manage the planting of crops, weeding, and harvesting. Women also prepare palm oil, clean rice, and sell fruits and vegetables in the markets. Children assist with all tasks from about six years on and are particularly responsible for frightening birds.

Littlejohn has written that "the basic unit in Temne society is the *makas,* an exogamous patrilineal lineage, three to five generations in depth. It is by virtue of membership in this group that the individual has rights to land, residence etc., and in royal *makas* to chieftainship. All land is divided among *makas,* and cannot be alienated from the *makas.*"[3] *Bonshaw* is the name for composite lineage groups, made up of the *makas* and the *makara,* on the mother's side. The *buna* is the Temne clan consisting of all those people with the same surname and said to be descended from a common ancestor.

Temne political institutions vary somewhat, but the usual method used to install the chief in a particular chiefdom determines the nature of the political institutions of that chiefdom. In the Temne chiefdoms to the South and East, installation of Temne chiefs is carried out by secret societies, mainly Ragbenle but also by Poro and Ramena. In the North and West of the Temne country, where Islamic influence is strong, installation is carried out by Muslim ceremonies. To the Muslim, secret societies are abominable and installation of chiefs by secret societies is not found among them. Unlike the more secular chief of the Mende peoples, the Temne chief has often been described as a priest-king with extensive ritual power protected by numerous prohibitions and taboos called *ma-sam*. Where secret societies install the chiefs, officials form inner councils for running the chiefdoms.

The Temne supreme deity was known as Kuru; he was associated with the sky, and sacrifices and prayers were made to him. With the advent of Islam, the Temne conception of God changed from Kuru to Allah, while many of the former functions of Kuru were transferred to ancestors of the lineage groups and to the various devils or spirits called *ay-krifi* that inhabit all natural features of Temne country. Temne perception of their world can be thought of temporally in terms of *daru*, which is the everyday world that everyone sees, and spiritually in term of *Ro-krifi*, which is the abode of the dead that ancestors inhabit and of *Ro-seron*, the world of witches. *Ro-socki* is the power that enables an individual to see beyond the everyday world of *daru*.

The births of Temne children are attended by old women; males are not allowed to be present. Weaning takes place when a child is between two and two and a half years old, and no parental sexual intercourse is permitted within that period. Supplementary food is given in the form of starchy liquids from six months onward. It is lack of protein in this sup-plementary feeding that, as Gelfand noted,[4] is widely held to be the cause of *kwashiorkor*. *Kwashiorkor* is very common among Temne children. The baby is carried on the mother's back up to the age of five and up to two years of age is always in very close contact with the mother. The baby is treated with much affection until weaned, after which he is subjected to considerable severity in disciplinary measures, and toilet training is, from this stage, very strict. Gamble noted such cases in Lunsar: "A small girl was given fifty strokes with a rod for taking some meat."[5] He goes on to explain that:

> Behind the punishment lay the theory that a devil, *krifi*, had entered into the child and must be beaten out, and the girl is thrashed until a long litany of a confession is repeated after the mother, the child being then ready to confess anything. Other mothers completely lost their tempers with children and in uncontrollable rages inflict extremely heavy blows on their off-spring. A child may be beaten with a piece of bicycle tube for "crying for nothing." One small boy was made to do a knee bend with his arms crossed on his shoulders 100 times for failing to go and draw water. When he stopped after about 50 times he was made to start again and it was only after another 30 when he could scarcely stand that an elderly woman intervened on his be-half. On the other hand if anyone other than the parent or guardian were to raise a hand against a child, the mother would fly into a great rage about it—a fact of which some children take advantage. One the of main results of the severe treatment of the children is that they in their turn delight in

being cruel to animals, tormenting dogs and monkeys, pulling insects to pieces, and in hitting children smaller than themselves when they can get away with it."

This observation also applies to the treatment of small children by their larger brothers and sisters.

Gamble goes on to point out the contrast between the treatment of Temne children and the treatment of Mandinka and Fulbe children in villages in Gambia where he has also carried on considerable fieldwork: "In Mandinka and Fulbe villages in Gambia . . . if a child was being punished there was a tendency for the other parent, a grandmother, or some relative, to step in, prevent the punishment being too severe, and comfort the child afterwards."

Questionnaires were used to obtain information of a qualitative nature about Temne and Mende child-training practices. Mende fathers are generally reluctant to punish their children. Mende believe that, if the father brings up the child in his house, that child will not be well trained. Little[6] stated, "the Mende fear that their children will be spoiled if they stay too long at home." Mende children are thus often sent to close relatives or good friends. Generally children remain with their guardians until they are initiated at twelve to fourteen years of age. If the father does not send his children to relatives, it is necessary for him "to pretend to forsake the child so that the child will treat the father as an ordinary person." Rather than "flog" the child, the father usually prefers to punish misbehavior in other ways—withdrawing food and similar deprivations. When the child is under training, there are certain punishments administered for certain "crimes." For stealing, pepper is rubbed into the face. When a child urinates in bed, a mixture of urine and mud is put on him. For beating other children, he is tied up and the beaten child allowed to hit back. If the child leaves home without permission, he is confined to the house for some time. If he should eat his food too greedily, he is made to sit while others finish.

In all studies of personality carried out in our samples, Temne subjects were significantly more disturbed than Mende subjects. In addition, external ratings of job efficiency and personality on prepared rating scales evinced similar differences. It is impossible to determine exactly whether or not the higher level of psychological disturbance observed among Temne in the urban situation is connected with the severity of Temne child-training practices, but there does appear to be a relationship. It is possible that Temne values, emphasizing as they do the desirability of aggressive characteristics, are oriented toward the past when, in the days of intertribal warfare, Temne were always regarded as excellent warriors. It appears that traditional Temne values have been carried into the urban situation, where there is no socially acceptable outlet for traditional Temne aggressive behavior. It is possible that this situation may then be the source of Temne psychological disturbance in the urban environment. In order to obtain more information on tribal value systems and on how different tribal groups perceive themselves four scales were constructed, one of which will be described here.

This scale listed, on the left hand side of the page, all the tribal groups of Sierra Leone, together with European national groups, Americans, and members of other African countries. Twenty-one characteristics were listed across the top of the page, while the numbers one to twenty-one were placed opposite each group of people. Subjects were asked to check five characteristics they thought typical of each group. The scale was administered to both literates and illiterates in all areas of Sierra Leone. Results of this scale for ratings of themselves by Temne, Mende, Creole, and Limba are set forth in Table 1.

Table 1—Self-Ratings of Tribal Characteristics

Temne	Percentage of total	Mende	Percentage of total	Limba	Percentage of total	Creole	Percentage of total
Always want to fight	75.95	Very friendly	67.02	Honest	63.6	Very clever	82.22
Strongminded	51.90	Hard workers	64.89	Quiet	47.37	Honest	71.11
Hard workers	45.57	Good farmers	61.70	Hard workers	47.37	Quiet	62.22
Very clever	44.30	Very clever	58.51	Good farmers	42.11	Friendly	57.78
Hot tempered	43.04	Honest	47.87	Very clever	36.84	Rich	51.11
Fight with bottles	39.24	Very generous	34.04	Chop monkeys	31.68	Very generous	42.22
Are thieves	25.32	Rich	31.91	Are drunkards	31.58	Hard workers	33.33
N	158		188		38		90

The seven most frequent self-ratings for each tribal group are arranged in rank order from the top of the table. The aggressive content of the Temne ratings confirms the hypothesis regarding the orientation of Temne values toward the past. Traditional Temne values have therefore not shown much change in the urban environment. Of the seven most frequent ratings made by Temne, only those that refer to "hard work" and "cleverness" can be regarded as compatible with such urban processes as education and industrial training. Mende perception of themselves appears, however, to be more compatible with the values of the emerging society and the urban and industrial role. These Mende values appear to have facilitated the process of Mende adaptation to the urban environment. Independent ratings for personality, job efficiency, and absenteeism, all favor Mende at the .01 level of confidence, while leadership potential reaches the .05 level. It is interesting to note that ratings by Limba, Mende and Creole of Temne agree almost exactly with Temne self-ratings, except that "very clever" and "hard workers" are replaced with "stab people" and "are very unfriendly."

The evidence available indicates that Temne are having much more difficulty than Mende in adjusting to the urban situation. Temne values appear to be less compatible with the needs of the emerging society, and psychological disturbance among Temne reaches a higher level in the urban situation. It is possible that difficulties in Temne individual adjustment arises from the severity of Temne child-training techniques, which appear to be more oriented toward the past than toward the present situation. It is impossible, however, to determine empirically whether or not this severity is the precise cause. Whiting and Child,[7] in their cross-cultural study of the relationship between child training and personality, hypothesized "that fear of others arises by generalisation from fear of the parents acquired as a result of the severity of socialisation." They obtained some confirmation but concluded that the hypothesis had to be set in a context of conflict theory. They concluded that, of the hypotheses they considered regarding the origins of fear of others, the projection and displacement of aggression were much more consistent with the whole range of their findings.

Mechanisms involved in the displacement and projection of aggression in African society involve witchcraft and similar social sanctions. All Temne who are associated with practice of witchcraft and who are liable to be accused in social crises of being witches are people who deviate, either physically, socially, or psychologically, from accepted Temne norms. Witchcraft activity and the consequent displacement of aggression is much more common among Temne than among Mende, who are more concerned with ghosts. For example, physical deformity among Temne is associated with witchcraft. Deformed Temne babies are allowed to die for this reason, but similarly deformed Mende babies are allowed to live. It is possible that the greater amount of witchcraft activity found among Temne stems from what Whiting and Child have termed "fear" of others, arising from generalization of the fear of parents resulting from the severity of socialization. This explanation implies, not a psychological explanation of a sociological phenomenon, but rather that while such social sanctions as witchcraft safeguard law and order and maintain society as a functioning entity, they also serve as individual outlets for aggression.

Of the other tribal groups in Table 1, Creole ratings have very little aggressive content and are in accordance with Creole social structure and cultural values, which have been subject to strong educational and Christian influence since the early nineteenth century. Limba, situated to the North of Temne country, are the third largest tribe in Sierra Leone with a population of 190,000. They have not been exposed to education and urbanization as have the other three tribes and must be regarded as more traditional. Limba have always had a reputation for hard work and honesty, and this reputation is reflected in their self-ratings, although the Limba sample is rather small. Many characteristics of Limba society are similar to those of the Temne, but quite obviously their values are rather different. One of the traditional occupations of the Limba is palm-wine tapping. The tapping of palm wine has been institutionalized in many aspects of Limba culture, which is why they refer to themselves, although well down the list, as drunkards.

§ Marampa and Lunsar

The iron-ore mine at Marampa was established in the early Thirties, and production started in 1933. Mining was begun on an open-cut basis on the large mountain of iron ore that the Temne call Massoboi Tanka. A smaller hill of iron ore nearby is called Gbaffle. On December 31, 1961, the company employed at Marampa and at Pepel, the shipping port fifty-two miles away, a total of 2553 Africans, most of them Temne. There is a company program to train apprentices for all trades; in addition, the company offers training for promotion and literary classes. Company training programs are in operation in Freetown and at Fourah Bay University College, and selected personnel are also sent to the United Kingdom for both university and technical training. More than 485 employees, 25.58% of the Marampa work force, live within the company compound at Marampa in company-owned accommodations, while 950 employees or 50.1% live in Lunsar about two miles away. The remainder live in nearby Temne villages, although some live as far as eight miles away.

The indigenous tribal group of the area, the Temne, forms 58.05% of the work force, while Limba from the North are next largest with 12.33% and Mende from the South, who are the largest tribal group in Sierra Leone, make up 12.17%. While the majority of Temne and Limba are employed at laboring and semiskilled tasks, a higher proportion of Mende are apprentices, artisans, and clerks. As more jobs have become available in other parts of Sierra Leone over the past ten years, migrant labor at Marampa has decreased. The work force at the mine is relatively static, with a mean length of service for the total mine labor force of about six and a half years.

Temne form the largest single tribal group of mine employees living in Lunsar with 66.63% of the total, followed by Limba with 9.26% and Mende with only 6.74%. When the mine was first established, Lunsar was only a small Temne village of some twenty houses; today the population is approximately 14,000. The town has suffered somewhat in its development; it has never been a large administrative center, a prerequisite for the rapid development of roads, water supplies, electricity, and other services. Water is available at central points, and electricity is coming, however. There are numerous shops, mostly run by Syrian and Lebanese traders—a chemist, a new shoe shop, a large market, and numerous palm-wine bars—and a new town hall, which was an independence gift to Lunsar from the mining company. There are two Christian primary schools, which take about 1200 pupils between them, and a Muslim school of 300 pupils. Beside the health center at the mine, there is a mission hospital just outside Lunsar and a government dispenser and midwife in Lunsar itself.

§ Therapeutic Functions of Traditional and Semitraditional Societies in the Urban Situation

Both Temne and Mende secret societies have always played a major role in the traditional treatment of the mentally ill and maladjusted, treating patients either individually or on a group basis. Direct treatment of the individual has been carried out mainly by society practitioners, while indirect treatment has been available through the group functioning of a society, which permits satisfaction of individual needs by virtue of membership in a social group. Where Islamic influence has become strong, as in the North and West of the Temne country, these traditional functions of secret societies have gradually passed to Muslim *alfas*. Islam has satisfied individual needs on a group basis by providing a cohesive guiding force, while individual *alfas* have taken over the role of both "holy men" and "doctors," carrying out treatment of the psychologically disturbed.

Traditional secret-society methods of direct and indirect psychiatric treatment were designed to fulfill a social function, by ensuring that those members of society who deviated psychologically from group norms and accepted standards of behavior would be redirected in paths of normal behavior. To some extent, witchcraft as an institution and as a social sanction has fulfilled a similar role, since psychological deviation from normal Temne behavior sets the individual apart, which cannot be tolerated if a society is to maintain cultural continuity. The deviant, whether his "difference" is physical, or social, is likely to be thought of in terms of antisocial—witchcraft—behavior. If social stress precipitates a group situation requiring some outlet for aggression, the individual who differs from Temne norms is most likely to be accused of witchcraft. The accused individual can then be reintegrated into society by a process of confession and punishment.

The institutions of witchcraft and secret societies fulfill a similar function to the use of oaths in that all three function to a large extent as social sanctions to maintain traditional Temne society. Perhaps one reason why social sanctions appear more active in the urban situation is because of the breakdown of traditional society and the social problems inherent in the urban environment. Social sanctions are thus used more actively in the attempt to maintain the stability of the group in an extremely unstable situation.

In such an unstable situation, the structure and content of secret societies have been modified and adapted to meet the needs of the emerging society. Semitraditional societies have, to a large extent, taken over the functions of traditional secret societies, although the societies continue to exist in a limited form. As these traditional societies served a functional purpose in maintaining conformity with group behavior by the provision of physical, social, and psychological treatment for their members, so have the new semitraditional societies provided similar integrating facilities to encourage individual identification with familiar patterns of group behavior but in forms adapted to the new society.

The employment demands of the mining company and associated projects have resulted in a tremendous influx into Lunsar of migrant workers, which has in turn created severe social problems of adaptation and integration. Different tribal groups tend to adjust to these stresses according to their cultural backgrounds. Mende and Creole have solved the problems to a large extent by creating in the company compound their own communities based on tribal affiliations. Temne from distant chiefdoms tend to settle mainly in Lunsar, and as Temne make up 69.9% of Lunsar's population, they have, to a large extent, in-group status.

The next two largest immigrant tribal groups are the Limba and Loko, with 8.8% and 5.4% of the population respectively. Both Loko and Limba have close cultural affinities with Temne people and therefore tend to settle in Lunsar rather than in the company compound. To a large extent, the social problems created in Lunsar by the migration to the area of both distant Temne and other tribal groups have been overcome by the adaptation of traditional tribal institutions like the secret societies into voluntary organizations. Little, writing on the role of voluntary organizations in West African urbanization,[8] states that "from the point of view of social organization one of the most striking characteristics of these modern towns is the very large number and variety of voluntary organizations." In the modern West, medical and psychiatric treatment tends to be an individual process; in West Africa, such treatment is essentially a function of social groups. The traditional societies that have always performed therapeutic functions in the indigenous society are displaced in the process of urbanization by the voluntary organizations, which fulfill similar therapeutic roles and provide, within an alien environment, individual security and satisfaction of the psychological need for identification with familiar group patterns.

Banton[9] estimated that in Freetown in 1952, there were 123 registered societies of a total of 203 registered and unregistered societies, of which 26.11% were Temne and only 2.46% were Mende. Although in 1952 there were 19,000 Temne and 11,000 Mende in Freetown, the marked difference in numbers of the voluntary organizations formed by each of the two tribal groups must reflect differing methods of adaptation to the urban environment, which are determined to some extent by differences in traditional social structure and cultural orientations. Banton emphasizes that Mende kinship ties are not so strong as those of the Temne. Mende systems are based partly on patrilineal descent and partly on inheritance and show greater emphasis on locality, as opposed to the Temne emphasis on descent. He considers that the less rigid nature of the Mende system is one reason why Mende have been more subject to Westernizing influence.

The Mende chief is a more secular figure than the Temne chief, who is often described as a priest king. The strong traditional Mende societies, Poro, Wunde, and Sande, possess ritual and symbolic power that the Mende chiefs lack. The position of the Mende chief is in fact controlled by these traditional societies, which are thus the center of political as well as ritual power. These traditional societies are common to the whole of Mende country, and consequently are more powerful than those of the Temne. Almost every Mende in Freetown would be a member of

Poro; some would also be members of the even more powerful Wunde. The awareness of belonging, which the Mende derive from common membership in the very strong traditional Mende societies may explain why they have formed fewer voluntary organizations in Freetown than have the Temne. Furthermore, as Banton[10] has pointed out, the Temne, the largest tribal group in Freetown and the original owners of the Freetown and Colony area, initially suffered from a position of low prestige and only reasserted their tribal consciousness by the formation of essentially Temne voluntary organizations. Too, the Temne have been psychologically more vulnerable to the processes of social change. The very large number of Temne voluntary societies formed in Freetown and other urban areas may thus reflect strong Temne needs for social and psychological adjustment to the urban situation on a group basis.

Banton[11] suggests further that the voluntary associations "develop partly in response to the need for role differentiation—for developing in a confused situation a new structure of roles and status." Temne had always achieved psychological and social adjustment through membership in traditional societies. In developing the new roles and statuses necessary to provide new Temne role identifications, the degree of need for societies to help the individual adjust to the stresses and problems of the Freetown environment is partly a function of structural differences between traditional Temne society and that of Freetown. For example, the traditional society for women, Bundu, which is universally found throughout Temne country, is very strong in Freetown. But traditional male societies are limited in Temne country according to the influence of Islam in a particular area. Additionally, such societies as Poro, Ragbenle, and Gbangbani differ considerably in organization and function. Because of their variety, these societies cannot satisfy the needs of Temne to identify with a single group in Freetown, for such a group would have to offer simultaneously an Islamic identification, a traditional identification, and a set of group behavior patterns essential to satisfactory adjustment in the new environment.

One of the most effective Temne societies formed in Freetown is the Ambas Geda, branches of which were later formed in Lunsar. Banton[12] reports that the name "Ambas Geda" is derived from the Temne *ambas* for "we have"; *geda* is the Krio form of the English "together." Such societies as Ambas Geda were called *compins* from the English "company." Banton noted that the term "Ambas Geda" expressed the feeling that "we, the Temne, have the people and must collect them in." In this way, the individual psychological needs of the Temne migrants, which are in part a function of adaptation to the new emerging society, seek expression in a typical Temne cultural form. Such a society collects Temne together and provides the traditional means by which individual Temne adjust to group norms, which are themselves adjusted to the demands of the new environment.

The function of voluntary organizations of this nature in the emerging society is to minimize individual anxiety and psychological disturbance by providing group identifications. The traditional therapeutic function of societies becomes an essential characteristic of these social groups in urban surroundings.

The semitraditional societies are those that have essentially African characteristics but have largely been formed in Lunsar in a direct response to social change.

The main semitraditional society in Lunsar is the Oje, which is of Nigerian origin, having been brought to Freetown by the Yoruba. The Temne of Freetown took over from the Yoruba certain aspects of Oje ritual and eventually formed Temne Oje societies. The influence of Oje has spread to other Temne centers of urbanization. A branch was formed in Lunsar, where the society has a very large Temne following. Oje has society devils, the two main devils being Ogugu and Iyogbo. These devils are used for hunting witches, although the essential functions of the society are drumming and entertainment. Initiation is required for membership, as well as knowledge of various Aku words used in society ritual. A semitraditional society like this modified form of Oje has particularly strong appeal in the urban setting. Those Temne who have been partially divorced from their traditional culture have a strong need to identify with a semitraditional organization that offers both membership and group characteristics adjusted to the realities of the new urban environment. The functions of the society are both traditional and semitraditional. Gamble[13] reports that members of Oje tend to come from higher socioeconomic levels—fitters, drivers, electricians, clerks, and traders. Oje thus typifies the traditional and semitraditional characteristics with which the more educated and industrially trained worker feels that he can identify while still maintaining levels of prestige appropriate to his new position. These educated workers tend to reject membership in the more traditional societies as incompatible with the educational levels they have attained. This rejection of the traditional was discussed by Littlejohn,[14] who commented on the conflicts that occurred in the middle 1950s in Lunsar between the "owners of the country" and "strangers." The "owners of the country" are those Temne who are indigenous to the Marampa-Masimera Chiefdom and who, together with the chief, have their own land with a consequent share in traditional political power, which is essentially a hereditary right. "Strangers" are residents of Lunsar and surrounding villages and include both Temne from other chiefdoms and migrant workers from other tribal groups. Those Temne who have been educated in Freetown and who hold higher positions with the mining company, even though they may originally have come from this area, have, as a function of their educational and career achievement, psychological and social needs essentially different from those of the traditional "owners of the country." These differences increase the degree of psychological and social distance between the two groups and increase proportionately the townsmen's degree of "strangeness."

The trade union formed by the mine workers is an example of an essentially nontraditional society whose role of worker representation is in direct conflict with the traditional functioning of Poro. Littlejohn[15] reports that the "Poro secret society, which in ordinary conditions helps to maintain law and order, in these conditions helps to destroy it." Conflicts have arisen between the two groups, and some Temne who were either devout Muslims or educated have been forcibly initiated into Poro. There are unsubstantiated reports that some young educated employees of the mine have been threatened with forcible initiation by Poro and have gone to Freetown rather than submit. In the course of an analysis of etiological aspects of case histories at the Kissy Mental Hospital in Freetown, we found two educated male patients who had reported severe emotional disturbance following forcible initiation into Poro, while one female patient reported similar emotional disturbance after forcible initiation into Bundu.

Littlejohn, in describing the attitude of Poro to the formation in Lunsar of the Oje society reports considerable hostility between these two groups.[16] He states that an Oje member was beaten to death for singing a Poro song, the words to which Poro regard as their sacred trust. As the chief and tribal authorities refused to do anything about the murder, Oje members tried to burn down the chief's compound. As a result of these activities, Oje was disbanded for a period.

It appears that the role of traditional Temne secret societies in the urban environment has not been compatible with the psychological and social needs of immigrant Temne and workers from other tribal groups, who have attained, by virtue of education and industrial training, higher socioeconomic positions in the urban society. It has therefore been necessary for these educated workers to seek social and psychological satisfaction and adjustment in the urban environment by identification with social groups compatible with their new role identifications. The traditional secret society Poro, feeling itself threatened by the semitraditional and nontraditional societies, had endeavored to prevent both the formation of these societies and their continuing activities.

Membership in traditional societies diminishes with increasing educational and occupational achievement. Individuals who have rejected the traditional societies turn to social groups like Oje whose characteristics reflect the realities of the emerging society.

The other type of semitraditional society found in Lunsar is the *kompin*, a dancing society similar to the *compins* in Freetown. Such societies as the Ambas Geda were formed in Freetown to meet the social and psychological needs of urban Temne to identify with their own tribal group. Unlike Oje, Ambas Geda and other societies of this nature have very few ritual functions, although certain of their characteristics are in fact traditional. These societies have organized a system of contributions from which entertainments and dances are paid for and some provision made for social welfare and bereavement benefits. Most of the dancing societies in Lunsar have been of a transitory nature, enrolling large numbers of members generally from the younger age groups. Jolly Boys is the largest such *kompin* in Lunsar. Generally the dancing societies become considerably more active at such festival times as Christmas and at the celebrations to mark the end of the Muslim period of fasting, Ramadan. At such times, they join in the processions with their society devils. The *kompins* in Lunsar fulfill the needs of an essentially younger age group, which has need of its own organizations prior to and just after marriage. Migrant workers in urban areas are particularly prone to stresses resulting from isolation from individual and social interaction with members of their own cultural group, and this sense of isolation is heightened when the individual is single or newly married. The *kompins* provide peer-group activity. Interaction with others of similar interests and tribal affiliations, particularly during this period of social isolation in an alien environment, offers emotional satisfaction at a crucial time.

Ninety-nine per cent of female residents in Lunsar belong to the strongly traditional female society of Bundu. The Temne and other Sierra Leone tribal groups consider the training given by this society essential to the attainment of complete womanhood. Muslims, who themselves reject secret societies in most cases, will not marry women who have not been through Bundu training. They do not consider Bundu a secret society but a training school in which initiates are taught the domestic, dancing, and singing skills necessary to every-day existence. In this character, it is compatible with Islam.

Since a large company of Sierra Leone police was established in Lunsar in 1955, criminal activities have been considerably limited. One group that is still criminally active to a considerable extent is made up mainly of adolescent Temne males and young adults who wear the cowboy clothes they have seen in Western films. These "cowboys" usually come from unsettled homes, and, generally because of emotional instability rather than lack of intelligence, they have failed in school. By identification with their cowboy heroes they endeavor to compensate for their failures in school and in interpersonal and social relationships. As the formation of voluntary organizations fulfills the needs of migrant workers isolated socially and psychologically from their own cultures, so does the formation of "cowboy" groups fulfill similar needs for young men who have, because of social problems stemming from urbanization, been isolated socially and psychologically from their own tribal groups. These groups were not initially formed to function solely as criminal organizations but rather as peer groups in which the antisocial value system that these boys had evolved could find group acceptance.

More specialized societies have been formed to protect particular aspects of social functioning. For example, the Temne Ragbenle has been responsible for the maintenance of incest laws and, through application of Ragbenle therapeutic methods, for maintenance of normal physical and psychological functioning. In addition, Ragbenle oaths have been used to govern social behavior. The Mende Humui is similarly concerned with the regulation of incest laws and the maintenance of normal physical functioning, while the Mende N'jayai has ensured normal psychological functioning and the preservation of those personality characteristics that Mende regard as desirable. Although, in the urban setting, some traditional societies have not provided new norms of behavior compatible with the new role identifications of the educated and industrially trained workers, they have continued in varying degrees to fulfill the described functions.

§ Traditional Psychological Treatment
in Lunsar and Other Urban Areas

Lunsar, with a population of 14,000, has a very large number of diviners, in Temne called *o-men*, native doctors called *bulomba*, and *alfas* or *mori*-men, who are the Islamic holy men, each of whom specializes to some degree in an aspect of healing or diagnosis, usually treating both the physically ill and the psychologically disturbed. When someone becomes sick, the first step toward a cure is for an *o-men* to determine by divination whether the sickness is purely physical or whether there are social complications. If the sickness is ascribed to the activities of a witch, *a-ser*, it is then necessary to locate the witch and obtain a confession, by which act the witch's hold over the life force of the sick person will be broken. If no social complications are divined, then treatment will be carried out by a *bulomba*.

Generally the more educated mine employees attend the Marampa Mine Health Center. Those not employed by the mine may attend the government health center in Lunsar. There are also a Roman Catholic mission hospital two miles up the Makeni Road, where the more seriously ill can be taken, and a fully equipped government hospital at Port Loko about twenty-two miles away. Even among educated and industrially trained workers, however, suspicions of social complications in any physical or psychological disturbance will cause a sick person to consult a native doctor. The patients in such cases often exhibit symptoms of marked anxiety that make it difficult to treat them in a health center. They and their relatives feel that only African doctors can successfully handle the variables.

The following case, which occurred in Lunsar, demonstrates the need to understand the cultural variables involved. The Temne wife of an educated mine employee had lost her second baby. The loss of her first child had been followed by a dream in which she, as a witch, had given her baby to be ritually eaten by the witch cult in the meeting place of witches, *ra-serong*. Two nights after the loss of the second child, the wife exhibited extreme symptoms, screaming, shouting, and wailing, together with physically violent behavior. The native doctor was called; after divination and questioning the mother, he accused her of responsibility for the death of her child through witchcraft and told her that she must confess. She started to confess, saying that, when asked by her confederates in the witch cult to sacrifice her infant, she had at first objected but had been forced to make her contribution. She had taken part in the ritual eating of children of other members of the cult, so that she had to agree to give her child. Both of her children had been offered to the cult in this way. After making her confession, the woman was told by the native doctor that she had been cleansed, after which her violent and hysterical behavior subsided. She was then required to make *a-sathka*, a sacrifice (the Temne translate this as a "charity").

In the course of our work in Lunsar and surrounding villages, four cases were encountered in which the patients had had precisely the same type of dream following actions involving real or imagined neglect or wrong-doing. In three of these cases, those involved were mothers who had lost children. This type of dream is often referred to by Temne as *o-worap a-ser*—"I dream a witch"—and can be regarded as a culturally stereotyped reaction to conscious or unconscious feelings of guilt in which the person does indeed become a witch. The events that take place in dreams seem to them synonymous with reality; following such a dream, a woman firmly believes that she has become a witch. The loss of the second child in the case described had precipitated an emotional outburst resulting from these initial guilt feelings and reinforced by the dream, which had firmly convinced the mother that she was evil and indeed a witch. After the accusation of witchcraft made by the native doctor, there followed the confession, which is also culturally stereotyped, always following an accepted pattern with only slight individual variations. Only by making this cathartic confession can the symptoms be relieved and the person cleansed and consequently reintegrated into society. Temne say that, if a person is a witch and has done something wrong, he can be saved only by confession. The individual is thus cleansed, putting an end to his antisocial behavior and restoring him to accepted patterns of behavior. The institution of witchcraft therefore functions as a social sanction, and those individuals most likely to be accused of witchcraft are those who, by abnormal physical, social, and psychological behavior deviate from accepted Temne norms. If the mother had not confessed, the husband might have taken out a general oath against the person who had been responsible for the death of the child. When the mother next became ill, if she still did not confess, the native doctor would not have treated her, and the Temne say, she would have died.

When such strong traditionally determined behavior is present, treatment of physical symptoms is very difficult until these guilt feelings can be alleviated in the traditionally accepted way. In this instance, the native doctor had immediately recognized the culturally determined aspects of the case and knew that accusation and confession were required to obtain catharsis. This cultural awareness enables the native doctor to detect the extent to which such social complications as witchcraft and oaths are involved. When patients exhibit characteristic symptoms of extreme guilt and fear following antisocial acts that have invoked the use of oaths or witchcraft against them, the native doctor will then define a course of treatment to counteract the effects of these social complications.

The medical officers at the mine health center report that very few true psychotics have come into their hands over the past five years. There was one schizophrenic about whom little was known, but he was removed by relatives to be treated by a Muslim *alfa* in Kabala. The senior medical officer noted that he had seen only two depressives in six years; they were also removed to be treated by native doctors. In 1961, a seventeen-year-old apprentice began to have periods of persecutory delusions in which he made wild, unsubstantiated statements against both Africans and Europeans. When his behavior became worse, he was removed by his relatives for traditional treatment at Makeni. There is only one known epileptic in the mine population; originally employed in the mill, he was placed in semiclerical work because of the danger involved should he have an attack in the mill. Medical officers in the mine all agree that the incidence of neurosis and mental illness in general is not high. In 1953, Carothers remarked that hysterical symptoms are perhaps the commonest neurotic manifestation in Africa.[17] In the Marampa Health Center, there are occasional hysterical patients. Some apprentices occasionally report physical symptoms when there is some particularly hard work to be done but recover quickly when given sick leave without pay. At Kissy Mental Hospital in Freetown, patients manifesting violent psychotic behavior have been brought in, with the violence subsiding rapidly after the patient has been admitted. These patients usually have been hungry and homeless. The same thing has happened with a number of people who have committed criminal offences, particularly murder; they apparently manifest psychotic behavior in order to gain admittance to Kissy and escape punishment.

In the Lunsar population of 14,000, there is only one true psychotic, a chronic schizophrenic Temne aged about forty. He is bearded, wears ragged clothes, and spends his time walking through the town, where he is a source of much amusement to its citizens. The townspeople, however, provide him with food and give him clothes. He sleeps in the town market and does not exhibit any violent behavior. It is said by the Temne that he only really becomes excited at the full moon. One person who knew him before he became sick gave this history: "I knew Molai before he is crazy. He was a good intelligent man and he was a straightforward man, because he has been doing trade for my brother, and he is also a good barber and he is always serious in his trade and as far as I know I don't think anyone will say bad against him for Molai has not done any bad against anyone. It was for his money that they harm him, because they find out that Molai is trying very hard, that is why they give him the sickness. And he has only one wife, that is when he is not yet crazy and it was June, 1958, that the sickness hold him. His mother has tried all her level best but still no success. And I also heard that Molai's brother is crazy." The phrase "they give him the sickness" seems to refer to those evil forces that are precipitated by some action of the individual concerned (like seeing a bad devil) or by witchcraft or oaths against him. One category of deviation from normal behavior includes people who try too hard or become too wealthy. In such cases, they become vulnerable to social sanctions. Another informant had in fact stated that, because Molai was successful in his business, "they" had turned witchcraft on him and made him as he is. Molai reports seeing and talking to devils, which makes him *ro-sacki*, that is, able to see beyond the every-day world, and this ability gives him power.

There is also in Lunsar a Temne transvestite aged about forty-five, who carries on work normally done by Temne women and who wears women's clothes. Although not a true psychotic, he has schizoid tendencies. Gamble, reported in 1962 that in Kenema a number of Temne traders selling women's clothes wear women's clothes as well.[18] Mills in 1959[19] encountered only six mentally defective subjects in Lunsar and estimated the rate of mental deficiency as 6 per thousand, compared to eight per thousand for England and Wales (quoted by Gelfand).[20] The Temne allow physically deformed babies to die, and this factor probably contributes to the low rate. Schlenker[21] reported that Temne deformed children were burnt or suffocated by people called *pa-ra-sam*, which means a "sacred" or "holy thing." Temne believe that deformed children are associated with devils, *ang-krifi*, and should therefore be destroyed. The Temne value system cannot tolerate those who do not conform physically, precisely as it cannot tolerate social and psychological deviation. A Temne who becomes crippled through illness or accident is called *gbeba*, a cripple, or *wuni te lesur*, one who is not complete. Such a person is different; because of this difference, he may be accused of being a witch should a socially accepted outlet for aggression be required during a particular crisis. One other factor that complicates the sampling of both mentally defective individuals and psychotics in a town of Lunsar's size is that psychotics and mentally defectives tend to migrate to larger urban areas where they have much greater opportunities to obtain food, clothes, and shelter.

Jahn has pointed out that "no aspect of African culture has so alienated Europeans and Americans as the so-called practice of magic."[22] He goes on to state that "the fundamental objection to the therapy of the 'medicine men' came from the circles of pragmatic European medicine— arguments which were also appropriated by the missionaries." It had always been assumed that the mystical, unscientific approach of the native doctor could not possibly be effective in curing disease. It is undoubtedly true that native doctors in Lunsar cannot cure many of the more serious diseases, but they can, with their extensive range of herbs, cure most minor and some serious illnesses. Curing illness, however, is not their main field of operation. The traditional methods of native doctors are most effective when there are psychosomatic and other psychological disturbances that have been precipitated by some social complication. Treatment is based to a large extent on prestige, reassurance, and suggestion; some physical remedy is always used, and, in addition, social complications are analyzed. This extensive therapeutic assault commands enormous confidence and respect from the patient, who is as ready to respond to therapy as he is to the use of oaths and witchcraft. Where symptoms are complicated by social issues, the native doctor is likely to be most successful with his treatment; the greater the psychological content in the illness therefore, the more effective the treatment by the native doctor.

There are approximately twelve native doctors in Lunsar who among them deal with most of the physically and psychologically ill requiring traditional treatment. One of the most successful of these doctors whom we shall call A, holds high office in the *Poro* society. In therapeutic situations, it is very obvious that patients place considerable confidence in A's ability. He has the full range of Poro herbal medicines, and, by means of his strong and commanding personality, he has acquired considerable prestige. He carries out diagnosis by divination, sacrifice, and questioning, for which he is paid a small fee. If the patient requires further treatment, he charges according to the treatment given. A does not treat "crazy people" but only those he describes as "small crazy." To treat such a person, he goes to the bush and selects the necessary herb after carrying out the "celebration" to the spirit owning the herb. The herb is mixed with water, with which the patient is required to wash himself every day for a month. Anxiety states and other psychological disturbances resulting from the use of oaths and witchcraft are treated by counteroaths and confession. Typical results of the use of oaths include impotency, called *ferrata* by the Temne, when that part of the body is said to die. A specific root is obtained, boiled, and given to the patient, and, in addition, a confession, usually to adultery, is obtained, and the oath is removed. Dreams are interpreted, and their contents are used in arriving at diagnoses. When a dream is interpreted as warning of impending danger, a sacrifice must be carried out to mollify the appropriate forces and to show recognition of what is called "God's warning." This sacrifice is carried out using a kola nut and an egg to ward off the harmful effects. The majority of A's patients are female, generally from older age groups. Mine employees often say that, although they themselves attend the mine health center, they cannot take the same risk with their families, who must attend native doctors. This explanation partly accounts for the fact that more females than males visit the native doctors in Lunsar.

Furthermore, the education the mine employee has received probably makes him feel that he should attend the mine hospital, but his wife who has no education has greater faith in native doctors, and therefore she and her children patronize a traditional practitioner.

The other major practitioner in Lunsar, B, is head of the Ragbenle society. As head of this society, he has hereditary knowledge of its herbal medicine and traditional methods of treatment. There is only one other Ragbenle practitioner, but, as an *a-men*, his activities are confined to predictions. He is also an employee of the mine but has a rather limited practice. B's herbal medicines are more highly regarded than A's, but A has a more commanding personality and is attached to a stronger society. B makes a small charge for prediction and diagnosis and then a further charge depending upon the treatment given. His treatment of psychological disturbances is very similar to that practiced by A, involving inquiry and divination of fundamental causes.

Psychosexual disturbances usually result from severe anxiety induced by fear and guilt reactions following an adulterous or incestuous union. Such anxiety often results from the knowledge that certain oaths and other forms of sanction are designed to inhibit sexual activity. Its treatment always follows the same pattern, designed to obtain a confession and consequent removal of the oath but always in conjunction with some physical treatment. To treat such a "brain mix up" physically, some leaves, *ma foi bana*, are selected. These leaves are boiled and applied with hot water to the head, "to get the heat," "to drive the bad people away and free the head." After a week, the patient should recover. Many of B's therapeutic methods for treating neurotics and psychotics involves the application of heat to the head. He claims that he can induce psychotic behavior by the use of an oath involving an herb called *ang-po*. In addition, he claims another herb, *ka-karra*, will counteract the effects of *ang-po*. The *ka-karra* leaves are mixed with hot water, and the patient is required to wash with the mixture, while the *ka-karra* flowers are also mixed with water and given to the patient to eat.

If an employee from the mine wants to increase his salary, he goes to B and is given an herb called *ang-amara*. This herb is obtained from the bush and mashed. Some scent is placed in it and then mixed by hand, while, at the same time, the client must say what is on his mind. Finally, the mixture is rubbed on his face before he goes to work. This herb is often purchased and used by mine employees who wish to consolidate their positions. Requests are often made to the native doctors for something to increase salary, to pass examinations, or to make the boss more favorable. In the last instance, it is necessary for the client to obtain some piece of personal property belonging to the boss, which is then used to make up a charm, *sebe*, which will influence the boss in his favor. Similarly, if the employee wants to harm his boss because of some wrong the boss has done him, he must have something belonging to the boss, which is used to make an oath. The more personal the item, the more effective will be the *ang-sasa*. Other methods are used to obtain benefits at work and in examinations. Talismans, rings, and other types of charm are purchased from overseas and other African countries through the advertisements that appear in many magazines circulating in the area. One such advertisement for blotting paper, priced at one pound, serves to illustrate: "Datto Ellis blotting paper for examination. Blot your answer with it and gain the sympathy and luck of the examiners who will undoubtedly give you credit and first position." This advertisement was taken at random from a catalogue and is only one of many similar ones. Individuals who buy these charms are generally less intelligent and would probably fail their examinations anyway but seek to tip the balance in their favor by influencing those mystical forces that determine fortune. The fact that an individual buys a charm does not, however, mean that he works less hard than he otherwise would. The relationship between hard work and success is clearly understood. But an attempt is made to control those forces that determine the balance between success and failure and to ensure that they will assist rather than block individual efforts.

The next most successful of the native doctors in Lunsar is the *ya bai*. *Ya bai* is the term used to describe the female members of the society that controls the most powerful of all oaths, the thunder-and-lightning oath called *ang-bom*. Male members are called *o-sok*. Membership is passed from father to son and from mother to daughter. This oath is so powerful that it cannot be used without the permission of the chief. Its prestige has diminished somewhat since an incident in the diamond-mining area, when it failed to catch a thief who stole a particularly valuable diamond. In order to be vulnerable to the effects of the oath, the thief would have to be a participating member of the culture and thus aware of the potential power of the oath. In this case, it is possible that the thief was from another country. Even so, *ang-bom* is a powerful force, and a payment of two pounds is required before it can be invoked. It is significant that the society with the most powerful oath should also have the largest number of patients in Lunsar with symptoms of acute anxiety. This oath not only inflicts injury and damage by thunder and lightning but can also make a person sick and if necessary "crazy." If someone has committed an antisocial act for which this curse is taken in revenge, unless the deviant individual quickly manifests a psychosomatic reaction, the first real organic illness he acquires will be attributed to the effects of the curse. This illness is enough to send him to the *ya-bai* to confess and have the curse removed. As among the other practitioners, psychological disturbance is treated physically as well as psychologically and socially. Special leaves are taken from the bush, boiled in water, and placed in a bowl between the patient's legs. A blanket is placed over his head, and he is required to inhale the fumes. This application of heat to the head is also one of the main methods used by Muslim *alfas* in the treatment of psychotics. The *ya bai* also treats patients suffering from physical illness. In addition, she endeavors to locate and prevent the activities of witches causing physical or psychological illness.

The *ya bai* is the only native doctor I saw in Sierra Leone who achieved anything approaching the states of dissociation described by Field in 1960[23] and manifested by shrine priests in spirit possession. She achieves this state both in the ceremony invoking the thunder-and-lightning curse, in the ceremony to remove the curse, and in the treatment of psychological disturbance. When she is invoking the curse, she dances naked, except for a cloth at her waist, to the accompaniment of the rhythmical beating of a drum. She dances with a sword in her hands, which is symbolic of the powerful forces of the thunder-and-lightning curse. As she attains a state of dissociation, her eyes become fixed and staring, and she relaxes temporarily. At trance-like state, she makes the pronouncement concerning either the invocation or the removal of the powerful forces of thunder and lightning. In the treatment of a disturbed patient, she indicates that the forces causing the disturbance have been removed. Where *ang-bom* has been used specifically to make a person "crazy," "that person will start to dance with a naked body" in exactly the same way that the *ya bai* dances when she invokes the curse.

Occasionally, some patients are brought to the *ya bai* who have actually experienced periods of dissociation similar to her own. These attacks usually take the form of violent fits, in which the victim can hardly be held to the ground. These fits are apparently periods of hysterical dissociation resulting from extreme guilt and fear reactions precipitating the precise psychological condition the *ya bai* had predicted. It will happen to anyone afflicted by the *ang-bom* curse after being detected in his criminal activities. Messing[24] noted that "in most societies which have developed specialised healing patterns for mental ailments, patients and doctors enact certain roles which govern the frequency, intensity, and meaning of their interaction . . . Even the disturbed patient knows something of the performance expected of him when he falls ill. Indeed, his first task in the new role of patient is often to demonstrate his sickness, e.g., spirit possession, so that society in general will accept him in this role." The person against whom this thunder-and-lightning curse has been directed, by his manifestation of periods of hysterical dissociation, fulfills the role of victim laid down for him by the *ang-bom* society. The person involved will develop symptoms of physical illness, emotional disturbance, or hysterical dissociation. The only way the affliction can be removed is through complete confession and payment for revoking the curse. In this way, the thunder-and-lightning cure functions as a social sanction inhibiting antisocial behavior and criminal activities. When such a person is detected by the power of the curse, guilt and fear of the consequences precipitate a public recognizable stereotyped reaction that can only be relieved by confession and reintegration into society. The *ya bai*, like all African native doctors, has the dichotomous role of executioner and savior.

Histories of other individuals who have had periods of hysterical dissociation have been encountered in schools and training colleges in Sierra Leone, in every case where the school has been residential. The socially intimate environment of a residential institution may perhaps be ideal for this type of reaction. The cases encountered, however, appear to have arisen out of strong conflicts between traditional obligations and responsibilities and the desire for education. The following account was reported by a Mende teacher at a teacher-training college. "I noticed he was a bit queer, one student saw him running away towards the swamp. The students caught him and brought him back somehow, but he didn't throw this fit until the second period at 8 A.M., just outside the dormitory. The students held him down but he was fighting with his arms and legs and they really had to hold him. Once they let go he fought so that they had to hold him down again. He started to come round, someone called his name, he looked very distant eyed. He started to struggle again and he was taken to a lorry and then to hospital for a sedative which quieted him down. He said afterwards that the devil had got into him as he hadn't made certain sacrifices. He was sent home for two weeks, he made his sacrifices and he has been all right ever since. When I was at Koyama this sort of thing happened at least once a term. They are playing with black magic." The student was a twenty-year-old Mende, a Christian, and a member of Poro. The teacher-training college is in Temne country, a considerable distance from his home, and it appeared that he was required to carry out sacrifices in the Poro bush at certain times. Having neglected his obligations because of the distance involved in returning home (he was in his first term and could not obtain leave), he became extremely anxious and afraid of the consequences of his neglect. This anxiety and fear culminated in the attack of hysterical dissociation, which may have been a conscious or unconscious attempt to gain attention and thereby to obtain leave or alternatively a culturally stereotyped reaction to his own neglect. Information about Poro rites indicates that they involve periods of dissociation and that self-hypnosis is used to induce analgesia when knives are thrust into the body during public demonstrations. I have witnessed these public ceremonies, and that does appear to be what happens. As the student would be aware of the behavior characteristics of individuals possessed by the devil, it seems likely that his neglect had precipitated this culturally stereotyped reaction. In addition to this particular attack, the Mende teacher described others at Koyama, which he stated were all to do with Poro. A Temne female student at the college, a member of Bundu, had had a similar period of hysterical dissociation some time before the reported young man. Four students were required to hold her down during the attack. After returning home for a few weeks, she returned to the school fully recovered. There was no explanation forthcoming in this instance except that "it might have had something to do with Bundu."

The spirits, or devils as they are more often called, of these traditional secret societies in Sierra Leone appear to be more demanding than those of the Xhosa in South Africa reported by Mayer,[25] who stated that "The spirits (Xhosa) 'understand' and 'know what things are like in town.' Thus far do they sanction conformity with urban requirements and submission to the powers that be. They demand recognition of themselves within the migrant framework, but not at the cost of destroying the framework itself." The strong traditional demands made by the secret societies of Sierra Leone have already been noted in connection with the conflict in Lunsar between the traditional secret societies on the one side and the semitraditional societies and the trade union on the other. The society spirits have not sanctioned the emergence of urbanization in Sierra Leone as have the Xhosa spirits in South Africa, and there is therefore, considerable individual psychological conflict.

Little[26] notes that among the Mende, Poro is much less susceptible to processes of social change and other modern innovations than is the Sande, the Mende equivalent of the Temne Bundu. Referring to modern methods of teaching girl initiates, Little writes that "the *Poro* elders have generally been very hostile to analogous forms of educational experimentation in their own 'school' on the grounds that the *Poro* function is to be regarded as symbolical rather than utilitarian." The symbolic aspect of Mende Poro as the center of Mende ritual makes the society much less flexible in situations of social change. On the other hand, the utilitarian role of Sande, like that of the Temne Bundu, accounts for its strong survival characteristics in the urban environment. In addition, Islamic acceptance of Bundu as a "trade" rather than as a secret society is due to the utilitarian role of Bundu, compared to the symbolic role of Poro.

THERAPEUTIC FUNCTIONS OF MUSLIM ALFAS

The practice of native psychological medicine in Lunsar is confined to the treatment of neurotic and psychosomatic disturbances. The native doctors themselves do not attempt to treat the more severely psychotic disturbances. Apart from the Mende N'jayei and the Sherbro Yassi societies, there are only two centers—in Kabala and Freetown—where traditional treatment of psychotics is practiced. If, for example, someone in Lunsar were to develop a severe psychotic disturbance, the native doctor would advice the relatives to take the patient to the Muslim *alfas* at either Kabala or Freetown, although Kabala is preferred. Kabala, is a center for cattle and other agricultural activities in the extreme North of Sierra Leone. Situated on the edge of Limba country, Kabala borders on Yalunka and Koranko country. Foulahs have settled there in large numbers, although their home is to the North in Guinea. They are strict Muslims and have been largely responsible for bringing Islam to many parts of the North of Sierra Leone, particularly to the Temne. Many Foulah Muslim *alfas* in Kabala have been trained in the arts of healing at a special training center in Futa Jallon in Guinea. Psychotics are brought to these Muslim *alfas* from all over Sierra Leone. These healers also have a wide reputation for making people "crazy," and, like the *ya bai,* are regarded as both executioners and saviors. This dual role is an essential characteristic of the African native doctor. Medical practice is thus inextricably bound up with the preservation of social institutions, for it is through the native doctors that social sanctions are exercised in order to maintain conformity with norms of society.

Muslim *alfas* are also concerned with making various protective devices, which are regarded as the most effective charms available, providing protection against the effects of devils, witches, and misfortune. Much of their protective power stems from the association of the *alfa* with the Islamic god. Charms are actually made from passages of the Koran written out in Arabic on pieces of paper or board. Such charms, called by the Temne *ma-nesi,* are then placed over windows or doors to protect households from all forms of possible misfortune and evil.

Actually, a variety of charms can be seen under any roof in Lunsar, usually close to the front entrance. Each *sebe,* as the Temne call a charm, is designed and purchased to fulfill a particular protective function. A Temne must take these normal social precautions if he is to maintain his prestige and status within the community, for a man who has failed to provide the necessary charms is considered neglectful of his duties as head of a household. The charms use appears to be cyclical. In 1960, there was a spate of charms set up in houses outside Lunsar as protection against thunder and lightning. Each consisted of three wooden sticks forming a tripod with palm fruits resting on the apex. The charms were installed after excessive thunder and lightning had been predicted for that year. The power of the charms made by Muslim *alfas* is, however, greater than that of these more temporal devices, for the *ma-nesi* is associated with God. The Temne say, "The Muslim *alfas* use the power of God to drive craziness away."

The five *alfas* at Kabala who regularly treat psychotic patients usually take between five and eight patients each. They generally keep the patients for periods ranging from one month to two years or more, depending on the degree of recovery achieved and the resources of the relatives. When a patient becomes too violent, he is chained outdoors to a tree or log or to some support inside. Treatment is carried out daily and consists initially of verbal inquiry and examination. At this stage, the emphasis is on locating any source of fear that may be present in some offense the patient may have committed. Where such an offense is found, the Muslim *alfa* will attempt to unravel the social complications in the same way as do the native doctors. After he completes the initial inquiry and examination, the *alfa* prescribes a course of treatment; he prays to God for success. Treatment in its physical form is fairly standard for the different psychotic conditions. It includes prayers and daily washing in water that has been poured over a board inscribed with passages from the Koran. Special herbs are administered orally. Other herbs are boiled in water and the bowl placed between the patient's legs as he sits on the ground. A thick blanket is placed over his head and over the bowl. He then inhales the steam from the container. This treatment was called by one patient "perspiration of the sweats." The boiling water is replenished from time to time, the aim of the treatment being to raise the body temperature by applying as much heat to the head as possible. This method is in fact "induced pyrexia," rather similar to that used in the West for treatment of syphilitic brain disease and first carried out by Wagner-Jauregg in 1917 when he inoculated patients with malaria, a treatment based on the belief—later disproved—that *dementia paralytica* was extremely rare in those countries in which malaria was endemic; the pyrexia was regarded as the potent agent. It seems possible that the Muslin *alfas* may have made some similar observations, perhaps at a much earlier date. Possibly they noted remission of symptoms after bouts of malaria and endeavored to improvise some method that would raise the temperature. It is interesting to note that the alfas place emphasis on replenishing of boiling water and application of heat to the head rather than on inhalation of the herbs. The question, however, is whether induced pyrexia is effective against other forms of mental disorder or only against cerebral syphilis. If it is effective only against cerebral syphilis, to what extent is cerebral syphilis found in Sierra Leone? Finally do the Muslim *alfas* receive a sufficient number of these cases to warrant the claims made by both themselves and other native doctors for the effectiveness of the treatment.

Malaria is endemic to Sierra Leone, and patients suffering from it form the largest single hospital inpatient and outpatient groups. In 1957, 28,684 cases of malaria and only 622 cases of syphilis were treated at Sierra Leone government hospitals. As Carothers[27] pointed out, however, it is extremely difficult to diagnose syphilis in Africa. "Attempts to measure the extent of syphilization by blood tests are somewhat vitiated in Africa by the existence of certain other endemic diseases (especially yaws, leprosy and malaria) which sometimes give a positive reaction." As yaws is also endemic to Sierra Leone, the high number of positive Kahn tests obtained by the laboratory in Freetown, in 1957, registering 2600 positive out of 6647 Africans tested, must represent a large number of yaws cases in addition to syphilis. In 1957, 3902 cases of yaws were diagnosed and treated in all government hospitals. Because of these complicating factors in the diagnosis of syphilis, it is difficult to determine the exact incidence of infection and even more difficult to obtain information on cerebral involvement. Tooth[28] noted that in Ghana, "The fact remains that G.P.I. is rarely diagnosed during life although it is sometimes revealed in Asylum patients at autopsy." In 1957, ten cases of G.P.I. were diagnosed in Sierra Leone government hospitals. Since, however, in cases that show symptoms of mental illness, patients tend to go to traditional practitioners rather than to hospitals, it seems possible that a larger number of undiagnosed patients were being treated by Muslim *alfas*. The *alfas'* claims for remission of symptoms may be valid in such cases. It seems doubtful that other forms of mental disorder would respond to treatment by induced pyrexia, although Tredgold[29] did state that symptoms were improved in some forms of mental disorder after febrile illness. In addition to the improvements obtained by Muslim *alfas* with physical treatment, other instances of recovery have been

noted, usually involving social complications with no organic involvement. In such cases, the *alfa* uses his prestige to very good effect. The
methods used in Kabala are also used by the three Muslim *alfas* in
Freetown, each of whom averages four to five patients at a time. The
alfas in Kabala have a greater reputation than those in Freetown and
thus receive many more patients, although Kabala is 250 miles up country.

THE HUMUI SOCIETY OF THE MENDE

The Mende Humui Society's functions are similar to those of the
Ragbanle among the Temne. Like other Mende societies, Humui is
concerned with the maintenance of moral prohibitions, in this case
against incest, and with the maintenance of physical well-being. Prohibitions on sexual relationships are extensive, including sexual relationships with any relatives on the patrilineal side, any descendants of one's
own mother, a nursing mother, a pregnant woman, and any woman at
all in the bush either during the day or at night. There are also extensions
of these prohibitions, which actually form rules of sexual hygiene.

Although the prohibitions governing sexual relationships are much
stricter than those enforced by the Ragbenle, about 27.9% of the male
Mende population of the mental hospital at Kissy have histories of
psychosexual abnormality, compared to only 9.1% of the Temne, 12.5%
of the Limba, and 9.3% of the Creoles. Possibly the greater severity of
Mende prohibitions on sexual relationships results in a greater number
of infringements of these laws, although often only of minor prohibitions,
and consequently in strong feelings of guilt about sex, which would play
a major role in the dynamics of their psychoses. It is also possible that
restrictive Mende sexual prohibitions have in fact increased the possibility
that psychologically unstable Mende will manifest their instability in
this area.

If a Mende becomes ill after breaking a Humui rule, he attends a
soothsayer, who will divine the cause of his illness by the use of stones
and very close questioning designed to extract a confession. The patient
must then be initiated into the society in order to receive the treatment
that will cure him of his illness. In cases of physical illness where no
contravention of law has occurred, it is possible for the patients to be
treated by individual Humui practitioners without having to be initiated
into the society.

Hale is the Mende word for medicine, which Little[30] believes can
include any common object that derives special powers from the fact
that *hale* "represents a special kind of supernatural power or quality
which becomes attached to the object through the influence of *Ngewa*

(God) because a connection with *Ngewa* is implicit in the notion of *hale.*" Each Mende society has its own *hale.* Mende secret societies use their medicines like their curse as social sanctions. When breaches of a society's specialized prohibitions occur, the illness that follows can only be treated by confession and consequent initiation into the society. In order to treat any physical illness among the Mende, the practitioner must always consider the possibility of complicating social issues.

THE GENII OF THE MENDE

Genii are the Mende equivalent of the Temne *ang-krifi.* The *genii* are spirits that inhabit all Mende natural features. Little[31] states that Mende *genii* "are specifically recognisable in anthropomorphic terms and possess, apparently, well-marked human tastes, emotions, and passions." Mende consider that relations with a *genie* are a matter of individual responsibility rather than the concern of the group. Little goes on to say, "the person who deals with them must act boldly. Either he obtains power over the *Genie,* or the *Genie* takes control of him." The Mende concept of a *genie* involves an interpersonal relationship in which the Mende must maintain his superiority and outwit the *genie* he meets. Little notes that "the methods of regarding and treating these spirits are an expression of some of the values which motivate and guide the Mende in their personal relations with each other."

Hofstra describes two main groups of Mende spirits, "the ancestral spirits and the spirits, who in a former existence, have not been human beings."[32] For the latter group, Hofstra uses the Mende term *dyinanga,* distinguishing between good and evil *dyinanga.* The good *dyinanga* brings good fortune; the evil *dyinanga* worries and disturbs people. Some Mende believe that attacks by evil *dyinanga* may be dangerous and may even lead to a form of mental disorder. Evil *dyinanga* can be driven away by native doctors, although the Islamic *mori*-men are considered best at this treatment. It is thought that, if the *mori*-men take no action to protect themselves against the *dyinanga,* the *dyinanga* will injure them in some way.

One such case reported by Hofstra involves the seventeen-year-old son of a *mori*-man. This particular *mori*-man had been noted for his ability to drive away these evil spirits. His son had been considerably disturbed since the death of his mother about eight years earlier. Since then, the boy had complained that he was being worried by a particularly evil *dyinanga,* and all attempts by his father to drive away this evil spirit had proved unavailing. The spirit had continually urged the son to kill his father until finally the boy succumbed to the *dyinanga* and killed his father with a machete. Details of the case history indicated hallucinated phases and catatonic states lasting for some days at a time.

An analysis of the delusional and hallucinatory content in the illnesses of male patients at the Kissy Mental Hospital showed that, while Temne were concerned with the activities of witches, Mende were much more concerned with spirits and devils. In a number of cases, Mende patients actually attributed their illnesses to the actions of evil *dyinanga*. One Mende patient described dreams in which a *dyinanga* had incited him to assault people in return for which he was to be made Paramount Chief. In another case, the Mende patient claimed that he had been told by a *genie* to kill someone in order to become Paramount Chief. This man had killed his wife for infidelity, and his claim that he had been incited by a *genie* was probably a form of rationalization.

Mende show concern for the necessity to maintain satisfactory relationships with *genii* by conforming to accepted patterns of Mende interpersonal behavior, for otherwise a *genie* is likely to overcome individual defenses and make a person act against his own will. In such specific cases, the Mende say, mental disorder can follow, and the person will become "crazy." Before an individual can become vulnerable to such a *genie*, however, he must first have infringed some law of the N'jayei secret society.

N'JAYEI AND YASSI SOCIETIES

The N'jayei and Yassi secret societies are unique in Sierra Leone, restricted as they are to two functions: the treatment of mental illness and, secondarily, the maintenance of agricultural fertility. Although N'jayei is Mende and Yassi is Sherbro, the societies have marked similarities in both structure and function.

Psychological abnormality, both neurotic and psychotic, is attributed among the Mende to some infringement of N'jayei laws. These infringements include trespassing on N'jayei bush, seeing the sacred N'jayei stones, or seeing the dead body of an important member before ritual purification. When such a breach of N'jayei law occurs, initiation into the society is regarded as the only cure unless the individual is already a member of the Humui society, whose function is to treat physical illness, in which case he can be treated by N'jayei without initiation. Little noted two other ways in which membership was obtained: by dreaming of the N'jayei medicine or by committing some wrong against an elder of the society.[83] In addition, there are also some who have membership by virtue of descent. The society also supplies medicine to make farms fertile and certain other medicines designed to strengthen self-confidence and character. Little notes that these medicines are used by candidates for election to the chieftaincy.

§ Some Characteristics of the Kissy Mental Hospital Population

The Kissy Mental Hospital in Freetown is the only residential mental hospital in Sierra Leone, drawing patients both from the Colony area (since independence renamed the Western Province) and from the Protectorate, consisting of the Northern, Southern, and South Eastern Provinces. The hospital contains four wards, three for males and one for females. For men there is an admission ward, a chronic ward, and a curable ward. A new female ward is to be completed, at which time the curable cases will be moved, and the chronic cases will occupy the present female ward. The hospital has no psychiatrist, but two medical officers visit during the week. There is a trained psychiatric nursing staff and a psychiatric welfare officer. On the basis of the estimated population of about 2.26 million in Sierra Leone in 1958, the incidence rate of the institutionalized mentally ill is .93 per 1000 of population.

The sex ratio of the 1962 Kissy Hospital population was 2.58 males to each female. Temne, the second largest tribal group, form the largest male hospital group with 28.95%, the Mende, the largest tribal group in Sierra Leone, constitute only 17.11%. Creoles, who had an estimated population in 1958 of 32,500 in the Colony area, form the second largest male hospital group with 28.29% of the male hospital population.

Of the 152 male patients in Kissy, no fewer than 101 have been admitted from the two main urban areas of Sierra Leone. It is therefore tempting to hypothesize that the social, physical, and psychological stresses in these urban areas have contributed to the high incidence of institutionalized insane. There are, however, too many other variables involved to permit any conclusions regarding the stresses of urbanization and the incidence of psychological abnormality. It is not possible to determine the incidence of psychoses in traditional villages, and thus no comparison can be made. In addition, those personality characteristics that originally motivated migration to urban areas may also increase susceptibility to psychological breakdown. Individuals who become psychotic in urban areas are also more likely to come under official notice, be certified, and be admitted to Kissy.

§ Conclusions

Traditional treatment of all abnormalities in Sierra Leone is essentially a function of social groups. Where abnormality is too extreme, as with the deformed Temne babies, society has found it necessary to remove the deviation. Where less severe offenses have been committed against society, social sanctions have been used to ensure the guilty person's reintegration into society by a process of confession and treatment. Treatment is not merely a "doctor-patient" relationship but a form of social reintegration through the medium of social groups like the highly specialised N'jayei Society of the Mende. African medicine therefore plays a dual role designed to maintain the continuity of society as a functioning whole. Deviant behavior is eliminated by social sanctions, but, at the same time, the very act of elimination is part of the cycle that ensures the reintegration of the individual into society. In situations of social changes, as in Lunsar, traditional social sanctions appear to be used even more actively in order to create a stable social situation. The treatment of physical and psychological illness is still complicated by such social factors as witchcraft and curses, even in urban settings.

It is also difficult to draw any definite conclusions about the incidence of psychological abnormality in the urban areas. Numerous cases of individual psychological conflict have been noted, but even when the statistical incidence of psychological disturbance in urban areas is established, it is impossible to compare it with that in traditional villages. In the same way, it is impossible to draw any conclusions about the incidence of institutionalized insane resulting from urban stresses because of the difficulties in getting information about the numbers of psychotics receiving traditional treatment in villages and other rural areas. As has already been pointed out, migrant workers who become psychotic in urban areas are much more likely to be certified and admitted to Kissy. Furthermore, patients are usually admitted to Kissy only after traditional treatment has failed, and thus the cases in Kissy, particularly those from the Protectorate area, tend to be of a more organic nature. The distribution of institutionalized mental illness between the sexes shows interesting differences in relation to the educational achievement of each tribal group, but again no conclusions can be drawn because of the absence of information about the incidence of mental illness in rural areas. When such census information becomes available, it may then be possible to control for these variables and to determine incidence rates more exactly.

Although it has not been possible to draw conclusions about the incidence of mental illness and psychological abnormality in urban areas, it is possible to draw some conclusions about the psychological susceptibility of the different tribal groups to processes of social change. In Lunsar and Marampa, the settlement patterns of the different tribal groups are related to the extent of the cultural difference between the immigrant groups and the indigenous tribe of Temne. Distant Temne and other tribal groups culturally related to Temne, like the Limba and Loko, tend to settle with the indigenous Temne in Lunsar, where they have varying degrees of in-group status. On the other hand, the Mende and Creoles, who are completely unrelated to the Temne, have created their own cultural environment within the mine compound. Although the Mende, as a migrant group settling in Marampa, have been exposed to greater urban stresses than have the Temne, the indigenous tribe, testing and objective ratings by external observers show greater personality disturbances among the Temne.

Severe Temne child-rearing practices appear to be unsuited to the needs of the new urban environment, although it is very difficult to determine whether or not the higher incidence of Temne psychological disturbance in the urban environment is attributable to child-rearing practices. Temne values, oriented as they are toward the past, have no socially accepted outlet in the urban environment, and this lack appears to offer a further source of conflict.

In addition, Temne psychological susceptibility to social change seems partly related to the incompatibility of the Temne value system with such urban processes as education, industrial training, and a new authority system. These hypotheses are supported by the numbers of Temne in the mental hospital—sixty Temne, compared to thirty-three Mende, although the Mende are the country's largest tribe. This difference still holds when such variables as educational achievement and place of last residence are controlled. Another difference noted between these two tribal groups was the strength of the traditional Mende societies. Temne tend to form a larger number of voluntary associations than do the Mende, which may reflect their greater need for psychological and social interaction in the urban situation.

The Temne thus appear to be compensating for difficulties of adjustment in urban areas by forming these social groups. As we initially postulated, these social groups have been formed in part to take over the therapeutic role of the more traditional secret societies. They have been modified and adapted in the urban environment to satisfy individual psychological and social needs for identification with familiar group patterns in an otherwise confused situation. Thus Temne in Freetown have created social groups that have restored their tribal consciousness and have given the individual Temne the opportunity to identify with his tribal group. These social groups formed in the urban environment thus fulfill their traditional therapeutic roles by maintaining norms of behavior through social sanctions—and individual security through group membership. Social sanctions are exercised by the new voluntary associations and semitraditional societies to the extent that, for an individual to maintain his identity with a social group, he must conform with their established patterns of behavior.

It is impossible to draw any comparative conclusions about the therapeutic benefits of institutionalised treatment of the mentally ill at Kissy compared with the traditional treatment of psychotic conditions. Patients at Kissy represent a larger number with organic psychoses and severe psychotic disturbance, and the discharge rate of long-term patients is very low indeed. In many cases, even when the symptoms of the long-term patient have subsided, relatives have either lost interest in the patient, or those into whose care the patient must be discharged cannot be traced. Diagnostic and therapeutic facilities at the hospital are limited, although this weakness will shortly be remedied by the appointment of a Sierra Leone psychiatrist. It must also be remembered that many of the cases in Kissy have been admitted after conviction for criminal offense and that one of the main functions of Kissy as a mental hospital is to protect the public from the criminally insane.

As Kissy evolves as a mental hospital, with a consequent increase in diagnostic and therapeutic efficiency, the facilities offered will become more compatible with the personality characteristics of the highly educated. Creoles, for example, whose society and cultural orientations are similar to those of the West, have no cultural awareness and belief in the benefits of traditional treatment. Creoles thus have no indigenous methods of treatment as part of their culture. The Creole mental-hospital population has characteristics and distributions of psychotic conditions similar to that of a typical European mental-hospital population, and Creoles require treatment compatible with their cultural orientations. On the other hand, for those literate or illiterate patients who have continuing awareness of their cultural heritage and who are thus vulnerable to the social sanctions of their traditional culture, treatment by traditional methods seems more effective.

This cultural awareness is precisely why the medical officer at Marampa has observed that patients removed from hospital are always those who exhibit symptoms of mental illness. Africans recognize that Europeans do not understand the social complications accompanying so many physical and psychotic disturbances and that these disturbances can only be treated by those native doctors, Muslim *alfas,* and societies that have complete understanding of the social complications involved. African medicine and psychiatry treat the complete man physically, psychologically, and socially.

Notes

1. Peter Kup, *A History of Sierra Leone, 1400-1787* (Cambridge: Cambridge University Press, 1961).

2. *Ibid.*

3. J. Littlejohn, *Report on Fieldwork in Lunsar, Sierra Leone* (Unpublished Ms., Department of Social Anthropology, Edinburgh University, 1956).

4. Michael Gelfand, *The Sick African* (3rd ed.; Cape Town, Juta & Co., Ltd., 1957).

5. D. P. Gamble, *Report on Sociological Survey of Lunsar* (Unpublished Ms., Department of Social Anthropology, Edinburgh University, 1961).

6. K. L. Little, *The Mende of Sierra Leone* (London: Routledge & Kegan Paul, Ltd., 1951).

7. John W. M. Whiting and Irvin L. Child, *Child Training and Personality* (New Haven: Yale University Press, 1953).

8. Little, "The Role of Voluntary Associations in West African Society," *American Anthropologist,* 59 (1957), No. 4, 579-96.

9. Michael Banton, *West African City* (London: Oxford University Press, 1957).

10. *Ibid.*

11. *Ibid.*

12. *Ibid.*

13. Gamble, *op. cit.*

14. Littlejohn, *op. cit.*

15. *Ibid.*

16. *Ibid.*

17. J. C. Carothers, *The African Mind in Health and Disease* (World Health Organization Monograph Series No. 17 [Geneva, 1953]).

18. Gamble, Personal communication to the author, 1962.

19. A. Raymond Mills, *The Effects of Urbanisation on Health in a Mining Area of Sierra Leone* (Unpublished doctoral dissertation, Edinburgh University, 1962).

20. Gelfand, *op. cit.*

21. C. F. Schlenker, *A Collection of Temne Traditions.* (London: Church Missionary Society, 1861).

22. Janheinz Jahn, *Muntu,* Marjorie Grene, trans. (London: Faber & Faber, Ltd., 1958).

23. M. J. Field, *Search for Security* (London: Faber & Faber, Ltd., 1960).

24. Simon D. Messing, "Group Therapy and Social Status in the Zar Cult of Ethiopia," Marvin K. Opler, ed., *Culture and Mental Health* (New York: The Macmillan Company, 1959), pp. 319-32.

25. Philip Mayer, *Townsmen or Tribesmen* (Cape Town: Oxford University Press, 1961).

26. Little, "The Mende in Sierra Leone," Daryll Forde, ed., *African Worlds* (London: Oxford University Press, 1954), pp. 111-37.

27. Carothers, *op. cit.*

28. Geoffrey Tooth, *Studies in Mental Illness in the Gold Coast* (Her Majesty's Stationery Office Colonial Research Papers, No. 6 [London, 1950]).

29. A. F. Tredgold and R. F. Tredgold, *Manual of Psychological Medicine* (3rd ed.; London: Balliere, Tindall and Cox, 1953).

30. Little, "Voluntary Associations."

31. *Ibid.*

32. Sjoerd Hofstra, "The Belief among the Mendi in Non-Ancestral Spirits," *Internationales Archiv für Ethnographie*, XL (Leiden, 1942), Heft 5-6, 175-182.

33. Little, *The Mende.*

Orhan M. Oztürk

with the Assistance of

Fuat A. Göksel, m.d.

Folk Treatment of Mental Illness in Turkey*

§ Introduction

Turkey's vast historical background and its numerous contacts with various major cultures of the Old World are well known. Since the beginning of history, Asia Minor has been the crossroads of many migrations, as well as an attractive land for settlers of many different ethnic origins. The material relics of the ancient civilizations of the Hittites, Greeks, Romans, Byzantines, Persians, Arabs, and Turks are still extant. In addition, common beliefs, values, and behavioral patterns are often found to be of ancient cultures.[1] Paganism, Judeo-Christianity, and the Moslem religion have all deeply influenced the societies of this area at various stages in history. The present ethnic group in Asia Minor is predominantly Turkish, and the religion of the great majority is Islam. The pagan Turks had accepted the Moslem religion before their migration from the East to Asia Minor, mainly between the eighth and eleventh centuries. Since then, the Arabic and Persian cultures have greatly influenced Turkish society in the economic, political, scientific, and aesthetic spheres. Until the second decade of the twentieth century, Islam was the major force for order in the society. The whole structure of the state in hierarchical layers was based on the Islamic code. The power of the Ottoman sultan, administration, property distribution, and penalties all followed Islamic principles dictated by the Koran. Individual lives (marriage and daily work activity, for example) and the total world-view (surrender to God and the concepts of life and death and

* I wish to acknowledge my deep appreciation to Drs. A. Kiev, R. Shuey, and D. Karan for their suggestions while preparing this paper.

343

of life after death) were also structured from the precepts of the Koran. Until the end of the nineteenth century, educational institutions (*medresehs*) taught only Arabic alphabet, theology, and jurisprudence (Islamic law). For many centuries, Moslem religion remained as an "unshakable" dogmatic force in the society.[2]

"Westernization," that is, the acceptance of Western science, modes of living, world-views, and philosophies, started with hesitant and weak attempts in the mid-nineteenth century. It was not until after the fall of the Ottoman Empire following the First World War and the establishment of a new Turkish government, however, that radical attempts were made to guide the social structure in a modern direction. Many religious and educational institutions and the caliphate (the religious leadership of the Moslem world) were abolished. The universities and schools were reorganized. The Roman alphabet was adopted in place of the Arabic. The state and its civil and penal laws were made entirely secular. Polygamy was outlawed, and women were given equal legal rights, including the right to vote. In spite of these serious attempts at changing the old cultural and religious systems, however, a considerable portion of the population is still untouched and unchanged in its beliefs and patterns of living. About 80% of the total population live in the villages. Sixty per cent of the total population and more than 70% of the rural population are illiterate.[3] The majority of the people, especially in the rural sectors, is devoted to the Moslem religion and applies its principles and laws as they have been applied for centuries.[4]

A typical Turkish village has a population of between 200 and 1500 people, and about twenty-four million people live in these small distributed communities, which are in general isolated from one another with limited contact with the urban centers.[5] A village is essentially a cluster of farm houses made of mud-brick, plaster, or wood, depending on what is available in the region. The typical villager is a peasant who makes a bare living by tilling the soil with a plow, threshing with a sled, and carrying the crops in oxcarts. Power-driven machinery is, however, used on large farms in relatively prosperous regions. The primary interests of the villager are his land, his crops, and religious activity. His thought content is predominantly determined by agriculture and religion, according to which his concepts of time and space, his social and work activities are shaped. For example, the seasons of the year are named according to agricultural activity (reaping season, hazelnut-gathering season, and so forth) and the months according to religious holidays (so many months or weeks before or after Ramadan). Daily work routine is also arranged according to the special hours of worship determined by the phases of the sun.

The villager lives a rather isolated life within the boundaries of his village and land.[6] The family unit is extremely compact, and its members are strongly tied to one another. It is not uncommon to find a whole family, including parents, sons, and their wives and children all living under one roof.[7] The father typifies the traditional concept of a patriarch. By the same token, the woman has a very low social position and does all sorts of work, including all heavy farm activity, as well as housework and child-rearing.[8]

The administrative organization of the village consists of a village chief (*muhtar*) and the village council (also known as the old-men's council), elected by the villagers. The chief and the village council act as agents who give advice, handle all sorts of administrative and economic problems of the villager, settle disputes and arguments, and act as interpreters between the villager and the government.

Child-rearing practices are not uniform in all of Turkey. We shall, however, describe certain fundamental and common aspects briefly. We have already referred to the social role of the woman, which naturally determines the type of child-rearing. In spite of their legal equality with men, women are still literally exploited, suppressed, and treated as subordinate to men. Self-esteem, time, energy, and security necessary for child-care cannot be adequately provided by a woman who must work continuously in the field and who must care for the farm animals and do all housework even at the time of birth. Conception, childbirth, and child death are believed to be inevitable phenomena determined by God. In general, babies are swaddled until they are about nine to twelve months old and are breast-fed for at least a year and not uncommonly for two or three years. Continued breast-feeding is not necessarily an indication of maternal generosity in love. In some areas it is practiced for economic reasons or from a belief that birth control is possible by continued breast-feeding. It is our impression that, in many areas, children are seriously deprived of adequate mothering during the first years of life because of woman's social position. Poverty, infectious diseases, and malnutrition are also additional important sources of biological deprivation. Mortality during the first year of life is 16.5%, according to the Government Planning Committee Reports of 1962. When the child reaches the developmental stage of walking and talking, the characteristic form of training can be described as coercive and constrictive. Obedience, compliance, and silence are rewarded. Activity, mobility, curiosity, and talkativeness are discouraged and even punished. During this stage of autonomy, as formulated by Erikson,[9] although no rigid toilet-training takes place, autonomous will and autonomous activity are prohibited. The child is rewarded if he behaves as an "extension" of his parents.[10] During the stage of initiative (Erikson) or the phallic stage, curiosity and aggressive intrusion in play and in other life situations are inhibited by the above-mentioned expectations of adults. Repeated frightening tales about the *jinns*, which are believed to be aggressive, mobile, autonomous, and changeable spiritual beings, are among important methods of punishment. Religious and mystical tales, which are loaded with *jinns*, fairies, and superstitions enter the fantasy world of the child as soon as he begins to comprehend. His fantasies become easily identified with those of the adults. We shall examine the *jinns* in greater detail later. Circumcision of boys is performed without anesthesia during this or the following period, usually between the ages of four and eight. The society recognizes the potential traumatic effect of the experience at this stage and provides many such compensatory and counterphobic devices as preliminary verbal preparation, ceremonies, gifts, and masculinity status.[11] The societal treatment of boys and girls is thus extremely differentiated from very early childhood. In certain areas, boys are breast-fed beyond the ages of two or three because of a belief that they will grow stronger with mother's milk. All children, however, are rewarded for obedience, silence, and loyalty to their elders. In addition, boys are specifically required to be courageous, not in the sense of aggressivity, curiosity, and work, but in the sense of physical strength, endurance of physical pain, and frustration. For example, boys will boast of not crying during circumcision. This emphasis may be related to the noted bravery and endurance of the Turkish soldier in the battle field, which is the major culturally sanctioned area for expression of aggression. Boys and girls start working with the parents of the same sex around age seven. Because the social and the geotemporal environment is greatly limited and constricted, the village child incorporates and assimilates rapidly the traditional "constricted self" (Lerner) of his parents.[12]

We have already indicated that the world of this "constricted self" is greatly shaped by agricultural and religious traditions that are authoritarian, stable, and unchanging. Stereotyped and monotonous relations with the soil and with God and their extensions constitute the major part of the phenomenal field of the villager. The dogmatic interpretation and practice of the Moslem religion with its monocausalistic and fatalistic attribution of all power and will to one supreme force have played a significant role in the establishment and maintenance of this stable world. As we shall see, many primitive folk practices have continued with little or no change. Superstition, magic, and religion find common meeting ground in this rural community, and there is considerable evidence of religio-magical practices for therapeutic purposes.

In this paper, we are mainly concerned with folk interpretation and treatment of mental illness. Our information is drawn from the literature and from a study of 100 patients admitted to University Hospital, Ankara, most of whom had previously tried various folk cures (Table 1).

Table I—Distribution of Patients[a] According to Diagnosis and Their Verbal Reports of Contacts with Folk Therapy

Diagnosis	Used folk therapy	Did not use folk therapy	More than one visit to hodja	Verbal exchange with hodja[b]	Partial or temporary improvement[c]	Total number of patients
Organic disorders	11	16	7	1		27
Schizophrenic disorders	22	4	8	5	3	26
Anxiety reactions (neurasthenias included)	16	6	10	10	5	22
Conversion reactions	5	3	3	1	1	8
Depressive Syndromes	3	4	3	1	1	7
Manic reactions (M.D.P.)	1	1				2
Hypochondriasis		2				2
Character disorders	1	1				2
Paranoid reactions		1				1
Obsessive-compulsive neurosis	1			1		1
Undiagnosed		2				2
Total	60	40	31	19	10	100

a. Randomly selected from the Psychiatric and Neurological Clinics of the Faculty of Medicine, Ankara, Turkey.

b. This category refers to those hodjas who listen or make explanations to their patients. Obviously, the majority of hodjas prescribes treatment without much verbal exchange with the patients.

c. Naturally, there are many patients who never reach the clinics. Therefore the real therapeutic efficacy of these folk treatments cannot be reflected in this study. Of sixty patients who visited hodjas, all received muska, praying, and breathing. Twenty-one received conjured water and ten fumigations as well. Thirty-three patients stated that their illnesses were explained on the basis of jinns or sorcery. Twenty-seven patients reported no explanation of illness made by the hodja.

The writers' own experiences and observations were included only if they were confirmed by the study and the literature.[13] Obviously, there is no one single institutionalized method to be elaborated. As would be expected, thanks to the variety of influences on the present culture, the variety of beliefs and practices is wide. Nevertheless, certain generalizations can be made. Many concepts and practices are not specific for the culture. We shall not endeavor therefore to make detailed explanations of the origins and essentials of these practices as they are encountered in Turkey.

One fact should be emphasized here. In 1925, all religious and quasi-religious educational and therapeutic institutions were abolished, and the practice of magic and religion was outlawed. In spite of many prosecutions and punishments, the practices do continue to some extent and still have a place in the lives of the traditional majority.

§ Psychiatric Illness in Turkey

Although there are no adequate statistical studies to indicate the incidence of mental illness in Turkey, it is quite apparent to all those interested in medicine and psychiatry that mental illness is not a minor problem in this country. All sorts of psychotic and neurotic reaction encountered in the Western countries (Europe and the United States) are common, with some minor differences in the incidence of the types of reaction, as well as in certain culturally determined aspects of symptomatology. The general agreement among psychiatrists is that neuroses (neurasthenias, anxiety reactions, conversion reactions, and grand hysterias) are very common in Turkey. The most common psychotic reactions are the schizophrenias and manic-depressive illnesses. There does not seem to be a striking difference between the incidence in urban and rural populations.

Psychiatric illness in Turkey carries the usual stigma among the majority of the people. Cruel and inhumane treatment of patients has, however, never existed to any remarkable degree in this part of the world. Mental illness has usually aroused pity and sorrow, and patients in general have been treated accordingly. In Turkey, the first hospital ward for the mentally sick was reportedly established in the sixteenth century,[14] and the care of the patients was conducted in accordance with the Islamic medicine of the Middle Ages. During the last three centuries, however, while the Ottoman Empire declined in every respect, medical science and patient care, including the care of the mentally sick, made little or no progress. The first asylum was founded in 1860, and since then three state hospitals with a total population of about 5000 patients have been established. There are three university psychiatric hospitals for the training of psychiatrists, and they also function as acute treatment centers. There is a growing interest in psychiatry within the medical profession, as well as among the public. This interest is suggested by increasing numbers of applications for training in psychiatry, as well as by the waiting lists for admission to the hospitals.

§ Folk Interpretation of Mental Illness

Understanding of and attitudes toward physical or mental illness are changing as modern medical facilities and communication media are becoming more and more available to the rural people. It is therefore difficult to achieve a clear sample of the folk interpretation of illness. Within any given village, there are people who take their patients to medical doctors, while there are others who rely only upon traditional healers. In general, patients with bodily complaints are more readily taken to medical doctors than those patients with mental illnesses. Our examples of folk treatment methods show clearly, however, that many of them are utilized for the treatment and prevention of both bodily and mental illness. Folk beliefs and ideas about illness are usually nonspecific and are applicable to all sorts of illnesses. Still, a few specific etiological and therapeutic concepts do exist and provide the basis for a minor degree of specialization.[15]

The criteria for folk diagnosis of insanity are not clearcut. The difference between a person who is *deli* (insane) and a *veli* (saint) has apparently long posed a problem, as noted in an old expression, "Some said he was *deli*, some said he was *veli*."[16] In our observations, the general criteria for the diagnosis of insanity include essentially *aggressiveness* (whether directed toward oneself or others), *instability*, and *nonconformity* (as opposed to the passivity, stability, and changelessness of the constricted self). *Deli* also means "aggressive and destructive" or impulse-ridden. A person may be hallucinated or delusional, but as long as he is not destructive or very unstable he may not be considered insane, particularly if the content of his hallucinations or delusions is religious and mystical. Such a person may sometimes be considered to have a supernatural capacity for communication with the spiritual world and may therefore be regarded with reverence and awe. It appears that external manifestations of a socially unacceptable nature are more important criteria for insanity than are harmless autoplastic thought disturbances. Clinically, when patients express fear of becoming *deli*, they invariably define a fear of losing control and becoming destructive. On the other hand, in folklore, it is not uncommon to find insanity viewed as a manifestation or result of hopeless and unrequited love. In most cases, however, whether a patient is considered insane or not, similar therapeutic methods will be attempted.

We have already hinted that the villager does not distinguish among superstition, magic, and religion. He believes that his understanding of illness is in accordance with his faith, that is, with what is written in the "book." The average villager, however, actually knows very little about the meaning of the Koran, which is in the Arabic language; what he knows is usually certain common rules and rituals for daily worship. Because of this ignorance, we find discrepancies between what the villager believes and what the Koran "really" says. Beliefs in sorcery, magic, evil eye, and so forth are among such discrepancies. It appears that the Moslem religion as it is practiced in the village is considerably modified by local social and psychological characteristics. An elaboration of the authentic Islamic interpretation of illness is beyond the scope of this paper. It is a well known fact that during the Middle Ages science did advance with the expansion of Islam, that medicine became a practical science,[17] and that patients (including the mentally ill) were treated kindly and with humane interest. It is also very clear that, although the Koran does not deny the existence of sorcery, it does not approve it either and does not attribute supernatural powers to mankind.[18] Miracle cures by men are not accepted. In our opinion, however, it does include concepts that can easily nourish any tendency toward magical thinking and practices. The Koran states that all evil and good come from God,[19] and God is therefore the literal provider of health and sickness in the eyes of the villager. "God gave an illness" is a common expression, which the villager uses concretely. God is the foremost etiological agent. How and why God gives an illness are not explained and are considered beyond human curiosity. As long as the patient is not depressed, he does not feel or consider that his illness is a punishment from God. God knows better, and there is no need to ask questions of him, but one can wish and hope from Him and Him alone. The Moslem religion accepts the existence of spiritual beings like the *jinns* (equivalent to demons), the angels, and the fairies. The *jinns* are capable of taking the shape of anything (human, animal, or plant). They are invisible, extremely mobile, and usually aggressive beings that dwell in ruins, woods, rocks, caves, deserted houses, fireplaces, chimneys, and so forth. They can be either male or female. Beside having sexual relations with each other and having children of their own, they can seduce human beings and make love to them. Children who are too independent, curious, or disrespectful toward their parents are frequently frightened by *jinn* tales. From early childhood, the *jinns* are recognized as aggressive, mobile, deceptive, and punitive agents. Villagers commonly believe that mental illness in particular is a result of being possessed or "mixed-up" by the *jinns*. Possession or being "mixed up" is believed to occur usually by accident—but sometimes as punishment for violation of certain taboos or for performing daily activities without ritual precautions against the *jinns*. Cursing bread, failure to take a ritualistic bath after sexual activity with ejaculation (whether heterosexual, autoerotic, or dream activities), and repudiation of parents or of God are some of the violations of taboos that may incite *jinns* to strike. Numerous daily activities like urinating, pouring waste water, sitting, and so forth are preceded by verbal expression of *destur* ("excuse me," used specifically for the *jinns*) to ensure safety from the evils of the *jinns*. The *jinns* may be "seen" accidentally or following such incidents, or one may get an immediate "strike" or the "breeze" or the "holding" from the *jinns*. The result may be aphonia, aphasia, strokes, epileptic attacks, or certain "mixed-up" states known in psychiatry as schizophrenic reactions, manias, and severe delusional depressions. We have observed that many patients with free-floating anxiety or repetitive anxiety dreams often claim that "they are frightening me," referring to the *jinns*.

The evil eye is another extremely common belief, not only among the illiterate, but also among many sections of the literate population. Many illnesses, failures in life, and physical or personality defects are explained by reference to the evil eye. Certain people (most likely those with blue or green eyes) are believed to have the capacity to look with evil eyes. Successful, progressing, healthy, and attractive people are particularly vulnerable to the evil eye. Such people are believed to arouse envy and hostility in others whose eyes have the power of inflicting various diseases by a mere glance. It is the envy-hostility behind the glance that causes the ailment in the victim. Paradoxically, it is sometimes believed that the eyes of the closest and dearest person may have an evil influence. For example, some people believe that mothers are not supposed to praise or to look at their children with admiration. Villagers usually hide their babies from the eyes of other people in order to protect them from evil influences. Verbal and visual influences seem to be equally powerful. If one does not wish his eyes to have an evil influence on someone he admires, before he looks with admiration or says something complimentary, he must say *masallah* (God protect him). This verbal utterance counteracts the evil eye or the evil wish behind the praise.

Although sorcery is banned both by religion and law, there is considerable belief in it as a source of mental illness. Such conditions as inability to concentrate, physical weakness, restlessness and agitation, headache, hallucinatory and confusional states, sexual impotence, and loss of love for one's spouse are attributed to the influence of a sorcerer hired by an enemy. This enemy may be a rival, an in-law, a spouse, a neighbor, or some unknown person. There are numerous ways of performing sorcery. Hiding amulets in the house of the victim, reading from the "book," tying knots, and putting pork fat or hair on household materials are some common methods of sorcery. It appears that the actual application and practice of sorcery are much less common than the belief in them or actual antisorcery practices.

§ Beliefs About the Prevention and Treatment of Illness

These beliefs and practical measures are essentially based on the etiological concepts already described. They are numerous. We can mention only the general categories of treatment and prevention that are most common.

Individual praying is considered to be both preventive and curative. If praying is done by men of religion—the *hodjas, sheiks,* and *dervishes* —it is undoubtedly more effective. Praying is often accompanied by other methods like sacrifices; visiting certain holy places, tombs of saints, and *hodjas;* or visiting certain other places like caves, rocks, or fountains to which supernatural healing power is attributed. Special words or prayers are used to ward off the *jinns* while passing certain places or performing certain daily activities. Beside praying, "writing" is also used as a therapeutic device, for it is believed to be holy and powerful. This belief is not surprising when one considers that for many centuries a monopoly of reading and writing was kept by the priests, who could establish contact with the God's wishes and powers. Copies of the Koran or even of the Bible are highly revered in a Moslem community. Although this reverence is usually present toward religious writings, we have encountered patients talking about boiling the doctor's prescription sheet and drinking the water, which is believed to absorb the curative power of the writing. This belief in the power of written material is reflected clearly in the technique of *muska*. A *muska* is an amulet inscribed by the *hodja* for the treatment or prevention of such evils as illness, evil, and sorcery. Sometimes, however, *muskas* are used as a means to apply sorcery. On a piece of scroll, various *surahs* from the Koran are inscribed, and certain ill defined ritualistic signs and numerical figures are added. The scroll is folded into a triangle or a rectangle and covered with cloth or leather to protect it from dirt and keep it from becoming worn. This practice is the most common, and one can see *muskas* worn like necklaces or tied under the arms beneath the clothes of physically or mentally ill patients. They are also extremely common among healthy people for preventive purposes.

Since belief in the evil eye is popular, methods to combat it are very popular also. Eye-shaped blue beads or unattractive objects (bone, animal excreta) are hung on the clothes of children or put on valued objects. As the evil eye is supposed to be directed particularly toward something attractive and perfect, imperfection, unattractiveness, inconspicuousness, or hiding from other people are also preventive measures. Fumigations, various phrases (*Masallah*), prayers, and certain ritualistic actions like spitting and knocking on wood are also utilized against the evil eye.

Ritualistic praying, breathing, laying on of the *hodja's* hands, animal sacrifices, fumigations, special phrases, tying pieces of cloth on consecrated places (*odjak, yatir,* and tombs of saints), and plants (no specific plants) are other common methods of treatment. Melting lead and pouring it into a cup held over the body of the patient is another common method of exorcism of the *jinns,* sorcery, or the evil eye. The ambiguous figure of the melted and frozen lead stimulates speculations on the type and shape of the *jinns,* the sorcerer, or the person with evil eye. Such animal excreta as stork feces are used as specifics against sorcery.

Although these methods are the most common and major practices, each individual practitioner has his own style. The main therapeutic practitioners are the *hodjas,* the *sheiks,* the *dervishes,* and the *odjaks* and *yatirs.*

The *hodjas* are the priests of the Moslem religion. In the past, they were both priests and teachers. The word *hodja* is still synonymous with "teacher." They conduct the religious ceremonies in the mosques, at funerals, and during religious marriages. For many centuries, *hodjas* were trained and educated in the religious schools called *medresehs.* When those schools were abolished with the establishment of the Republic, *hodjas* apparently were trained through apprenticeship. About thirteen years ago, there was a partial revival of the old schools with some additions of modern science to the curricula. Among the *hodjas,* some are believed to have inherited from their masters capable "hands" or particular styles of praying or writing. They are considered to have real *keramet,* a supernatural power to heal and to strengthen. Some are believed to have "armies of *jinns*" at their service, which they use against other evil-producing *jinns*. When the *hodja* is the leader of a particular sect, he is called a *sheik* or a *dervish*. All *hodjas* are male. There are occasional female healers who utilize similar methods, however. Our personal observations and the study of patients who have visited such practitioners indicate that the great majority of these *hodjas* has no particular skill or specialized ritual. Many of them have no religious training or function but introduce themselves as men of religion and wisdom and use a good deal of quackery.[20] Their practices are rather stereotyped, in that they write *muska*, pray, breathe or lay their hands on patients, massage, and pray to the water and offer it as a conjured drink. These practices are usually carried on without first asking anything about the patient's problem. Only a few seem to be closely and genuinely interested in the individual problem of the patient. They listen to the patient's complaints and occasionally to his dreams. There are *hodjas* who continue seeing their patients in fifteen- to twenty-minute or longer daily sessions for weeks and, rarely, for months. The process in each session does not vary and includes the methods already cited. The following case is illustrative of an uncommon practice that has some relevance to psychotherapy.

A thirteen-year-old schoolboy, the son of a bookseller was taken to several psychiatrists, but his father was not satisfied with their recommendations for medication and psychotherapy. The father and the son then made a long trip to see a recommended *hodja* in a remote village on the Black Sea Coast. The boy was suffering from acute anxiety attacks, which at times seemed to suggest serious decompensation in the form of a schizophrenic reaction. The father and his son were welcomed by the *hodja* in his village home, and they lived there for two weeks, during which time the *hodja* applied his method of intensive treatment. The *hodja* had a family and lived a very ordinary village life but was highly respected in the vicinity. Every day, in two or three sessions that lasted altogether between two and three hours, he and the patient sat facing each other on pillows on the floor. The *hodja* started by praying, reading from the Koran, and breathing on the patient. Then he drew an irregular incomplete circular figure on a piece of paper. On one side of the figure, there was an opening, an "exit." The patient was asked to look carefully at this figure and to try to recall the *jinns* he had encountered in his recent life. The *hodja*, with his particular commanding and awe-inspiring tone of voice insisted that the patient see these *jinns* within the circle as images of real people. With much excitement, fear, and crying the patient produced certain images (the *jinns*) in the circle. He was then asked to cut these *jinns* into pieces and burn them one by one. In every session, this process of recalling the *jinns* and burning them on pieces of paper continued until the *jinns* were eradicated. Every time a *jinn* was destroyed, the exit on the circle was closed. After fifteen days of such treatment, the father and the patient returned to Ankara, and both believed that there was marked improvement. A psychiatric interview supported this belief. About a month later, however, the patient was brought again to the clinic because of recurrence of his symptoms.[21]

It is extremely difficult to locate and investigate such *hodjas* as they seem to be more sophisticated and more capable of carrying on their practices in secrecy since legal prohibition. The fact that some data have been obtained on a few suggests that they probably are more common than suspected.

The other group of common treatment agents beside the *hodjas* are the *odjak* (literally, the hearth) and the *yatir* (the laying one). The *odjak* may be a living specialized *hodja*, or it may be a tomb, a secret convent, a tree, a rock, a fountain, or any other place where magical influence is present to ward off evil and sickness. One frequently hears of a malaria *odjak* or a jaundice *odjak* or an *odjak* for mental illness. When the *odjak* is a living *hodja*, the methods are no different from those described above. When it is a location, people simply come to pray and sacrifice an animal—a sheep, lamb, goat, or rooster. Animal sacrifice in Turkey is conducted according to the principles of the Moslem religion. On a certain religious holiday most people who can afford it are expected to sacrifice a sheep or a goat. Sacrifice is also made when health is regained or sought. In all conditions, the meat of the sacrificed animal is supposed to be distributed to the poor. Before leaving the location, the people tie a piece of cloth on the tomb, rock, tree or whatever serves as *odjak*. The *yatir*, literally translated as the "laying one," is not radically different from the *odjak*, except that it is always a highly honored, revered, and spiritually gifted dead *hodja*. Many villages have their own *yatirs* buried nearby, around whom much elaborate fagulation is constructed. The villager believes that the buried *hodja*, who is equivalent to a saint in this case, has the power to cure illness. The villager has a rich inventory of fabulations to support this belief. The sick villager visits the *yatir*, brings gifts to the keeper of the tomb, prays there, and sacrifices animals.

All these ceremonies are usually conducted on an individual basis. Group therapeutic rituals[22] are seldom seen in Turkey except among certain sects or under certain conditions. For example, *mevlevi* rituals are carried on for mystical purposes by the whirling *dervishes*. *Mevlud* is another group ritual, in which a poem is sung about Mohammed's birthday. The performance is given periodically as a requiem in memory of a dead relative. These group rituals excite a good deal of emotional discharge, praying, and weeping, usually among women. *Mevlud* may or may not have a therapeutic influence in mourning, but the performance is not given for any specific therapeutic reason.

Finally, we should add that there are many other types of folk belief and idea about mental illness in Turkey. Among both illiterate and literate people, certain common-sense explanations for mental illness are typical. Life's miseries, frustrations, conflicts, fears, fatigue, and loss of love objects are frequently accepted as causes of neurotic and psychotic disorders. Rest cures, baths, certain spas, good nourishment, herbs, and marriage are among the most common recommendations for the treatment of such disorders. Stereotyped interpretation of dreams based on folk symbolism is also used for foretelling the future. These recommendations or dream interpretations are made among the people themselves. If they come from a *hodja*, however, they are considered more reliable and effective.

§ Discussion and Conclusions

Unlike relatively homogeneous primitive cultures, Turkey's traditional society does not lend itself to clear cross-sectional study because of its heterogeneity and the fact that the stability of its traditions has been shaken. It is very difficult to localize and describe Turkish folklore in time and space, for its long documented history is spotted with numerous contacts with other cultures. Folk beliefs and practices concerning illness are known to have antique origins. Evil spirits (the *jinns*), the evil eye, and sorcery as causes of illness and amulets, prayers, sacrifice, laying on of hands, animal excrements, and so forth as therapeutic agents are ageless beliefs and practices of man. In this article, our purpose has not been to indicate the specific origins and other universal aspects of these beliefs and practices in Turkey. A comparative study of ancient beliefs and customs about illness clearly reveals the fact that these practices and beliefs have universally common roots and characteristics.[23] We are interested in the authentic meanings and functions of these beliefs and practices for the Turkish villagers. What needs do they meet, and how have they been perpetuated under the conditions in which people live? In what ways are they related to psychotherapy?

In our brief presentation of the historical and sociocultural background and of the specific conditions of existence and childrearing, the writer has tried to point out certain traits of a traditional people. Reference was made to the well documented study by Lerner on the characteristics of the "constricted self," and their development was described in terms of psychosocial stages of early childhood. In this traditional group, human life, instead of being well regulated and subject to secure human care, is generally more exposed to chance and to the mercies of the natural and the supernatural—the soil, the sun, the rain, illnesses and all other evils, and God. Children apparently can learn to adapt themselves to many modes of care and to be satisfied within limits with what they are given by their earliest providers. It can be assumed that the village child learns to modulate his needs and frustration thresholds and learns to live with what can be given. Erikson has written:

> the amount of trust derived from earliest infantile experience does not seem to depend on absolute quantities of food or demonstrations of love but rather on the quality of the maternal relationship. . . . A traditional system of child care can be said to be a factor of making for trust, even where certain items of that tradition, taken singly, may seem unnecessarily cruel.[24]

He also points out that:

> religion and tradition are living psychological forces creating the kind of faith and conviction which permeates a parent's personality and thus reinforces the child's basic trust in the world's trustworthiness.[25]

We suggest that, in the Turkish village, religion and tradition play a compensatory rather than reinforcing role in the establishment of internal security. That is, what is not provided adequately by the human and the natural environment is provided or is sought through faith and conviction in what is beyond the human and the natural. This compensation or reinforcement by tradition does not, however, seem to rule out the possibility of a nuclear deficiency in "basic trust" and of accumulation of aggressive impulses in accordance with the frustration-aggression rule. To be more specific, acceptance of helplessness and fatalistic-passive dependent expectations, on one hand, and accumulation of aggressive drives, on the other, become inevitably rooted during the oral-incorporative stage of childhood. These elements are further reinforced by the training attitudes and adult expectations during the following stages of childhood. In these training attitudes and expectations, we see predominantly a severe and diffuse suppression of behavior

modalities of autonomy and initiative, that is, of autonomous will and
activity, independent vigorous motility, intrusion, and curiosity. Granted
that such suppression exists in a "traditional system of child care," the
increase in aggressive drives in accordance with the frustration-aggression
sequence still persists. In this sense, the child-rearing methods can be
said to reinforce the process of accumulation of aggression, which can
only find its expression usually in culturally sanctioned areas. To summarize, it can be said that the passivity, that is, "the helplessness in
the face of drive demand,"[26] accumulation of drives, and ever-increasing
social need and demand for powerful mastery over one's own drives
become essential areas of conflict within the villager's ego.

Freud and subsequent writers have pointed out the homeostatic
significance of magical and animistic thinking associated with such concepts as evil spirits, the evil eye, sorcery, amulets, and prayers. Freud
has written:

> Magic must serve the most varied purposes. It must subject the processes of
> nature to the will of man, protect the individual against enemies and dan-
> gers and give him the power to injure his enemies.[27]

He concludes that:

> spirits and demons were nothing but the projection of primitive man's emo-
> tional impulses.[28]

Along the same line, Erikson wrote:

> The belief in demons permitted persistent externalization of one's own un-
> conscious thoughts and preconscious impulses of avarice and malice as well
> as thoughts which one suspected one's neighbor of having.[29]

More specifically, sorcery and magic have been shown to be institutionalized instruments of covert aggression.[30]

The homeostatic significance on psychological and sociological levels
lies not only in provision of socially sanctioned means to project, to
displace, and to express aggression, but also in mastering the unknown.
Vague and intangible threats are rendered recognizable and concrete
through beliefs in evil spirits, evil eye, and sorcery in the same way that
the concretization process takes place in individual symptom formation.[31]
In his description of middle European superstitions of the Middle Ages,
Erikson writes:

In all magic thinking, the unknown and the unconscious meet at a common frontier: murderous, adulterous, or avaricious wishes . . . are all forced upon me by evil-wishing neighbors. . . . In a world full of dangers they may have served as a source of security, for they make the unfamiliar familiar, and permit the individual to say to his fears and conflicts, "I see you! I recognize you."[32]

Although the villagers described in this paper are not typically and altogether primitive, they have characteristics of living and thinking in common with primitive man. This similarity is most pronounced in their concepts of illness and other natural phenomena that remain unknown. In describing the perplexing and potentially catastrophic aspects of illness for primitive man, Ari Kiev has written:

Given the threat to his existence and relative inability to cope with his environment, it seems likely that the primitive would be subject to anxieties more frequent and of greater magnitude than contemporary Western man. In addition, we should expect that the diffuse states of tension caused by a loss of regulation and a consequent upset in libidinal and aggressive controls would magnify and sometimes even create the illusion of an outer danger. Owing to his marked anxiety or fear the primitive would seem to be unable accurately to evaluate and objectify the external forces of disease. Accordingly we should expect primitive medicine to be more subject to influence of personality factors than to the immediate realities of the illness situation.[33]

The attribution of active, aggressive, changeable, and seductive characteristics to the *jinns* seems to parallel the need for denial of comparable needs in the villager. This observation is supported by the fact that behavior motivated by such needs is discouraged or punished in childhood. The extremely common belief in the evil eye shows conscious understanding of the destructive potential of hostility and envy. All glances and therefore all wishes can be destructive, but as long as one can take precautions one does not have to feel guilty about one's own eyes. The belief that demonstration of love and admiration should be preceded by a precautionary word or phrase indicates the presence of hostility behind these pleasant demonstrations. As institutionalized projections, sorcery and magic serve a similar purpose. It is interesting to note that a strong denial of guilt is probably connected with this diffuse denial of aggression. When "God gives" an illness or when the *jinns* "strike" or "take hold of" a person, there is usually little or no implication of consciously accepted guilty action or fantasy. Human will and responsibility have nothing to do with anxieties and fears.

In brief, then, the prevailing beliefs about illness in Turkey serve as institutionalized channels for the projection, displacement, and indirect expression of aggressive and other undesirable associated impulses, as well as attempts at mastering the unknown.

The healing and protective principles based on these etiological agents contain elements converging with what we have described of the villager's ego and the conflicts therein. On one hand, there is the passive-dependent expectation, and, on the other, there is the need for adequate mastery of one's own ever-increasing internal aggression. The therapeutic measures seem to take advantage of these two facets, and they may persist for that very reason even though their results are not always satisfactory. It has been pointed out that "the medium through which a mental cure is achieved is the psychological apparatus of the recipient."[34] J. D. Frank argues:

> the core of the effectiveness of methods of religious and magical healing seems to lie in their ability to arouse hope by capitalizing on the patient's dependency on others.[35]

The fatalistic passive-dependent expectation already described is seen in the villager's attitudes toward God, the state, parental figures, *hodjas*, and medical doctors. The *hodja's* social role is actually structured with this aspect of the individual's psychology. To quote Frank:

> the patient's expectation of help is aroused partly by the healer's personal attributes, but more by his paraphernalia, which gains its power from its culturally determined symbolic meaning.[36]

In the case of the *hodjas* or the *odjaks* and *yatirs*, this element is automatically supplied by the diffuse passive-dependent expectation of the villager.

The other facet, that of accumulated aggression, is handled by the therapeutic measures through reinforcement of the projections, displacements, and concretization. For example, the villager who suffers from an anxiety attack believes that he is being "frightened" by external forces (the *jinns*). He expects cure from the *hodja*, who reinforces the belief that the *jinns* have taken hold of him. The defense-strengthening aspect of this approach is obvious. The next step is dependence on the *hodja's* attributed powers to fight the *jinns*. Even in the example in which the *hodja* provided the patient with images to destroy and led the patient to express his aggressive feelings and fears, aggression and fears were displaced to objects on a fantasy level. As Fenichel has pointed out:

> The magical power, projected on to the doctor, does not necessarily need to be used directly as a prohibition of neurotic symptoms. It may also, as in cathartic hypnosis, be used for an annulment of certain repressions. However, any recovery achieved in this way remains dependent on the patient's passive-dependent attitude toward the doctor. The patient's ego instead of being enabled to mature is definitely established as immature.[37]

Finally, a few statements should be made about the guilt-reducing value of these beliefs and practices. We have already implied that, as long as the general tendency is to project all that is internally undesirable and all responsibility onto the institutionalized external forces, there is little or no awareness of guilt associated with one's own impulses or responsibilities as long as one complies with the rules and rituals of these forces. Certain atonement devices are also provided in daily religious ritual—daily prayers and worship and annual fasting and sacrifices. The commonly utilized therapeutic methods do not have gross self-punitive elements. It appears that there is more guilt-denial than guilt-reduction within the therapeutic and preventive framework of these beliefs.

Notes

1. Village administrative organization and agricultural techniques, weekly village markets, some annual district festivals held around ancient Greek ruins, folk interpretation and treatment of illness, circumcision rites, rain-making rites, to name a few. Some of these patterns will be elaborated in this paper.
2. A. Adivar, "Interaction of Islamic and Western Thought in Turkey," T. Cuyler Young, ed., *Near Eastern Culture and Society* (Princeton: Princeton University Press, 1951).
3. *Census of Population* (Ankara: Central Statistical Office, 1961).
4. We do not wish to give the impression that the revolution has failed. As Daniel Lerner has shown in "Modernizing the Middle East," *The Passing of Traditional Society* (New York: The Free Press of Glencoe, 1958), a considerable portion of Turkish society is in a "transitional" state, and the changes are still continuing. We feel the need to emphasize, however, that the "traditional" group is still the majority, and it is this group about which our article is written. The forces impeding change and the reasons for adherence to the past are many. Above all, the changes have been (and have had to be) instituted in a matter of a few years on a legal and ideological basis through rapid changes in the religious and educational spheres. Little could be done to change the basic land problems and economic conditions of the villager. Atatürk's "communication revolution" was carried out by an intellectual minority, but its spread to the villages requires much land reform and such communications prerequisites as roads, schools, radio, and so forth for 40,000 villages, which could not be supplied within this short period. Beside, it has been difficult

for the rural people to co-operate fully in the efforts of the state in view of their traditional suspicion and hostility toward a body that had previously only collected taxes and recruited soldiers. The psychosocial aspects of these impeding factors will be seen in this article.

5. The total population of Turkey is about twenty-eight million, with a high annual increase of 3%. There are more than 40,000 villages.

6. Migrations from rural areas to cities have increased rapidly for economic reasons, which means a continued expansion of the "transitional" society, but the percentage is small, and the acculturation process is slow and not too apparent. Although this migrant group seems to adapt itself to the medical facilities available in the cities, the beliefs and practices described in this paper continue to obtain.

7. D. D. Crary, "The Villager," Sydney Nettleton Fisher, *Social Forces in the Middle East* (Ithaca: Cornell University Press, 1955); N. Erdentug, *A Study on the Social Structure of a Turkish Village* (Publication of the Faculty of Languages, History and Geography, University of Ankara, No. 136 [Ankara: 1959]); and M. Makal, *A Village in Anatolia*, Paul Stirling, ed., Sir Wyndham Deedes, trans. (London: Vallentine, Mitchell & Co., Ltd., 1954).

8. For detailed and excellent descriptions of village life, we refer the reader to M. Makal, a native villager and village schoolteacher who wrote "passionate autobiography and descriptive sociology," according to Lerner, *op. cit.* M. Makal, *op. cit.*

9. E. H. Erikson, *Childhood and Society* (New York: W. W. Norton & Company, Inc., 1950).

10. R. Shuey, Aid educational adviser to Turkey, in a personal communication to the author.

11. O. M. Oztürk, *Psychological Effects of Circumcision as Practiced in Turkey.* Paper presented at the Second Middle Eastern-Mediterranean Paediatric Congress, Ankara, 1961.

12. The term "constricted self" refers to the lack of curiosity, of initiative, of empathy, and of changeability described by Daniel Lerner (*op. cit.*) as characteristic of traditional society in Turkey. In our extremely brief account of child-rearing practices in Turkey, we have also referred crudely to Erikson's concepts of early psychosocial stages in order to understand the development of this "constricted self."

13. O. Acipayamli, *Türkiyede Dogumla Ilgili Adet ve Inanmalarin Entolojik Etüdü* (Ankara: Türk Tarih Kurumu Basimevi, 1961); V. C. Askun, *Sivas Folkloru* (Sivas: Kamil Matbaasi, 1940); M. H. Bayri, *Istanbul Folkloru* (Istanbul, Turkiye Basimevi, 1946); M. Kardes, *Turtumda Halk Inanmalari, Adetlar ve Taslamalar* (Istanbul: Ekin Basimevi, 1961); Makal, *Memleketin Sahipleri* (Istanbul: Varlik Yayinlari, 1954); B. N. Sehsuvaroglu, *Turkish History of Medicine in Anatolia for Nine Centuries.* Paper presented at the Eleventh General Assembly of the World Medical Association, Istanbul, 1957; F. N. Uzluk, *Genel Tip Tarihi* (Ankara Universitesi Tip Fakültesi Yayinlarindan, Sayi 68 [Ankara: 1959]); A. S. Ünver, *Tip Tarihi* (Istanbul: Istanbul Universitesi Yayinlarindan, 1943); and F. Yenisey, *Bursa Folkloru* (Bursa, 1955).

14. R. Adasal, *Ruh Hastaliklari*, II Cilt (Ankara: Ankara Universitesi Tip Fakültesi Yayinlarindan, 1955); and Sehsuvaroglu, *op. cit.*

15. The passages about social hierarchies in *Kutadgu-Bilig* (a book written in the Turkish language in the eleventh century A.D.) are interesting in this respect. They indicate that at the top of the social hierarchy there was the *hekim* (the physician), who treated physical illness with medications. Next came the *efsuncu*, who treated mental illness by warding off the *jinns*. See Ünver, *op. cit.* This distinction suggests that, in the past, there was probably more specialization among folk practitioners than there is now.

16. Adasal, *op. cit.*

17. G. Sarton, "Islamic Science," Young, *op. cit.*

18. M. M. Picthall, *Koran, An Explanatory Translation,* CXIII (New York: New American Library of World Literature, Inc., 1953), 4.

19. *Ibid.,* IV, 78.

20. An official statement by the Minister of State indicates that there are about 60,000 men of religion in Turkey. Of these men, only 5,000 have had any schooling or training. The other 55,000 are illiterate and have been reared in *dervish* convents or secret local Koran "schools," where they have learned to memorize certain parts of Koran without much understanding of true meanings. *Cumhuriyet Gazetesi,* August 19, 1962.

21. We wish to thank Dogan Karan, M.D., of the Department of Psychiatry of the University of Ankara for his follow-up information on this patient.

22. A. Kiev, "Psychotherapy in Haitian Voodoo." Paper presented before the 3rd World Congress of Psychiatry, Montreal, 1961.

23. W. Bromberg, *The Mind of Man: A History of Psychotherapy and Psychoanalysis* (New York: Harper & Row, Publishers, 1959); R. Calder, *Medicine and Man* (London: George Allen & Unwin, Ltd., 1958); B. L. Gordon, *Medicine Throughout Antiquity* (Philadelphia: F. A. Davis Company, 1949); D. Guthrie, *A History of Medicine* (London: Thomas Nelson & Sons, 1958); and J. M. Schneck, *A History of Psychiatry* (Springfield: Charles C Thomas, Publishers, 1960).

24. Erikson, "Growth and Crises of the 'Healthy Personality,'" C. Kluckhohn and H. A. Murray, eds., *Personality in Nature, Society, and Culture* (New York: Alfred A. Knopf, Inc., 1953), p. 195.

25. *Ibid.,* p. 196.

26. D. Rapaport, "Some Metapsychological Considerations Concerning Activity and Passivity" (Unpublished, 1953).

27. S. Freud, "Totem and Taboo," *Basic Writings* (New York: The Modern Library, 1938), p. 868.

28. *Ibid.,* p. 878.

29. Erikson, *Young Man Luther* (New York: W. W. Norton & Company, Inc., 1958), p. 60.

30. A. I. Hallowell, "Aggression in Saulteaux Society," Kluckhohn and Murray, *op. cit.;* Kiev, *op. cit.;* and J. W. M. Whiting, *Becoming a Kwoma* (New Haven: Yale University Press, 1941).

31. S. Arieti, "A Re-examination of the Phobic Symptom and of Symbolism in Psychopathology," *American Journal of Psychiatry,* 118 (August, 1961) No. 2.

32. Erikson, *Luther,* p. 60.

33. Kiev, "Primitive Therapy: A Cross-Cultural Study of the Relationship between Child Training and Therapeutic Practices Related to Illness," W. Muensterberger and S. Axelrod, eds., *The Psychoanalytic Study of Disease* (New York: International Universities Press, 1960), p. 191.

34. Bromberg, *op. cit.,* p. 9.

35. J. D. Frank, *Persuasion and Healing. A Comparative Study of Psychotherapy* (Baltimore: The Johns Hopkins Press, 1961), p. 62.

36. *Ibid.*

37. O. Fenichel, *The Psychoanalytic Theory of Neurosis* (New York: W. W. Norton & Company, Inc., 1945), p. 562.

Jozef Ph. Hes

The Changing Social Role
of the Yemenite *Mori**

I N THIS CHAPTER, we are concerned with mental illness among
Yemenite Jews in Israel, its cultural background, and the practices utilized by their *moris* (native wise men). We want to direct our attention
to the changing role of the *mori*, especially in his relation to the emotional and mental problems of his community.

In Yemen no doctors or hospitals, either general or psychiatric, were
available. The only source of medical care was the native practitioner,
the *mori*. This *mori* fulfilled many functions: He was a teacher, a judge,
a religious leader, a ritual slaughterer, and a healer.

Since their immigration into Israel, the Yemenite Jews live in a
modern society, which offers extensive medical care in the form of
hospitals, outpatient clinics, private physicians, public health nurses, and
other medical and paramedical institutions.

One of the questions we asked ourselves was, What is the impact
of immigration and acculturation on the role and function of the *mori*
as healer and counselor?

In order to gain some insight into this matter, we conducted interviews with fifteen *moris*, talked with Yemenite patients, and studied the
relevant literature.

The significance of this study lies in its clarification of some of the
ways that psychiatric help is given to the patient and his family. Often

* This investigation has been aided by a grant from the Foundations' Fund for
Research in Psychiatry. The author also wishes to express his appreciation to Johebad
Re'ani, M. Sc.; Rose Shuval, M. A.; Awraham Zloczower, M. A.; Aaron Antonovsky,
Ph.D.; and Prof. H. Z. Winnik, M.D., for their collaboration in collecting the data
and preparing the paper for publication.

the psychiatrist does not extend his care outside the mental hospital. Social workers, frequently overburdened in their attempts to supply the basic physical needs of newly arrived immigrants, have neither time nor historical understanding of the emotional needs of ailing Yemenites. The general physicians are too busy to pay attention to the psychological aspects of their patients' illnesses. It is in this void that we might expect the *mori* to fulfill an important function.

§ The Background

The Yemenites comprise about 4% of the population of Israel. Although few in numbers, they have been more intensively studied than other groups, for several reasons. The Yemenites can look proudly back at a long history in which they did not allow themselves to become assimilated to their Arab environment, in the sense that they preserved a tradition of learning: Illiteracy does not exist among them, that is, among the males—an outstanding contrast to conditions among Jews from other Middle Eastern countries. The Yemenites maintained their relationship with Zion and the Land of the Fathers throughout the centuries.

Exact data in regard to the immigration of Jews into the southern part of Arabia are not available.[1] Many legends, however, cast some light on this problem. In one of them, it is told that the Queen of Sheba had a son, fathered by King Solomon (about 950 B.C.). The Queen invited teachers for this son, and these teachers were the first Jews to enter Arabia.

Another legend tells us that forty-two years before the destruction of the first temple (in 587 B.C.) more than 75,000 Jews emigrated to Arabia.

In the year 432 B.C., Ezra the Scribe invited all Jews of the Diaspora to come to Palestine, in order to restore the state and to rebuild the temple. After being informed of the Yemenite Jews' refusal to come back, he cursed them. From that time until today, the name of Ezra is seldom given by a Yemenite father to his son.

Through the ages, the Yemenite Jews knew periods of relative prosperity and of persecution, hunger, and drought, regardless of whether Christians, Arabs, or Turks were in power. At times they were forced to accept Islam; at other times they were plagued by dissension among themselves over false Messiahs. It is known that they always had contact with Jews in other parts of the world, either through letters (from the famous scholar Moses Maimonides, for instance) or through travelers' tales.

Toward the end of the nineteenth century, conditions in Yemen became almost unbearable. Hunger and disease decimated the population. Arab hatred of the Jews increased. It was at that time that emigration to Palestine began. Rumors of Lawrence Oliphant's intervention with the Turkish government on behalf of persecuted Russian Jews filtered through to Yemen. Oliphant, a British friend of the Jews, tried to obtain the Turks' consent for an autonomous Jewish settlement in Palestine. This intervention was interpreted by the Yemenite Jews as the first sign of the coming of the Messiah, and soon many of them decided to return to the Land of the Fathers. Inhabitants first of Yemen's capital, San'a— mostly silversmiths, potters and other craftsmen—and later the villagers started the long difficult journey, which was taken partly on foot, partly by ship. The majority of the Yemenite Jews, however, arrived in 1949- 1950 *via* Operation Magic Carpet. In 378 flights almost the entire Yemenite Jewish community of 47,400 people was transferred to Israel. The total number who have immigrated to Israel since 1880 is 65,400.[2]

§ The Yemenite Jews in Israel[3]

Some of the early urban immigrants remained in Jaffa, the port of arrival; most of them, however, settled down in Jerusalem in the narrow Jewish quarter of the old city. In 1886, the first Yemenite settlement was erected, and many more were to come. New Yemenite quarters in Jerusalem appeared necessary.

Although most of the first immigrants worked at the crafts they had learned in Yemen and thus performed functions that had belonged from time immemorial to the Palestinian Arabs, there was a tendency to shift to agriculture. An organization was formed to train Yemenites for farm jobs.

Its members corresponded with the Organization of Zionists in Odessa on this subject. They also made contact with Eliezer ben Jehuda, the reviver of Hebrew as a modern language. These early contacts between Yemenites and Ashkenazim (European Jews) were based on a common love for the Land of the Fathers, a wish for the revival of Hebrew as a national tongue, and dreams of a return to agriculture as an ideal and heroic occupation.

Although sharing these ideals and goals with the Ashkenazim, the

Yemenites did not want to mix with them and preferred to remain in their own schools and synagogues in which the services were conducted in Yemenite fashion, and married only within their own group. This behavior seemed to be a continuation of the life pattern in Yemen, where the Jews lived in Jewish quarters exclusively and had only economic relations with the surrounding Arabs.

The first years in Palestine were very difficult. Infectious diseases and high infant mortality ravaged the early settlers. At that time only 40% of their marriages were with non-Yemenites. They organized the Association for Life and Peace, which recommended, among other measures, mixed marriages (with Ashkenazim) in order to escape the complete extinction of their community. Medical conditions, however, improved only after the British conquered Palestine in 1918.

In 1907, thirteen Yemenites decided to make the trip to Palestine, followed by 100 more in the same year and 220 in the next year. These rural immigrants settled down in villages, which have since become towns—Rehovoth, Petah-Tikvah, and Rishon l'Zion—and earned their livings as farmhands. They lived in closed groups like their predecessors of the Eighties and were discriminated against by their Ashkenazi employers, who apparently identified them with Arab laborers. The Yemenite farmhands were in great demand because of their industry, their modesty, and their willingness to accept low wages. In order to encourage the immigration of Yemenite farmers, an expert by the name of Shmuel Javnieli was sent to Yemen by the Jewish Agency. As a result of his activities, more than 1500 Yemenite Jews immigrated in 1911-1912 and settled down in Palestine, in circumstances much more convenient than those that had greeted the early settlers.

In the post-World War I years, thousands of European Jews were pouring into Palestine, and the Zionist organization paid little attention to the Yemenite Jews who were waiting in Aden. Many of them had to wait there for years until the end of World War II, when European immigration came to a standstill. Most of those who succeeded in emigrating to Palestine joined existing Yemeni settlements or founded new ones like Kfar Marmorek (1930) and Kfar Elishav (1933). Others populated Yemenite quarters in Tel Aviv.

The mass immigration of the years 1949-1950 required special measures. Two immigrant villages were erected, one located at an old British army base, Rosh Ha'ajin, which received 10,000 Yemenite immigrants In addition to the two villages, thirty-nine new settlements were set up.

One is in constant danger of generalizing about the Yemenites in Israel. First it should be emphasized that the Yemenites are not a homogeneous group. To the outsider, they may seem to be homogeneous, a small, fragile, dark-skinned people, many of the males with side curls, many of the women wearing beautifully embroidered trousers instead of skirts. In fact, however, some come originally from cities and some from villages, some from the northern and some from the central and the southern parts of Yemen, each with a different set of habits and different organizations.

In addition to their different origins, they have followed different paths in Israel: Some have settled in urban quarters, others in villages, and a few in *kibbutzim* (collective settlements).

There is, however, a certain similarity between the lives of the Yemenites in Israel and their lives in Yemen.

They now feel themselves discriminated against by the Ashkenazim, as they had been by the Arabs. Yemenite Jews are clearly different from other Oriental Jews: They are darker and smaller. They are different too from Western Jews. They form a cohesive group among the Ashkenazim and the Sephardim. Among Yemenis, the Ashkenazim are frequently referred to in disparaging terms, which certainly stems from basic jealousy of a higher social group.

The Yemenites' inferiority feeling is based on many factors. Yemenite Jews were among the first pioneers who built the Jewish land. One of the reasons these pioneers were less appreciated than those who came originally from European countries is that the latter believed they were building a model socialistic society, while the early Yemenite settlers thought simply in terms of their Jewish homeland. The Yemenites had a religious ideal, the European immigrant pioneers a socialistic one, and socialistic ideals—at least forty years ago—had higher status than did religious ideals. One reason was that the European settlers knew this religious background from their fathers and from their own youth. To them, the religious emphasis implied passively waiting for the Messiah—prayer, rather than action. Socialism meant action and achievement.

When the first Yemenite settlers arrived more than sixty years ago, they were utilized as cheap laborers by the Ashkenazim. During the last waves of immigration in the Fifties and Sixties, it was the Yemenites who were sent to the dangerous development areas along the border, while the immigrants from Poland and Romania became the proud possessors of homes in newly built immigrant housing developments in urban residential areas.

This feeling of being discriminated against is partly justified: The urban housing was intended for professionals whose work was in the cities. Since those professionals were not found among the Yemenites, it is understandable that they were not selected for urban housing. But it seems very likely that nonprofessionals from Poland and Romania were also settled in urban areas.

Both discrimination by the Ashkenazim and continuation of life patterns from Yemen are conducive to the more or less isolated existence the Yemenite Jews currently live in Israel.

The process of acculturation took place in various ways. In some instances, the children were first to come in touch with Western ideas. Sometimes women who served as cleaning women for Western housewives were the first points of contact. At still other times, the men who had served in the army were the bearers of new culture.

One generalization, however, seems justified. Whatever the structure had originally been, there is no doubt that the Yemenite community changed profoundly as a result of immigration. The autonomy of the community disappeared very rapidly in the state of Israel, with its laws and regulations, its social welfare, and its health services.

The family structure was also altered, for children no longer were married at the ages of nine to eleven years. The period of puberty appeared therefore to be especially difficult for the girls, for they could not use their mothers as examples and identity objects—as their mothers themselves had never experienced such periods of sexual maturity before marriage and motherhood. Fathers too had difficulty understanding what their boys were doing and learning at high school at ages when they themselves had already specialized in trades and were bearing family responsibilities.

But what most characterized the decline of the classic Oriental family was the shattering of the authoritarian father image. Often the father was the only family member not adapted to the new circumstances: The mother would be employed as a cleaning woman and the children at school or in the army, but the father would be unable to find employment in his own trade or unwilling to learn another. Instead of being the sole provider for his family, he would often be dependent on his wife and children.

§ The Function of the *Mori* in Yemen

The structure and organization of Jewish society in Yemen had been very simple, in its urban as well as in its rural settings.[4]

The family was the cornerstone of society; there were neither bachelors nor spinsters. Small communities consisted of numbers of large extended or joint family groups. Children were married very early, between the ages of nine and eleven. The ideal was marriage to the father's brother's daughter or the mother's brother's or sister's daughter. Polygamy was not infrequent in villages and little towns. In bigger cities, monogamy seems to have been the rule.

In the face of many conditions, both threatening and joyful, a strong feeling of solidarity prevailed in the community. If a bride was in need of money for her wedding party and her parents could not afford it, friends and relatives joined forces and collected the necessary funds. When illness hit, friends stood by and were helpful, according to the saying, "*Zarath rabim hazi nehamah*" (company in distress makes the sorrow less).

Trade and industry were completely in Jewish hands, while agriculture was practiced exclusively by Arabs.

As far as relations with the Arab government were concerned, the Jews were represented by an official called the *nasi*. In all other functions like performance of marriage ceremonies and circumcision; in all matters of disease and sickness; in all matters of general hardship and catastrophe like continuous hunger or drought, the *mori* was the only person to turn to. He was the rabbi, the religious rainmaker, the doctor, the exorcist.[5] One can hardly think of a situation in which the advice of a *mori* would not be sought.

The word *mori* is derived from *mar*, the Aramaic equivalent of "master." *Mori* means "my master."[6]

Most of the smaller communities had at least one resident *mori* each; the larger the community, the more *moris* were available.

A person was chosen or prepared for these manifold tasks either by becoming an apprentice to another *mori* or by attending classes in a school for higher learning.

Most of the *moris*[7] possessed very considerable knowledge of the Bible and its commentaries, of the writings of Maimonides, of mystic and cabalistic literature, and of medicine and astronomy. In addition to filling his office, the *mori* practiced a trade like that of silversmith.

Among the *moris* today, some stratification according to status is observed. The highest in status is the *mori* who is mainly a judge and a scholar, the lowest the one who is a children's teacher (*mori 'ial*) and a slaughterer.[8]

As far as the practice of medicine is concerned, the *moris* are divided into two groups[9]: A minority of more scientific, organically oriented healers, is interested in precise diagnosis and appropriate treatment with herbs and drugs; the other and by far the larger group has a more magic-mystical orientation. Members of the majority believe in the evil eye and in *shedim* (spirits) as causes of disease in general and of mental illness in particular.

The organically oriented *mori* possesses a body of medical knowledge based on and derived from Arabic medicine. He uses textbooks and a pharmacopoeia that are often hundreds of years old.[10]

The magic-mystically oriented *mori's* treatment consists of the application of amulets in order to ward off the influence of the evil eye or the conduct of complicated rituals aimed at expulsion of the spirits.

There is a very interesting in-between group of *moris* who utilize both drugs and amulets, sometimes emphasizing drug administration, at other times the use of magic. The use of magic by these *moris* is often clearly a kind of accommodation to the needs of his simple clients. One of our informants told us about a *mori* to whom a man came complaining about the fact that his house was full of mice and requesting that the *mori* give him an amulet against mice. The wise *mori* wrote out a scroll for this special occasion, handed it to the client, and said, "Here is your scroll. Tie it to the neck of a cat, otherwise it won't help." The amulet was given in order not to destroy the faith of the client in this means; on the other hand, the *mori* succeeded in giving rational advice as well.

Another informant mentioned that the ink used for writing amulets was composed of medicinal herbs. The patients, who had to drink water in which the amulet had been immersed, believed that the solution of the magic words was the operating agent, although the *mori* knew that the herbs of which the ink was composed were the "real" active ingredients.

In Yemen, the *mori* did not ask a fee for medical advice; his subsistence was based on his profession as a craftsman. Many of the magically oriented *moris*, however, often requested considerable sacrifices from their patients—sheep, chickens, and so forth.

Most of the informants agree that the *mori*, as soon as he was called to a patient, went immediately, spent much time with him, and did not leave before he had "cured" him.

§ Mental Illness among Jews in Yemen

Most of the informants agree that mental illness in the narrow sense of the word—obvious cases of extreme agitation and suicidal or homicidal behavior—was very rare in Yemen. They are eager to explain that the climate in Yemen was healthier, the winters were not so cold as in

Israel, and the summers were not so warm. The air was not so dry as
in Israel. Beside, they add, the use of well water and of rain water is
much healthier than that of tap water. Others mention that food habits
in Yemen were different: One ate less than in Israel, and food did not
contain so much fat as food in Israel.

More sophisticated *moris* offer the explanation that absence of temptations of a sexual nature, of strivings for social and economic improvement
contributed to general mental health.

On the other hand, people apparently suffered more from the *'ajin hara*
(evil eye) and the *shedim* (spirits) in Yemen.

For this apparent paradox—that in Yemen there were more *shedim*
and less mental illness—I cannot offer a satisfactory explanation. A
possible answer is that, although more *shedim* existed in Yemen, the *mori*
also believed himself more effective in warding off their influence.

Most *moris* divide mental illness as follows:

> Group I: Disturbances accompanying febrile conditions
> Group II: Disturbances *not* connected with febrile conditions
> A. Diseases caused by the evil eye
>   1. anxiety states characterized by pallor, restlessness,
>   and lack of appetite
>   2. depression and sleeplessness
>   3. impotence
> B. Diseases caused by spirits
>   1. madness in which there are too many thoughts
>   2. madness in which the patient is too quiet
>   3. true madness in which the patient is agitated,
>   talks nonsense, and exhibits bizarre behavior
>   like undressing in public
> C. Others
>   1. falling sickness

SOME ILLUSTRATIONS

The details of these cases were gathered during interviews with *moris*
about their practices in Yemen.

Case 1. A woman, twenty-five years old became crazy shortly after
her wedding. Her husband got drunk at the wedding party. Later on he
traveled a great deal and was almost never home. The woman waited
day and night for his return until after some time she became crazy and
saw the image of her husband in front of her.

Comment: This case is an illustration of one of the causes of mental
illness, as interpreted by the Yemenites. Lack of satisfaction of erotic

needs leads to illness. Phantasied satisfaction of the patient's needs occurred in the visual hallucinations.

Case 2. A man, forty-five years old, suffered from wide swings in mood. Each summer he was elated, and toward fall and winter he became depressed. He was a merchant and always very busy in summertime.

Comment: As in cases of manic-depressive psychosis in other cultures, this patient belongs to the higher socioeconomic classes of the population. The informant tried to explain this case by saying that the patient wanted to continue his summer activities even after the season was finished.

Case 3. A woman became agitated after childbirth and was tearing her clothes. After her newborn child died, her condition became worse. The patient could not sleep and became agitated. In this stage of agitation, she entered a synagogue and frightened the rabbi. The rabbi later became tubercular.

Comment: Apparently a postpartum confusional state. Two things are relevant here: the view of the synagogue as a place where a cure could be obtained and the assumed ability of mental patients to have bad influence on others even to the extent of making them sick.

Case 4. A boy, fifteen years old, was beaten very much as a child. He could not talk or work.

Comment: Perhaps a case of mental deficiency.

Case 5. A woman had to wash her hands for hours and hours after touching things that were *tamé* (unclean according to religion).

Comment: A case of obsessive-compulsive neurosis.

ETIOLOGY

Some conditions like anxiety states, depressions, and nervousness, generally spoken of as the more uncomplicated cases, were supposed to be caused by the evil eye and, informants assured me, had nothing to do with the *shedim* (spirits). Disappointment in love was an important pathogenic agent; so was striving for power and possessions and for (forbidden) love objects. Sudden death of a parent or sudden noises could lead to anxiety states. Often this anxiety state was considered to be the beginning of mental disorder, its first stage. The second stage was characterized by decreased action and increased thinking, while the third phase was true madness, characterized by agitation, bizarre behavior, and verbal nonsense. This theory bears some similarity to the unitary concept of mental illness as defended, for example, by Karl Menninger.[11]

The group of magic healers often found magical causes for mental illness: hot water spilled at a "bad" time or passing dirt—a garbage can, for example—at a "bad" time. The first, the third, and the fifth of each month were "bad" days.[12] Contact with a menstruating woman was also considered an underlying cause of mental illness. And epilepsy was believed to be caused by drinking milk from a mother who had worked too hard during pregnancy.

TREATMENT

As indicated in our discussion of the *mori*, there were two different approaches to the treatment of illness in general and of mental illness in particular. One approach was based on precise diagnosis, which was often established by carefully examining the nails and the eyes of the patient, and treatment by administration of appropriate drugs. This approach we shall call "organic-naturalistic."

The other group of healers believed that most conditions were caused either by the evil eye or by *shedim*, and they acted accordingly. That is, their magical procedures were aimed at counteracting or undoing the action of the evil eye or expulsion of the evil spirits.

Many of the organic-naturalistic healers did not like treating mental patients and disliked their magical colleagues ("They cure people with flea's milk and door squeaking," either by impossible or useless means).[13]

Organic-Naturalistic Treatment. In case of melancholia: suppositoria of opium seeds or an ointment of opium seeds.

In case of madness from too much thinking: sennah leaves.

In case of anxiety and nervousness: healthy and sweet foods like almonds, raisins, figs, dates, and honey. One talks with the patient and does not leave him until he improves.

In case of nervousness and agitation: sedatives like *grun el-dallah* (unknown herb) and a diet of *kussah* (*Cucumis sativa L.*), a fruit similar to a small cucumber, which is thought to be food for the brain.

In case of agitation connected with a febrile condition: compresses of mustard oil on the head.

In case of true madness: *luban schachri* (*Boswellia carteri*) or *asat musa* (*Cassia fistula*).

Another treatment consists of three phases: inhalation of burnt gingiber roots; application of an ointment composed of saffron, salt, garlic, and fruits of caster; and a diet of sweet foods, *lisab* (Majorana), black pepper, cinnamon, and olive oil, made into a porridge and administered three times a day.

Magic-Spiritualistic Treatment. In case of nervousness and anxiety states: Immediately after discovering the influence of the evil eye, one should utter a magical formula like "Hear Israel, Adonai our God, Adonai is One" or "The Lord will keep you."

If this formula does not work, one should apply *pashta* (or *fashta*): With a razor blade, one makes three parallel scratches in order to extract some blood, then suddenly throws water from behind on the patient.

In another modification, once a patient is sitting down quietly and unsuspectingly, one throws or pours cold water on him from behind. Afterward one gives the patient clean clothes and the already mentioned diet of figs, dates, almonds, honey and raisins. This entire treatment is to be repeated three times.[14]

For conditions lasting longer than two months, it is of no use to say "Hear Israel" or to apply *fashta;* the only thing to do is to use *makwa,* a very popular or at least widespread custom. *Makwa* is the application of a hot nail to the site of the illness (head, stomach, back), causing a burn and enabling the evil spirit to leave the body.

In very severe and stubborn cases one applies *rassas.* It is not certain whether or not this procedure is specifically Yemenite, for it has been popular among Sephardic Jews in Palestine for scores of years. *Rassas* is a very complicated ritual in which metals (nails, keys, scissors, and lead) play an important role as means of expelling spirits. One applies *rassas* when it is no longer a question of the evil eye; on the contrary, *rassas* is for cases believed to be caused by evil spirits.

Another procedure for someone who seems to be losing his mind is to take an egg in which an embryo is hatching, burn the egg, and feed it to the patient.[15]

In the more severe cases, many means are available to expel the evil spirits. The spirits can be exorcised only by the most powerful and high-ranking healers, who are called *ba'alei hefetz* (masters of the will).[16] They have in their possession sacred books (*sifre hefetz*). Exorcism takes place in two phases: *jidschma* (or *lijma*)—assembling the evil spirits— and *yefruk*—separation of the evil spirits from the body of the patient. The most respected and highest ranking *mori,* who is well versed in the *kabbala,* invites the master of the spirits. The master asks, "Why did you call me?" Then the *mori* replies, "I request you to command the spirit who took possession of X to leave his body immediately. If not, I will condemn all of you to eternal wandering." During this whole procedure, the *mori* must not lift his eyes, in order not to expose himself to the evil spirits.

Another method used to exorcise the spirits is to take a sheep, dove, or chicken and revolve it three times around the patient. The *mori* then whispers to the spirits, "Masters, please have mercy upon the patient and take the sheep instead." Immediately afterward the sheep is slaughtered. One of the following phenomenon should then be observable as a sign that the spirit has left the patient:

1. The sign of the broken cup. If a cup containing fluid should break during the exorcistic ritual, it means that the spirit has left the body of the patient and entered the cup, which breaks as a result of this invasion.
2. The sign of the fire. A light or a fire where it has not previously been indicates that the spirit has left the patient and ignited the flame.

AMULETS

Most amulets are scrolls with magic formulas written in ink or a mixture of ink and a solution of medicinal herbs. Amulets are worn by women between the breasts and by men attached (with safety pins) to their undershirts. The scroll written in a solution of herbs should be immersed in water. The magic of the sacred words, combined with the power of the herbs, enters into the water, which is to be drunk by the patient. One of the magic formulas used for expelling *shedim*, is "Eretz beretz teretz we-katan hakatan hakatan difatek hakatan hakof awito shabehavvu" (remove from the body of X all *shedim* and evil spirits).[17]

Another amulet, which I have in my possession, is ninety-five centimeters long and four and one-half centimeters broad and is inscribed in Hebrew. It contains several illustrations: one of the human body, bearing the name of Lilith; three of daggers, bearing the inscriptions Kashtiel, Kastiel, and Pahdiel; one of the shield of David; and three monsters bearing the names of Sanui, Sansanui, and Samenglaf. On it is written a prayer requesting that all the evil eye in the world be removed, that all the evil spirits be warded off, and that medicine for the body and for the spirit be granted to Mrs. X, whose name is also mentioned on the scroll.

§ The *Mori* in Israel[18]

The person who stands as the symbol of assistance and counsel, as the link connecting the Yemenite past with the Israeli present, is the *mori*. But the *mori* is no longer the person he was in Yemen. He himself is a much threatened person. In many areas, his functions have been sharply curtailed. In other areas, such as the practice of medicine, his activities are even considered illegitimate. Instead of being self-confident and sure of his own authority, he has become uncertain, suspicious, and often hostile. Both *nasi* and *mori* have had to yield their places as community leaders to younger men, generally less religious and traditional than their predecessors.

The *mori* lost his function as a teacher when children were sent to schools maintained by the state. His legal activities have been taken over by judges appointed by the Ministry of Justice. Even in his religious domain, he has been partially replaced: The Yemenite religious leaders had to undergo "refresher courses" given by the Israeli chief rabbinate before they were allowed to carry on such duties as initiating marriages. These refresher courses were necessary because of different practices. In Yemen, for example, the practice of Yibbum levirate, in which a man's widow marries his brother, was favored, while the Israeli rabbis preferred *haliza*, which freed her from such a necessity.

Physicians and public health nurses equipped with patient clinics and sick funds have made the *mori's* services as healer superfluous.

What is left?

In addition to carrying out such religious duties as conducting services, initiating marriages, and performing circumcisions, the outstanding importance of the *mori* is his availability as a source of help in unforeseen circumstances or difficulties that cannot be remedied by any of the other professionals—mainly prolonged or incurable diseases; constant rheumatic pains; prolonged headaches and backaches; and above all mental illness. Questions about whether or not one will be successful in business or in love also belong to the territory of the *mori*. Many *moris* have ceased their therapeutic activities altogether and even deny having any knowledge of medicine. Among the latter are mainly the organic-naturalistically oriented *moris*, who rationalize their withdrawal from the healing role by claiming that in Israel the good and powerful herbs cannot be cultivated as well as in Yemen. These *moris* are serving now as regular rabbis —that is, as religious officials dealing with prayers, services, initiating marriages, and so forth.

The magically oriented *moris*, who generally have less education and knowledge are not eligible to be rabbis and have no alternative but to continue their service as folk-healers. Not only do they continue in their role, but they fulfill an existing need. Those Yemenites who feel themselves strangers in a hostile, Ashkenazi world turn to their *moris* for comfort. It is those uncertain people who are sensitive and not sufficiently flexible to adapt themselves to the new environment who suffer most from the evil eye and therefore turn to the *mori* for assistance. Not only the older immigrants but also some of the younger ones, those who have failed in matters of love or business or are otherwise handicapped, seek his help.

Now we come to the question of who uses the *mori* as a source of help in mental illness. Does requesting his visit depend on the severity of the symptoms? Does the degree of acculturation of the patient play a role? According to our informants, younger people who are acculturated first visit a sick-fund doctor or private physician. Only when their conditions turn out to be of a persistent nature do they feel themselves compelled—often at the suggestions of their parents or grandparents—to visit *moris*.

Not only Yemenites consult Yemenite *moris*. Once a *mori* is known, patients from other ethnic groups ask his advice too, although, to my knowledge, no Ashkenazim has ever consulted a Yemenite *mori*.

I know of cases where young, modern Yemenite patients have been in simultaneous treatment with a psychiatrist and a *mori*. Often patients visit a *mori* before they decide to go to a mental hospital or after hospitalization if some symptoms still remain. For example, after being hospitalized for withdrawal and delusions, a patient cured of these symptoms may consult a *mori* for persisting headaches or nightmares.

Most of the clients are evasive when asked for the names or the addresses of the *moris*. A patient will say his *mori* is dead, claim he has moved to another place, or pretend to have forgotten his name. It is not certain whether this attitude springs from feelings of shame or is aimed at protecting the *mori*; it may be a combination of both.

It is difficult to obtain clear information about the fee of the *mori*. In Yemen, the subsistence of the *mori* was based on his professional activities as a craftsman. He accepted fees only in kind—flour, chickens, doves. Some of the *moris* I interviewed still refuse to accept money, but I was told that if one leaves money accidentally in a *mori's* room, he does not object. Others have to make a living from their activities as *moris* and do not hesitate to ask large sums of money. Sometimes this practice even leads to blackmail: One client who had been under a continuous spell had to pay the *mori* a certain amount of money each month in order to get rid of the spell. This practice could lead to a considerable amount of hostility in the client and even to bodily attacks on or murder of the *mori*.

§ Mental Illness Among Yemenites
in Israel[19]

The rate of new admissions to psychiatric institutions is higher among Oriental immigrants and therefore among Yemenites than the Israeli national average. From this fact we deduce that the new Oriental immigrants quickly learn the path to the mental hospital. It is apparently not correct to state that in Israel they care for their own mental patients as they did before their immigration. We cannot draw any conclusions about the prevalence of mental illness in specific ethnic groups, for we have information only about the numbers of admissions, and ethnic groups are not comparable, partially because of different durations of their stays in the country.

If we look at the diagnostic breakdown, the following interesting facts appear: Oriental immigrants and Israel-born patients show more schizophrenia than does the average population, the exception being the Yemenites, who like the Europeans, show less. The frequency of psychosis among the natives of Yemen is the lowest among the ethnic groups. Admission rates for neurosis are higher than the average: 58.7 new admissions for neurosis per 100,000 inhabitants over fifteen years old, compared to Israel's average of 33.3 per 100,000.

The Yemeni rate of epilepsy is more than twice the national average: 7.8 and 3.1 per 100,000 respectively. All Orientals show less manic-depressive psychosis[20] than do the Europeans, but Yemenites show even less than other Orientals.

It is in the light of studies like that of Mabel Cohen[21] on the social factors in manic-depressive psychosis that we might explain why this disease is rare among Yemenites. She describes how parents utilize a gifted child in order to increase the prestige of the entire family. They feel that their family should be at least equal to and if possible should exceed the prestige level of their community. The child who is thus utilized by his parents as a tool to improve the family status in its environment is likely to become a manic-depressive patient. These findings have been confirmed by studies by Robert Gibson.[22]

In Yemen the Jews lived in closed quarters, and they had no desire to become assimilated to the non-Jewish environment. The Jewish community was stratified, and no social mobility was present: There were only the learned, the rich, and the poor.

§ Discussion

The role of the *mori* in Israel in the present period of transition can be understood better against the background of the system of beliefs prevalent among the Yemenites.

In Yemen, the Jews were very vulnerable: They were oppressed by the Arabs, suffered from poverty, and were subject to many illnesses. Their isolated life led to the development of two phenomena. The first was an impressive solidarity and cohesiveness. People took greater care of one another in case of distress and disease. The second was an increased tendency to projection. If an enemy is outside and all around, it is safe to accuse him of all the evils to which human flesh is subject. This tendency to projection finds its expression in belief in spirits and the evil eye. They are not only the causes of most diseases, but they are also responsible for bad luck and failure in love and in business. One also projects onto spirits and the evil eye his fear of his own drives. For example, if a man is attracted to a forbidden love object—a married woman, for example—he believes that she is bewitching him. The other person thus becomes the source of fear, and awareness of one's own instinctual needs is thereby avoided.

Many so-called primitive people do not differentiate between external and internal danger; for them, all fear is a sign of danger, and all danger is external. Destitution, injustice, and disease are all believed to be caused by external factors. Among these factors we find the *shedim* (spirits) and the evil eye.

It is on the basis of this belief in spirits and the evil eye shared by the *mori* and his client that psychotherapeutic help is provided. It may be helpful to differentiate among six types of approach.

Ventilation. The client has ample opportunity to air his troubles and difficulties, both past and present, in a setting of understanding without being judged. Even without receiving specific advice, he has the feeling that somebody is sharing his distress and supporting him in his fight against the evil forces.

Strengthening of Projection. The *mori* reinforces the patient's basic belief that all disease and pain are related to the influence of external evil forces. More than that, the *mori* knows exactly how to cope with each specific occasion and to give appropriate advice. When he gives an amulet as a curative means, the patient knows that it is prepared especially for him and for this occasion. The amulet contains the power and the knowledge of the *mori* in the form of the characters written on the parchment. It is a kind of extension of the *mori* himself, assisting the patient in his struggle against the spirits or the evil eye. This strengthening of the tendency for projective thinking is also found in the ritual of *makwe,* in which a burn is caused by a red-hot nail to enable the spirit to leave the body, or in the ritual of *fashta,* in which blood is extracted by means of a cupping-glass for the same purpose—namely to provide the spirits with an aperture by which to leave the body of the patient.

Suggestion. Linked to this strengthening of the projective tendency is the utilization of suggestion that the spirits abandon the patient. Suggestion is also the therapeutic technique for certain types of depression: The *mori* frightens the patient by unexpectedly throwing cold water on him. This alarm reaction is immediately interpreted by the *mori* as proof of the spirit's abandonment and the return of a state of health.

Active Mastery Instead of Passive Suffering. Once a man complained that his neighbor was influencing him by means of the evil eye. The *mori* advised him to draw a red line round the neighbor's house and to repeat it several times. This red line can be interpreted in at least two ways: as a means to ward off the influence of the evil eye emanating from the neighbor—as a message to the community that the neighbor was a source of bad influence, which could lead to his being ostracized. In this example, we see that the patient, instead of passively suffering as a victim of the evil eye, actively undertakes to defend himself.

Disposal of his aggression in a socioculturally accepted way. Ostracizing one's fellow man is of course not usually allowed, but defending oneself against the evil eye is permitted.

Regression and dependence in a socially acceptable way. The *mori*-client relationship is itself an example.

§ Conclusion

Immigration and acculturation have thus sharply affected the social role of the *mori*. Nevertheless, his function, although limited, is important in alleviating the stresses of immigration for the Yemenites in Israel.

In Yemen he had many functions and well defined responsibilities. He was the central figure in a rigidly organized society. After the emigration to Israel, the organizational structure of the Yemenites' society disintegrated. Family roles were shifted, in that the authoritarian father figure declined while the status of the mother and the children increased. Israeli schools substituted for the *mori* as teacher; doctors and health services replaced him as healer; judges fulfilled his legal obligations.

As a result of this displacement of responsibility, the duties of the *mori* became ill defined and were restricted to areas in which Israeli officials do not function. For example the *mori* takes over where the physician leaves off, in understanding the emotional needs of patients and in caring for certain types of patients with prolonged illnesses.

Although stripped of many of his traditional functions, the *mori* in

Israel still provides an important source of psychotherapeutic help for
persons suffering from emotional problems and troubles in living. This
kind of help is adapted specifically to the needs of his fellow men and
could not be easily supplied in more effective ways from any other source.

Notes

1. See Erich Brauer, *Ethnologie der Jemenitischen Juden* (Heidelberg: 1934), p.
18.

2. See Shimon Geridi and Israel Jeshaiahu, eds., *Miteman le-Zion* (Tel Aviv:
1938); and Keren Hayesod, ed., *Jeziath Teman* (Jerusalem: n.d.).

3. Hayesod, *op. cit.*

4. Brauer, *op. cit.*, p. 119.

5. Geridi, "Hazaddik hatemani wepe'ulotaf," *Niv hastudent*, Jerusalem, 1936.

6. S. D. Goitein, "Jewish Education in Yemen as an Archetype of Traditional
Jewish Education," Carl Frankenstein, ed., *Between Past and Future* (Jerusalem:
1953), p. 131.

7. Brauer, *op. cit.*, p. 284.

8. Joseph Kafih, *Jewish Life in San'a* (Jerusalem: 1961), p. 50.

9. This information comes from interviews with *moris* conducted all over Israel
by Johebed Re'ani and myself.

10. See Max Meyerhof, "Arab Medicine among the Jews of the Yemen," *Edoth,
Quarterly for Folklore and Ethnology*, III (1947-1948). Meyerhof describes a book,
which I saw and which was later in the possession of Johebed Re'ani, the *Kitab al-
mu'tamed fi'l-adwiya al-mufrada murattab 'ala huruf abjad* (The book of support on
simple drugs, arranged according to the [semitic] alphabet). The book is written in
Hebrew characters but in the Yemenite language. The name of the author is missing,
but he is known, from other data, to have been al-malik al-ashraf 'umar ibn Yusouf
ibn 'Umar, the third Rassulid Sultan of Yeman. The book is a compilation of five
older books and contains descriptions of 600 drugs. At the end of the text, there is
an appendix of nineteen large pages (seven columns each), listing remedies for all
kinds of disease, including mental illness.

11. See Karl Menninger, *et al.*, "The Unitary Concept of Mental Illness," *Bulletin of the Menninger Clinic*, 22 (January, 1958), 1.

12. Kafih, *op. cit.*, p. 270.

13. *Ibid.*, p. 269.

14. Cf. *la douche écossaise*, a form of hydrotherapy popular in the nineteenth
century.

15. Kafih, *op. cit.*, p. 270.

16. *Ibid.*, p. 269; and personal communication from Dr. Percy Cohen to the
author.

17. Kafih, *op. cit.*, p. 273.

18. The information set forth in this section was derived from four sources: a
sociological study of second-generation Yemenites in Rehovoth, carried out by the
author in behalf of the Department of Sociology at Hebrew University and the
Henrietta Szold Foundation in 1957; an anthropological study, conducted by Percy
Cohen for the Ministry of Health and the Israel Institute for Applied Social Research
in 1955; Geridi, *op. cit.*; and the author's own interviews with *moris*.

19. See H. S. Halevi, "Table XXVI—Admission to Mental Hospitals and Institutions for In-patients during 1958," *Mental Illness in Israel* (Jerusalem: 1960).

383

20. Jozef Ph. Hes, "Manic-Depressive Illness in Israel," *American Journal of Psychiatry* (July, 1960).

21. Mabel Cohen, *et al.*, "An Intensive Study of Twelve Cases of Manic-Depressive Psychosis," *Psychiatry*, 17 (1954), No. 2, 103-37.

22. Robert W. Gibson, "The Family Background and Early Life Experience of the Manic-Depressive Patient," *Psychiatry*, 21 (1958), 71-90.

L. Bryce Boyer

Folk Psychiatry of the Apaches
of the Mescalero Indian Reservation*

§ Introduction

During more than eighteen months of the last four years, I have collaborated with anthropologists in field work on the Mescalero Indian Reservation, an area of beautiful pine forests and grazing land ranging in altitude between 6000 and 12,000 feet, occupying about 461,000 acres in south central New Mexico. From the beginning, I was known as a psychiatrist, which the Apache translated into "white shaman." I was eventually asked by native practitioners to learn secret religious and medical philosophies and practices and even to accept a tentative new position as chief tribal shaman. In consequence, modern material was provided that has supplemented the monumental data previously obtained by others, notably Dr. Morris Edward Opler, to whom we are most indebted for dependable information about the aboriginal eastern Apache groups.

The Apache who now reside on the reservation number approximately 1200 and derive primarily from the Mescalero, Chiricahua, and Lipan tribes in that order.[1] Beginning perhaps a millennium ago, aggregates of nomadic, hunting and gathering, Southern Athabaskan-speaking Indians[2]

* The research that made this communication possible was partially supported by National Institute of Mental Health Grants M-2013 and M-3088. During the summer of 1958, Dr. David M. Schneider and I were assisted by Dr. Ruth M. Boyer (Grant M-2013). We conducted a preliminary survey to determine whether conjoint anthropological and psychoanalytic research was feasible on the Mescalero Indian Reservation. Dr. Harry W. Basehart and I were assisted in the field by Mrs. Boyer and Mr. Bruce B. MacLachlan for fourteen months of 1959 and 1960. The purpose of our investigation was to study the interactions of social structure, socialization processes, and personality. My wife and I spent two further months in the field in 1961. Basehart and the Boyers will continue collaborative work for the next few years (Grant M-3088).

migrated southward from northwestern Canada.[3] During the ensuing 700 years or so, the groups divided.[4] The segment most influenced by the sedentary Pueblos became known as the Navaho; the remainder developed into the Apache, who have been popularized in so much fictional and objective literature[5] and in television programs. Of the Apaches, Cremony wrote, "In point of intellect, in cunning and duplicity, in warlike skill and untiring energy, in tenacity of purpose and wondrous powers of endurance, (they) have no equals among the existing Indians in North America."[6] Schwatka, writing after the Gadsden Purchase, added:

> we saw the humiliating spectacle of two civilized nations, claiming rank among the nations of the world, sitting in solemn conclave to devise a common plan that would annihilate a batch of breech-clouted bandits whose whole numbers would not have made the hundredth city in either land, and to do this surrendering the highest prerogative of national sovereignty—the sacredness of their soil—to the soldiery of the other.[7]

Chittenden contributed:

> they have probably been the most troublesome Indians within the territorial limits of the United States. . . . In their whole career of more than two centuries, the Spanish and Republican governments never subjugated nor converted them, and, in fact, seem to have existed only by their sufferance.[8]

The three tribes claim large and somewhat overlapping areas for the pursuit of subsistence. In recent times, the activities of the Mescalero have radiated from the area of the present reservation, which was established in 1873. The Chiricahua, following the capitulation of Geronimo, were taken as prisoners of war in 1886 to Florida, then to Alabama, and subsequently to Oklahoma. The majority joined the Mescalero in 1913.[9] The Lipan roamed primarily over areas of Texas and northern Mexico until they were destroyed as a functioning group by other Indians (primarily the Comanche), Mexicans, and United States settlers and military forces. Their few known remaining members trekked to the Mescalero reservation near the turn of the present century. In early 1962, there were seven living, presumably full-blooded Lipan, the youngest of whom was fifty-seven years old. Although each group retains diminishing identity with its earlier affiliations, all now are members of the Mescalero tribe. In this essay, the word "Mescalero" will be used indiscriminately, unless otherwise designated. Basehart has reported differences in certain aspects of the social structure of the aboriginal Mescalero and Chiricahua,[10] but the similarities are sufficient to warrant blanket statements here. The fact that insufficient data exist regarding earlier Lipan practices to include them in the general statements does not handicap my theses, for their aboriginal ways have not preceptibly influenced current Mescalero social structure and socialization practices. In the material that follows brief statements will appear about past and present social structure, child-training practices, and personality configurations. In more detail, I shall present data on former and current religio-medical philosophies and practices. I shall attempt to demonstrate how the personality structure of the Apache has made and still makes it possible for shamanistic procedures to be effective to the degree that they were and are. The final section will constitute a comparison of Mescalero folk and Western psychiatric orientations and practices.

§ Social Structure and Socialization Processes

In the old days, kinship was reckoned bilaterally, and the significant kinship unit was the matrilocal extended family. Sociopolitical organization was strongly influenced by the need for mobility, stemming from subsistence practices. The largest political unit centered about a particular male leader. He and his followers formed a "band." Relatives of the leader formed the nucleus of each band; the proportion of relatives in such a group was a function of its size. The Mescalero had no superordinate tribal leader, no formal tribal council, no general tribal gatherings; nor did the tribe act as a unit with regard to offense or defense. The distribution of resources and variations of climate favored regular seasonal movements, with the result that Mescalero groups spent varying periods of time in different parts of their territory. Sacred places and rituals like the girls' puberty ceremony[11] brought small groups together. Individuals were not committed to permanent affiliation with any group. They could follow a leader for as long as they chose and go where they pleased. "Our country" was "our country" equally for all, and "trespass" was meaningless as far as tribal members were concerned.

> The only rules in this connection were rules of politeness, but if they were transgressed, the offenders were subject to no physical sanctions. Gossip and the weight of public opinion, however, were potent incentives for proper behavior.[12]

The necessities for subsistence were shared throughout the band. Family units became linked through a network of mutual economic obligations.

The men were responsible for hunting, warfare, and raiding and for training their sons in manly pursuits. The women gathered and prepared wild vegetable products and performed the duties associated with rearing young children and girls of all ages. They tanned hides, made clothes, and were primarily responsible for keeping family units together.[13] Their plant-gathering was a more dependable source of subsistence than were the activities of the men. Old people were respected and cared for. There appears to have been little overlapping of social roles. Effective leadership was the crucial element in assuring enduring band membership.

Farming was never popular and consistent in the old days.[14] Although men and women collaborated whenever planting was done, cultivating, weeding, and harvesting were women's work.[15]

According to MacLachlan's summary of Opler's data, in aboriginal Apache society seven major kinds of act would evoke "an organized negative sanction, i. e. a fairly well-defined response on the part of a particular person acting in the case as an agent of society."

Adultery and rape of a married woman were subject to limited punitive reactions by the appropriate spouse. Ordinary killing, theft, and rape of an unmarried woman were the province of the injured extended family: the "head" of the extended family group had no specific role behavior in such a case; the nantʔa [leader] of the "local group(s)" concerned might well intervene in an attempt at conciliation and at keeping the reaction within legitimate bounds, however he was not supposed to make commands or judgments. Witchcraft and killing of the nantʔa mobilized the whole "local group." It should be noted that all grossly deviant behavior, including notably incest and repeated trouble-making, was prima facie evidence of witchcraft. In witchcraft proceedings the nantʔa had no specified role behavior; it is likely that in some cases he voiced judgment or sentence, but this would be more an enunciation of the general consensus than his own decision.[16]

It appears that only witchcraft warranted capital punishment and that but inconsistently. Isolation from the group was the next most serious sanction.

In historic times, the Mescalero alcoholic drink was a brew of corn and sometimes other cereals called tulapai or tiswin. Usually, it was made in large quantities and was quickly used for group parties. As far as is known, before the introduction of Western alcoholic beverages, drunkenness did not cause chronic problems, although during periods in which there was drinking, quarrels occasionally blossomed into brief, violent outbursts of intragroup and unorganized interband hostilities.

Today, although kin ties continue to have fairly wide bilateral extension, the matrilocal extended family is no longer the critical kinship unit. Population concentration is limited to three reservation areas. Housing consists mainly of four-room frame dwellings complete with outhouses. Alternatives are privately built adobe houses and wooden shacks, dilapidated trailers, converted chicken coops and barns, and tents. The most common family unit is the nuclear unit. Common variations include additions of an adult relative or relatives, most frequently kin to the wife. In some cases, multiple families occupy the same dwelling, and there is gross overcrowding.

Political bodies, the tribe and the United States Government, provide the major sources of personal income. More than one-third of all income is unearned and is received in the form of cattle payments, unemployment compensation, welfare, and relief. Another third is distributed by the tribe, the Bureau of Indian Affairs, and United States Public Health Service agencies for performance of jobs provided by them. The average household income is about $3800. Impulsive spending and drunkenness, however, causes the majority of the Indians to live hand-to-mouth existences and to be always in debt. Husbands contribute higher percentages of income to their households than do their wives. Many men, however, have sufficient unearned income to permit them leisure for most of the year. In 1959, 40% of the men worked less than three and one-half months, and only 27% worked ten months or more. Almost all positions held by Apaches are unskilled in nature, and employment in the "white man's" sense is not a regular basis for prestige. The Apache man's means of gaining subsistence affords him scant esteem. The aged are no longer accorded respect, nor are they supported by their children, who may charge them for such personal services as rides to a store. The elderly are primarily dependent upon reservation welfare sources for their livelihoods.

Law enforcement on the modern reservation is delegated to three (or, at times, more) Indian policemen, employed by the Tribal Business Committee and the Tribal Court, composed of three elected judges. Although the jurisdiction of the court is restricted to minor offenses, Kunstadter states that:

the Mescalero population, even without counting the major crimes over which the federal government maintains jurisdiction, has known a crime rate about ten times that of the national average and five times that of the Mountain States.[17]

Drunkenness, which is often associated with violence, is the most common violation. Since almost every adult Apache has served a sentence in the "jailhouse," this form of punishment does not result in a major loss of status in the community. These Indians dislike restriction of their freedom, however, and "resisting arrest" is a charge frequently added to the more customary "disorderly conduct." Reservation enforcement agencies are particularly busy during the summer months, when drinking parties are common. The jail records reveal little distinction between the sexes in number of arrests, for both women and men enjoy "partying." The disposal of cases by the court and the activities of policemen are often attacked by tribal members, who allege that officials are biased in favor of kinsmen.

When sober, the Mescalero are gentle, courteous, fun-loving people whose rules of politeness are, in general, heeded. When they are intoxicated, however, their superegos appear to dissolve. The following example is typical of the behavior of Apache men: As I sat on his porch chatting with a drunken middle-aged Apache named Joe, his twenty-seven-year-old son, and boys of fourteen and eight, a thirty-five-year-old woman and her teen-age daughter plodded by, carrying groceries. Joe, who had been using English until he noticed them, turned from me and, in Apache, spoke to them in louder and louder tones that they could easily hear until they were a hundred yards away. He shouted to the older woman, "I know what you did last week when you were drunk down at Eddie's. I know you went out into the bushes and lay with those men. Why don't you come into my house, now. My wife isn't home. I'll take all your clothes off and I'll give it to you on the bed and on the floor and all over the house. Or maybe you'd rather we went into the bushes back up the hill. Come on and drink with me." The women walked by, pretending not to hear. Joe then offered to teach the younger one tricks she had not yet learned from younger men.

If an Apache woman has been drinking, it is assumed that she wants sexual relations, and she is considered fair game for any man or group of men. An intoxicated woman will challenge youths or men to prove their virility. Sexual relations, while the partners are under the influence, take place almost anywhere at all.

When Apaches are drunk, brutal behavior is common. The following examples, none of which was eventually punished by the courts, will suffice. 1. Two men drank together and began to fight. One of them passed out. His partner dragged him to a nearby fire and burned his arm and hand so severely that amputation was required. 2. A woman refused to comply with her brother's demand. He knocked her down, kicked her with his sharp-pointed cowboy boots, and raked her with his spurs. Her skull was fractured, and she was lacerated extensively. 3. A wife was caught in the act of cuckolding her husband. He, perhaps assisted by the seducer, beat her from head to foot with a club until she was literally a bloody pulp. Then he shoved the stick into her vagina and rectum, perforating the latter, and pushed her into a ditch to die.

Such drunken sexual and aggressive actions take place in the presence of children of all ages.

Apache men are proud of their federal military records. Not infrequently, an Apache, upon first meeting, will begin the conversation by relating his wartime experiences. Their memories for details of organizations to which they belonged, dates, and specific actions reveal considerable cathexis of interest. "Whites" who have served with Apaches report them to have been, in general, brave soldiers with great endurance, although few retained promotions received on the battlefield because of unruliness when not actually fighting. During recent years, the Apache have had a specialized fire-fighting crew known as the Red Hats. Although, apparently due to administrative difficulties, its reputation has declined, for the first several years of its existence, the bravery and resourcefulness of the Red Hats brought nation-wide renown.

Opler has written extensively[18] of ideal aboriginal child-training techniques, emphasizing that, "The rearing and training of children are among the most serious of adult preoccupations."[19] We have no data obtained from impartial observers of early Apache socialization processes.[20] Careful scrutiny of Opler's published material and our own research, however, suggest that, despite the official joyous welcome accorded pregnancy and childbirth, there was actually an ambivalence of attitude. Modern informants state that babies were not accepted as additions to the family until they were about eighteen months old; the death of a child prior to that time was treated with little concern. Infants could be left to the care of female relatives whenever their mothers chose to pursue other interests. Children were born about three years apart because of proscription of intercourse. Although today's old-timers present a rosy picture of aboriginal concern for the emotional states of children, contradictions in their claims and careful reading of Opler[21] lead us to question these formal statements. The general orientation then, as now, appears to have been that prelatency children "know nothing." No doubt, the small child had to learn some obedience—to be silent on command, for example—but latency children required admonishment. So far as we have been able to determine, training of children younger than about six years old proceeded very much as it does now. Then, however, two sets of mores were communicated that today are almost lacking. First, In the old days, there were strict rules governing relationships with relatives and in-laws.[22] Specific behavior patterns and special linguistic forms appropriate to different categories of kin had to be learned. Physical modesty was demanded where incest objects were concerned (although Opler's data are confusing and could. be interpreted to mean that absolute modesty became mandatory only with puberty). Premarital female virginity was strongly preferred, and sexual relations between siblings and cousins were taboo. Second, latency-period children began to undergo formal, increasingly rigorous training to prepare them for their adult roles. Boys were carefully and strenuously taught to become brave, predatory hunters, warriors, and raiders.[23] Not only did their fathers teach them the uses of weapons and encourage strength, stealth, endurance, and so forth, but special mentors were appointed.[24]

Today the ambivalence that greets pregnancy and small children is very obvious. Fifty-nine per cent of the mothers now under thirty years of age have had children premaritally. Prenatal-care facilities are ignored, and toxemia is the rule. Thirteen per cent of all Apache infants develop diagnosed chronic subdural hematomata,[25] probably reflecting a combination of physical traumata and dietary deficiencies due to gross neglect. Many Apache parents have given children away with scant evidence of more than superficial regret. In some instances, parents who have discarded a child forget they ever had it. Apache mothers who wish to shop, gamble, gossip, drink, or simply wander may leave their infants to the care of anyone at all. Fathers show no more concern for their children's welfare.

Apache babies sleep with their parents until, and sometimes after the birth of the next child, which now usually occurs perhaps a year and a half after the first. We heard several times of infants who had been smothered or crushed by sleeping drunken parents. Except when the mother impulsively decides to gratify some urge of her own, she is very gentle and physically affectionate in handling her infant. Bathing techniques are models of consideration and care. We are convinced that the usual Apache mother, however, has a minimal relationship with her infant, except as the child becomes a projection of herself—in which case, her ministrations provide her dissociated self (the baby) the treatment she as an adult wishes. The father's interaction with infants differs little from that of his wife. The latest born is king or queen of the household, within the limits set by the need of Apache adults to gratify immediately their own desires.

With the birth of another baby, the "king" is brusquely dethroned. Inconsistently, he is pushed away abruptly and brutally. During the first weeks, he cries desperately and tries to cling to his mother whenever she nurses or handles the new rival. It is not unusual to see such a howling child shoved away or even kicked in the face. After a time, he finds a crust of bread or his thumb. He quickly learns that he is not permitted to release his aggressions on the new baby. He can destroy the property of older children or attack them physically. He is passively encouraged to torture small animals. He usually turns to his father and older siblings for attention, which is given inconsistently.

Toilet training *per se* is practically nonexistent. An older child may take the younger to the outhouse, or the child may mess anywhere at all. Feces-laden diapers remain on some walking babies for hours or even days, or they may be thrown into a corner where they are soon covered with flies. No one heeds the stench. The child is not overtly rewarded for learning bowel control.

Except for the shoving described above, Apache discipline rarely involves physical punishment. It is the near-exclusive domain of the mother. An angry, drunken parent will strike out at anyone, however. The most consistent form of discipline is through threat. The protesting child of the past was told, among other things, that unless he stopped crying, *jajadeh*, the whippoorwill, would take him while he was asleep, carry him to a mountain recess, and either keep or eat him. *Jajadeh* is also one of the names of the Mountain Spirits.[26] Today, the whining toddler is told *"ashin,"* which means, "Here he comes." He who is coming is a ghost, dog, bear, or some other cultural bogey. The punishment to be expected consists of abandonment and perhaps being devoured. The child is thus taught simultaneously to project his aggressions and to develop institutionalized fears. A second powerful inhibitory disciplinary measure is ridicule, which is almost constant, albeit subtle at times. In more direct fashion, growing Apache children are taught that they must submit to the aggressions of the smaller and younger. In games between older and younger children, the latter always win. We have watched toddlers develop automatic responses to provocative behavior. These responses emphasize a stoical expression and limp passivity; in some instances, the behavior has become standardized by the time the child is three or four years old. Apache children of all ages eat constantly, suck their thumbs, and seek physical closeness with anyone who will tolerate their clinging, grasping, climbing, and crawling.

Although phenomena manifestly relating to the anal phase of development are common in Apache myths[27] the elements are infrequently connected with magic or power and usually involve laughter. Bourke, an army officer who lived among the Chiricahua, San Carlos, and Mescalero at various times during more than twenty years and wrote on scatological rites,[28] did not mention the magical use or fear of excrement among the Apache. Opler noted that the passing of flatus was taboo during the group peyote ceremony.[29] Currently, "witches' arrows" can consist of excrement. It is usual for an Apache child to be accompanied to the outhouse by an older child, especially after dark, when children do not dare to be alone. During the daytime, much sexual play goes on in the latrines. All sexual activities are referred to consistently by Apache as "dirty."

Dolls, today usually store-bought, are found in all Apache households in which children live. Girls play with dolls from the time they can hold objects throughout prepuberty. Preschool boys sometimes engage in doll-play, but usually they play house, very realistically, with girls of various ages. Jacobsen has written:

> Fantasies of pregnancy and delivery by the oral incorporation and anal re-birth of the mother appear to precede the phallic stage in little girls and boys: the wish for a baby is historically older than the wish for or pride in the penis. The wish for a child even seems to reflect, at first, only the mother-child situation without involving fantasies about the relationship between the parents.[30]

Kestenberg and Bradley have hypothesized that the doll, as a substitute for the fantasied baby, serves as an object onto which are projected vagina tensions.[31]

Each fall before school starts, children are taken to the hospital for "shots," which are generally given hypodermically into the upper arm. Soon thereafter, in almost every Apache household, mutilated dolls can be seen. Almost always, they will have holes ranging in size from one-quarter to three-quarters of an inch in diameter, *in the buttocks*. Bradley wrote:

> Comparison with the doctor-game as discussed by Simmel (1926) will serve to emphasize the *actual* value of the doll to the little girl. For just as that game is designed to help the child master the oedipal experience at the very time it is still an *actual* conflict, so the doll helps the little girl to master her *actual* vaginal sensations and impulses. Likewise, as the doctor-game provides all the participants with the possibility of realizing the primal scene in various roles, so the doll takes on many different meanings, not only that of a baby unconsciously representing projected vaginal sensations and impulses, but that of a penis, the child herself, a sibling, mother or even father.[32]

The Apache child is subjected to repetitive psychic traumata by the observation of sexual aggressive actions by his parents and other adults. Because of enforced fixation on the oral phase, with its attendant stunting of id and ego differentiation, his thinking continues to be heavily influenced by the primary process. He also interprets the behavior of the adults in terms of his phase-specific levels of psychosexual and psychosocial maturation, and his tendencies to interpret their acts in oral and anal sadistic terms is reinforced by their actual behavior. Apache children become preoccupied with certain classes of phenomena before such interest would be expected according to established analytic findings about chronology. As Anna Freud found among tiny girls reared in a residential nursery, an Apache female of eighteen months or a little older may already evince intense penis envy.[33] Fleiss has attributed such variance with analytic theoretical chronology to actual observations rather than to fantasies.[34]

Although we found little evidence of masturbation, we learned that relations that mimic adult sexual activity begin very early and frequently involve siblings and cousins. Such activities are officially banned but tacitly approved by the parents (who frequently openly condone premarital sexual relationships among adolescents). We have learned that preschool girls are seduced by older boys and that lads in their first years of grammar school are taught to have intercourse with pubescent lasses. As we would expect from the children's having seen and heard the aggressive-sexual actions of adults with such frequency, they tend to put themselves in the place of each adult and take on the excitements of both partners. The boys at least enter the oedipal phase with a bisexual identification.

There has been no differentiation in the behavioral requirements for girls and boys until this time. Both sexes have few household responsibilities. It will be recalled that, in aboriginal times, with the onset of latency, boys were formally trained for their adult roles. Now, most fathers have no contact with their children, except as unpredictable givers of physical affection or material goods, and do not take an active part in the education of their sons. Teaching of Apache lore is unusual today. Fathers have no honored adult role with which their sons can identify. Girls observe the reasonably well defined and consistent social roles of their mothers and become aware of the comparative strength and security of bonds among females.

Apache children are eager to enter grammar school, partly to get away from their homes. They have been taught, however, that they should be passive and uncompetitive, that they know nothing, and that whatever they do actively will result in shame and ridicule. Their white teachers frequently reinforce these expectations. We know that Apache children are bright, but they do poorly in school.[35]

Following formal education, Apache youth settles into the routine of the reservation. It is a rare Apache who is able to get along in some other area for more than a few months, regardless of government support. All return.

The basic personality type[36] of the Apache fits the Western diagnosis of hysterical and impulsive character disorder.[37] The psychosis of "choice" is one or more of the group of schizophrenias.[38] It appears that women are more secure than men, for the latter suffer from severe problems related to latent homosexual drives. The typical Apache is capable of only shallow emotional relationships to love objects.

I would hazard the opinion that the old-time Apache suffered from similar personality disorders. Training practices then, as now, produced strong aggressive drives. In former times, however, there was idealization of instinctual behavior,[39] and there were sanctioned outlets for unneutralized energies,[40] which were used in preserving life and social order. It seems reasonable to assume that there was also greater development of the conflict-free sphere of the ego.[41] Today, instinctual behavior creates conflicts and has no truly sanctioned outlets. The untamed energies are discharged primarily through drunkenness, with its attendant self- and social-organization-destruction.

§ Religion, Medical Practice, and Shamanism

Brinton has written, "There was no class of persons who so widely and deeply influenced the culture and shaped the destiny of the Indian tribes as their priests."[42] Although the influence of the aboriginal religion upon the lives of the Apache is ebbing, it can yet be perceived in every aspect of their thinking and action.

There is no way of determining to what degree Western European contact with the Apache has modified their mythology and philosophies.[43] The basic concept of Apache religion is that of vague, undefined, diffuse supernatural power. "This force floods the universe and renders even inanimate objects potentially animate."[44]

Features of the aboriginal concept of power, as described by Opler, are presented in the following quotations:

[Power] has no definite attribute of good or evil: its virtue is its potency. An

Apache who could control some of this power might accomplish things close
to his heart, it is felt. In contrast to the might of the supernatural stands
the human individual. Alone he is a pitiable object, a prey to sickness, to
enemies, to want, to the machinations of evil men. And so he hopes for
supernatural help . . .[45]

However, in order to become effective, it must "work through" mankind. Its
method is to utilize the animals, plants, natural forces, and inanimate objects familiar to the Chiricahua, as channels by means of which to get in
contact with men. After this contact has been made, the power appears in
a personified guise and offers a ceremony or supernatural aid to the person
approached.[46]

. . . the Apache, usually at a time of mental or physical stress, lies down and
believes himself to be approached and addressed by one of the agents to
which reference has been made above. . . . [He] recognizes it as a vision
experience. Whatever has come to this Apache speaks to him of his weakness,
of his need for something which will warn him of danger, which will be
ever at his call, which will help him cure the illnesses of his children, relatives and friends. The power offers him a ceremony, and, if he accepts it,
the songs and prayers which establish the rapport between the power and
the practitioner are revealed; the details of the ceremony, the uses to which
it can be put, and the evils against which it will prove efficacious are all
explained. If it is a bear that has approached this particular Apache, for
instance, those who are cognizant of his encounter with the animal will say
that their friend "knows" bear, or that bear "works through" him. Thereafter
anyone who becomes sick from bear may come to this man to have a curative
ceremony performed.[47]

Opler has written that in the earlier Apache conceptualization, supernatural power could be obtained by dream, hallucination, gift, or purchase.[48] The modern notion is that power makes itself available to any
individual only through "power dreams" or hallucinations. Ceremonies
can be learned from an "owner," and they retain some degree of power
despite the transfer. But most Apache now believe that ceremonies alone
have no more power than prayers. Opler has called the Apache a nation
of shamans, reasoning that any person who owned a ceremony possessed
supernatural power.[49] Yet Bourke has indicated that "small villages" had
no more than one or two of "their doctors,"[50] and, at the present time,
only thirteen Apache dwelling on the reservation are accorded the status
of shaman. Almost all adults and others as young as six years of age are
thought to possess ceremonies. In accordance with current Apache conceptualizations of shamanism, Basehart and I have defined the shaman

"as an individual who is considered to possess supernatural powers which support and are supported by the common values of his culture."[51]

Opler has written, "In the great enterprise of traffic with the supernatural there is no hierarchy of religious leadership."[52] It is not clear whether he referred to a hierarchy of supernatural powers or of shamans. Since he indicated that power conferred by the same source—like lightning—may be stronger when used by different shamans, he may have meant that the power source is not intrinsically important and that sun power, for instance, is *in itself* no more potent than mescal power.

Currently, there is no doubt that some shamans are considered "stronger" than others; even if two individuals have power from the same source, it may prove more effective when used by one of them. Most shamans agree that a power obtained from a celestial source (sun, moon, star, lightning, cloud, wind, and so forth) can be used to rectify a variety of ills, to ward off various dangers, to forecast the future, to determine whether an object has been lost or stolen and ensure its recovery, and so forth. A power from a terrestrial source (yucca, lizard, bear, waterbug, and so forth), however, can be used only to counteract sicknesses or misfortunes resulting from an affront to the "boss," *diyin* (spirit) or *nantʔa* (leader) of that source. Yet there is at least one area of confusion, for the *diyin* of the snake is considered the same as that of the lightning.[53]

In addition, there are celestial and terrestrial classes of power of varying strengths. According to Mescalero shamans, one who is entitled to call upon the "little whirlwind" or "little star" has "little power"; one who can summon the strength of the *diyin* of the sun or moon has "medium power"; one who can invoke the lightning, wind, or large hail has "big power." As far as I have been able to learn from the literature, the concept of hierarchy of bosses has not been described, although there is an allusion to it in Henry's study of the cult of Silas John.[54] The concept is ill defined, and informants' statements are contradictory about detail. Mescalero, Chiricahua, and Lipan shamans, as well as other informants, however, all state that each natural phenomenon has a boss of its own. The hierarchy resembles a military chain of command. He-Who-Created-Us, Yusn, (God) is the commander in chief. Three powerful *diyin* (angels) control events in the heavens, the earth, and the water. Lesser *nantʔa* concern themselves with individual celestial and terrestrial phenomena. For example, Thunderman, Thunderlady, Thunderboy, and Thundergirl have poorly defined roles related to the behavior and effects of lightning, thunder, rain, and snow. There is a boss in charge of land animals, another of land plants. A *diyin* governs water animals, another water plants. Lower-order bosses control faunal and floral families and, in addition, each living species has a *diyin* of its own. Large geographical features and stones of varying sizes, shapes, and colors are thought to have individual *nantʔa*. The *diyin* of sacred places may have more power than those of other inanimate objects.

I have written elsewhere:

> There is no clear reason for attributing the belief in the hierarchy of bosses to the aboriginal societies. Even if one did so, our data indicate the likelihood the belief was held only by the Mescaleros. It seems that acculturation is the most likely usable hypothesis. The hierarchy notion is consistent with Christian belief; reinterpretations of this kind are not uncommon as a result of contact.[55]

Also, large numbers of Apache have served in the United States military forces.

The concept of the Mountain Spirits (*ganheh, jajadeh,* Mountain Gods, masked dancers, devil dancers) was once very important, although today its influence is obviously waning. According to Opler:

> The Mountain Spirits are a race of supernaturals who dwell within the interiors of many mountains . . . There they are said to live and conduct their affairs much as the Apache used to do in aboriginal times. The Mountain Spirits conduct a dance and ceremony in which some of their men are masked and appear with their bodies painted in various patterns. Occasionally an Apache is fortunate enough to have a supernatural experience with the Mountain Spirits of a particular mountain, to witness the performance of these masked supernaturals, and to be influenced in the songs, designs, and prayers which belong to the rite.[56]

Such an experience, according to our informants, always involves an ordeal. Opler continues:

> After this Apache returns to the world outside, and to his own people, he masks and paints Apache men in imitation of the supernaturals he has seen, and sends them out to dance at times of widespread sickness or impending disaster. This procedure or rite is expected to establish rapport between the shaman and the aboriginal supernaturals from whom he has gained his power . . .
>
> . . . the real Mountain Spirits sometimes came out upon this world in person to punish those who have profaned their rite or to succor Apache in need of their assistance. Now it is said that only those appear who are "made" or dressed in imitation of the true Mountain Spirits.[57]

The "made" dancers, however, carried the same name as did the masked supernaturals. Opler was given to understand that all the masked dancers, or at least their leaders and the clowns, were shamans. During the period of our work, of all the leaders, dancers, and clowns, only one leader was accorded the status of shaman. The dancers and clowns were simply men who were selected, trained, and hired to perform the ceremonies.

Today, the general attitude toward supernatural power is that it is benevolent. Any person who possesses such power, however, will use it as he chooses or as his personality dictates, for good (collectivity oriented) or evil (witchcraft or sorcery) purposes. To own power is considered to be hazardous. A shaman who saves a life must at future time atone by giving up his own life or that of a relative. In the final analysis, the death of his relative is ascribed to his practicing witchcraft upon that loved one or passively permitting a death that has been caused by one of the agents that we shall describe.

Opler found that the old-time Apache attributed almost all misfortune and disease to the workings of witchcraft and ghosts.[58] Today, with the further influences traceable to acculturation, some credence is placed in the concepts of fortuitous mishaps and causation of diseases as taught by whites. Nevertheless, we met no Apache who was not still influenced by the aboriginal philosophies, and the great majority was obviously seriously involved with the old beliefs and teachings.

As already indicated, aboriginal conceptualizations of the means for acquiring shamanistic powers have changed. The present-day notion is that, in order to obtain supernatural power, one must experience a power dream or hallucination. Opler inferred that possession of supernatural power was mandatory for the performance of sorcery, and today each shaman is considered capable of witchcraft. The accusation is rarely leveled at more than half of them, however. One shaman is thought to practice witchcraft exclusively. Perhaps another dozen people are said to "witch" sometimes, although they are not thought to possess supernatural powers. They are considered to have learned actions or words that are themselves dangerous in the hands of anyone who knows them.

Aboriginally, various procedures could be employed to determine the identity of a witch. A shaman could have a patient look into a reflecting surface and command him to see a picture; the patient sometimes identified the person who had "witched" him. Indians who were sexually aberrant and those who committeed incest were assumed to have been witched or to be witches. Ideal behavior demanded an absence of intragroup trouble-making. No person was supposed to have possessions greatly in excess of those of his neighbors. The chronic braggart, trouble-

maker, or miser was thought to be a sorcerer. A person accused of being
a witch could undergo tests to prove his innocence. Examples of these
tests, reported by Opler,[59] include eating elk meat—a witch would vomit
the meat, which was relished by ordinary persons; hanging the suspect by
his thumbs over a fire—if a confession did not result within a certain
period, the individual was freed. Confession, on the other hand, constituted complete evidence of guilt, and the witch was burned to death. It
was possible, however, that people who had been thus declared not
guilty might still be killed by relatives of the supposed victims.

Schwatka observed a variant test of witchcraft guilt.[60] A woman was
stripped to the waist and suspended by her thumbs so that only her toes
touched the ground. Anyone in the group was at liberty to "flay" her with
sharp switches. If the woman confessed before her tormentors tired, she
was beaten and stoned to death.

Today, a person is diagnosed as a witch principally through his actions and personality. As a rule, he will be more than sixty years old.
Any person is suspect, however, if one or more of his forebears have been
known as powerful witches. If a person points at people with his finger
rather than his lips; is afraid to sleep indoors with others; eats only his
own cooking; dances naked in the woods; is paranoid, a braggart, or a
miser; or, above all, "talks mean," he is considered a sorcerer. On two
occasions, I heard that a woman was converted into a witch for refusing
to have intercourse with a man. There are no punishments beyond gossip
and some degree of ostracism, which encourages further intragroup
tensions.

Witches have three principal methods of operating: magical words
and gestures, calling upon their supernatural powers, and controlling the
actions of ghosts.

Sorcerers can use silent or spoken curses to harm individuals or entire
tribes. The current general drunkenness and decrease of water supply
on the reservation have been attributed to witchcraft. Should the witch
choose to bring "bad luck" to a person, he can cause that individual to
be in contact with a "witch's arrow." In past times, such arrows were
usually made of portions of cadavers or objects that had touched them.
The witch found a dead body and used its bones and hair to make a tiny
bow and arrow, which could be tipped with a piece of dried corpse flesh,
hair, a fragment of clothing, feathers, a spider, horsehair, a needle, or any
other object that had touched the corpse. The bow had magical powers
and could shoot the arrow into a given person at any distance. Today,
a favorite practice of a witch is to obtain hair, feces, urine, sputum, or
menstrual blood from the intended victim, imbue it with his evil powers,

and shoot it into or bring it in contact with the person to be harmed. Cursed herbs or a decoction of excreta from the individual to be witched may be put into his food or drink. A cartridge has often been used as an arrow in the past century.

Witches have traffic with ghosts of dead humans. They can change such spirits or living persons into any animate or inanimate object. The sorcerer can cause the disguised ghost or human to contact any person and cause him misfortune.

> Every ghost is potentially dangerous. The spirits of individuals who have died after "a full life" are feared less than those of people who have died "before their time," violently, or who were "mean" or witches. Ghosts of the satisfied dead are thought to go to some nebulous "happy hunting ground" (or currently, heaven). They must be very few. Others hover about in the darkness, waiting to frighten or inconvenience the living, ultimately to drive them crazy, that they might either suicide or foolishly lose their lives. In some cases, ghosts are thought to desire the deaths of loved ones, that their spirits will join the ghosts and remove their loneliness. In others, the ghosts are said to seek vengeance, to make others die before their time, that they, too, will be unhappy.[61]

Ghosts can become re-embodied voluntarily into various animals and birds. Informants have said that any animation or anthropomorphization requires the reincarnation of a ghost.[62]

Although any animal, bird, or plant can be used for the purposes of the witch, the owl and canines are particularly feared as agents of sorcerers and are sometimes called witches. If they are inhabited by ghosts, either through the choice of the spirit or the machinations of the sorcerers, they have the power of speech, which all animals had "in the beginning." An owl, dog, coyote, or fox has oracular powers. To foretell the death of an individual or a relative, it speaks the name and says "I am going to drink your blood."

Witchcraft, then, can cause an individual or a group to suffer any kind of disaster. Ghosts affect people with great fear and create psychic disturbances.

A third class of disorders results from negligent behavior of Apache to bosses. These disorders have a specific name, *itseh* (it makes sickness) or *nitseh* (it makes you sick). In the old days, before any living or inanimate object could be used safely by an Indian it was necessary that he perform a ceremony to appease its *diyⁱⁿ*. If mescal were to be gathered, the woman who did the collecting had to pray to its *nantʔa*, expressing thanks, promising that the food would be used for collective purposes, and requesting a good crop the next year. Should she fail to conduct the little rite, the mescal *diyiⁿ* would cause the plant she gathered to spoil, cook improperly, or fail to nourish her and her family and diminish the next year's growth. Ultimately, group starvation would threaten. If the boss of the deer, antelope, yucca, or any other food source were similarly affronted, like results were to be expected. If trees were to be cut or rocks collected for building purposes and their *nantʔa* affronted by such negligence, erection of the proposed dwelling would be made impossible, or it would fall down, once built. Herbs, other medicines, and sacred material that were improperly collected would not perform their appointed tasks, and their collectors would be punished in various manners. If the *nantʔa* of any object were seriously insulted, he might turn the offender into an animal, plant, stone, and so forth.

Certain *diyiⁿ*, when affronted, cause specific disease syndromes, all of which involve manifestations of acute anxiety. If an Apache steps on a spider and fails to apologize properly to its boss, he will soon suffer from spider sickness. The symptoms consist of cracks (or sensations as though there were cracks) in the skin, resembling the spider's web. If the *nantʔa* of the arachnid is not appeased by a shaman who has either a celestially derived power or spider power, soon the weblike cracks will involve the heart and kill the victim. Snake sickness results from touching a snake or a place it has recently touched. It is a disease in which some or all of the skin peels off as does that of the reptile when it is shedding. In addition, aches, pains, and crawling sensations occur on the surface of the body. If no shaman with appropriate powers treats the victim, the crawling will reach his heart and he will surely die. If an owl flies near camp and an Apache does not properly salute his *diyiⁿ*, he will suffer from tremulousness, sweating, great fear, contraction of the heart, spasms of the muscles, insanity, and ultimately death from suicide or "foolishness." Each syndrome caused by an affronted boss has its own name. Theoretically, according to one shaman, there are 60,000 such illnesses, many of which are named; few are evident today. Ceremonies consecrated to *diyiⁿ* of specific objects to be hunted or gathered are rapidly disappearing. The majority of Indians in their thirties or older still pray at least to God, Jesus, or the Virgin before they hunt or gather. Elderly Apache still frequently invoke the specific *nantʔa* as well.

It is clear from the preceding material, that any disaster or disease syndrome may have three different sources. The diagnosis of *goobinitseh* (snake-his-it-makes-you-sick, snake sickness), if the symptoms are classical, is not particularly difficult. But the shaman may be hard put to determine whether the sickness resulted from the actions of a witch, a ghost, or a boss. Apparently, in early times, there was a crucial need to differentiate among the three potential causes. If the sickness was the result of the actions of a ghost who had entered the reptile and then, as a snake, had touched an intended victim, the work of the shaman would be defined: to appease or exorcise the ghost. If the illness was determined to have been caused by witchcraft, the healer's job was to battle the specific sorcerer who had been hired or otherwise chosen to harm the sufferer. Should the sickness have been inflicted by the affronted *goobidiyin* (snake-his-boss), only a shaman with snake or lightning power was capable of influencing the *goobidiyin* to permit the offending Indian to live.

Of the treatment afforded by Apache shamans in the early nineteen thirties, Opler wrote, "the Apache shaman is not a credulous dupe of his own supernaturalistic claims and boastings, who undertakes to cure any ailment, no matter how hopeless."[63] The shaman was a shrewd and wary person who recognized and as a rule refused to accept responsibility for the cure of serious organic disturbance. Sometimes he resorted to *legerdemain* to demonstrate that his treatment would be ineffective. The shaman was quick to treat less serious indispositions, however, and to solidify his reputation by rendering prompt relief. He was "often interrupted by his 'power' while in the midst of his ceremonial songs and directed to dose his patient with some common laxative or emetic."[64] To be sure, the decoction was administered ritualistically.

Although the shaman usually refused to treat serious organic disorders, he sometimes accepted such cases. There were, of course, built-in safeguards. If he were convinced of failure in advance of or at some point during his treatment, he could claim his diagnosis had been erroneous because his client gave him faulty information, or he could state that his power had told him the Apache whom he was treating had too flagrantly insulted a boss. The curer insisted that a patient who sought his help have absolute confidence in the efficacy of the ceremony to be performed and the integrity of the practitioner. An Apache and his relatives had to humble themselves before the shaman from who they sought assistance. After he had magnanimously acceded to their pleas, the shaman of Opler's day would demand four ceremonial gifts for his "power":

A representative set of such gifts would be a pouch of pollen, an unblemished buckskin, a downy eagle feather and a piece of turquoise. Even after these have been presented, he has other orders to give. A special structure for the rite, with the door facing the east, is often demanded, and the close relatives of the patient are expected to furnish all the labor involved. By such requirements the Apache shaman takes pains to eliminate half-heartedness at the outset, and he proceeds on the assumption that for best results confidence in the technique he is to use, his ceremony and his "power," must be instilled. Accordingly, when all is in readiness and the ceremony is about to begin, the shaman's first act is to validate his ceremony, and to impress the patient and the assembled relatives with its potency and its source. He describes the supernatural encounter which led to the acquisition of the ceremony; he relates how he was led into the "holy home" of the "power" and there tested in every conceivable way, how the ceremony and its uses were unfolded before him, and how, through his ceremony, he has since been able to enlist the aid of his "power" in the curing of those who come to him in the proper fashion.[65]

Should the patient remain apathetic toward the shaman and the ceremony, the healer would sometimes terminate proceedings and blame his failure on the client. It was also usual for the shaman to invoke small taboos on behavior of relatives and clients—forbid them to scratch lice bites with their fingernails during the ceremony, for example. Breaches of conduct could then be blamed for failures.

During curing rites, shamans resorted at times to prestidigitation. As trick photography is used to create a pleasing illusion, "the Apache ceremony is designed to inculcate belief in the shaman's powers."[66] After the initial ritual, the shaman, who had much factual knowledge of the client's life beforehand, made a great display of enumerating significant events of the patient's past and present. He warned the sufferer that facts must not be withheld. Subjected to strong suggestion techniques, his memory jogged with data he had suppressed or repressed, the client would sometimes abreact associatively, and the actual event or trauma that had crystallized the tic or seizure was often recalled; in the course of such associations, the symptoms at times did disappear.

When the shaman had exposed the symbol of the patient's distress (bear, snake, lightning, and so forth), he attempted to determine *why* the embodiment of evil "bothered" his patient.

For the answer to this question he invokes his "power." He sings his ceremonial songs and recites his prayers in an effort to communicate with his "power," to obtain its aid in tracing down the forces which have made his patient ill and to gain its support in opposing those forces. The effort to enlist the co-operation of the "power" in this work is often a stirring spectacle. . . . In the end he announces, of course, his "power's" complete interest in the case and its determination to prosecute it to a successful conclusion.[67]

Then followed the dramatic battle between the shaman and his power(s) and the opposing evil machinations of witch or ghost. In the event witchcraft was diagnosed, the witch's arrow was ultimately sucked or grabbed from the sufferer.

> At the conclusion of the ceremony the shaman makes a final gesture which may in some cases have decided therapeutic value. He imposes upon the patient some restriction or taboo. It may be an injunction to eat no meat from the head of an animal, to eat no entrails, to refrain from picking up some object which has been dropped, etc. It offers, in place of a tic or compulsive symptom, a clever substitute. When it has served its purpose and become irksome, a short ceremony at the hands of the one who pronounced the taboo makes its continuance unnecessary.[68]

Today, the majority of physical illnesses are treated by the United States Public Health Service physicians. Those doctors are, however, considered completely unable to deal with disorders that the Apache, some with conscious and some with preconscious knowledge, prediagnose as psychogenic. For these types of disorder, the shaman remains indispensable. I was able to obtain incomplete records of the incidence of employment of ten shamans during a period of one year. A Lipan man, who did not divulge the source of his powers, chased a ghost from a house when death had occurred and performed two ceremonies to remove ghosts from sufferers of alcoholic hallucinosis. A Mescalero woman, who said she received her powers from the spirits of the long-ago dead, was hired fifteen times to remove ghosts, once from a child who had "doll sickness" and the rest from houses in which people had died and from sufferers of alcoholic hallucinosis. A Mescalero man, who claimed powers from numerous celestial sources in addition to bear, snake, and horse, was hired on "several occasions" to conduct witchcraft and to remove witches' arrows, to make "some" women fertile and sterile, to make a man potent, to perform love magic, or to remove ghosts from houses and from alcoholic hallucinotics. A Mescalero woman, who claimed star power, twice performed ghost-chasing ceremonies in the company of her Mescalero husband, who also owned star power. A Mescalero, the source of whose powers was not revealed, once performed a ceremony to prevent an Apache's conviction by a federal judge. A Mescalero woman, who did not tell the source of her powers, was hired many times more than anyone else on the reservation. As far as I could determine, she twice performed rites to enable Indians to be elected to office and otherwise mostly chased ghosts from houses and alcoholic hallucinotics. She was, however, also a renowned herbalist and treated many minor physical disorders. She may have used Silas John techniques. She also may have conducted

a rite to prevent a man's being convicted. One Mescalero man who owned
star and bear power was not hired at all. A Chiricahua, who did not reveal
the source of his power, performed a number of ceremonies for the treatment of tuberculosis, which was attributed to witchcraft. Although he
claimed to me that he only used an herb and prayers to God, other informants said that he dissolved witches' arrows through use of the
specific plants. One Mescalero woman who claimed star power was
hired only once, by me, when I suffered from a gastrointestinal upset.
She gave me very effective herbs but claimed the critical portion of the
treatment was her use of a root to dissolve a witch's arrow.

Today, the four gifts required for advance payment always include
smoke (tobacco to be used in rolling cigarets), a black handled knife,
and, usually, dress materials and money. Sometimes a shaman will ask
for a piece of turquoise. Black is the specific color most efficacious in
ghost-chasing. Ashes and pollen are always used, as in the old days. Fire
and its products are prophylactic against witches and ghosts. Pollen must
be employed in any sacred ceremony to ensure its success. No special
structures are used in contemporary ceremonies. Ceremonies remain
dramatic in nature. Peyote is rarely used to help the shaman or the
patient hallucinate the source of the difficulty. Hypnosis is sometimes
employed.

The interpretation and use of dreams have occupied men's minds
from the earliest times.[69] They have been part and parcel of the religion
and therapy of numerous primitive peoples.[70]

Although it is an individual matter, most Apache believe that dreams
foretell the future, in terms of good and bad luck.[71] Certain manifest
contents forecast illness or misfortune: Fire, floods, falling teeth, the
return of a dead person, a pig, the colors red or black, being chased
by a wild animal (particularly those with hooves)—in fact, any of the
usual cultural bogeys—tells the dreamer something bad will happen, provided he does not take preventive measures. Any dream that frightens
an individual has the same general connotation, regardless of its content.
A dream in which some action directly affects the dreamer prophesies
its opposite, however.

"If you dream you are going to be sick, that means you are going to stay
well." "If you dream that a snake bites you, that's good. It won't happen. If
you dream that you die, it means you will live a long time. If you dream
that your father, mother, brother or sister dies, it doesn't mean that one. It
means that someone outside the family is going to die."[72]

Other dream contents indicate the future occurrence of something good:

" 'If you dream about summer, about everything green, about things growing and fruits and pollen, everything is all right.' "[73] Deer, horses, mules, and burros are good luck symbols.

If one dreams of fire, he can prevent potential misfortune by building an outdoor fire. To prevent dreams about ghosts, one should not put clothing at the head of one's bed, especially in contact with one's pillow. Should one be frightened by a dream and know no countermeasure, a shaman might be consulted for a ghost-chasing ceremony or instructions. Not all shamans in the past claimed interpretive powers for dreams.

Among the Apache of today, no shaman inquires about his clients' dreams. If the patient spontaneously relates any vision, the curer interprets its occurrence or its symbology as we have outlined. At least one shaman hypnotizes clients with or without the aid of peyote in order to make a hallucination occur. The reverie is supposed to reveal the identity of the alleged witch or disclose the conflict about which the patient feels guilt. If it does not, the experience is used to impress the client further with the shaman's and the ceremony's powers and to forecast in general terms the outcome of the curative rite. Several shamans said that they examined their own dreams closely in order to determine whether or not they were in danger of being subjected to witchcraft practiced by rivals. They were particularly attentive to dreams and hallucinations that occurred before and during curing ceremonies. But their dream interpretations remained as nonspecific as we have suggested.

§ Interaction of Personality Structure and Shamanism

A significant aspect of the psychoanalytic theory of inherent maturational stages is the concept of phylogenetic influence on personality development. The biological effect of inbreeding on predisposition to develop personality configurations remains a moot argument. If such a formulation is valid, it may well apply to the Apache. The observable socialization phenomena alone would, however, appear to explain adequately the growth of their typical personality structure. The narcissistic attitude of Apache mothers toward their infants stunts id-ego differentiation and constitutes, in my opinion, the fundamental factor of greatest importance in their psychosexual and psychosocial unfolding. The typical Apache retains faulty id-ego differentiation throughout his life, a phenomenon that must contribute to the specific kinds of psychotic breakdown to which these Indians are subject: variants of the group of schizophrenias. Such early traumatization of their potential psychic maturational capacities is compounded by abrupt displacement by younger rivals and drastic observations of sexual and hostile behavior by adults. In the case of the males, a fourth serious psychic injury is provided by the absence of an esteemed masculine role with which to identify. The female, more fortunate, has a model for adulthood role-assumption that has remained more nearly intact. Although she too remains psychologically immature, her psychopathology appears to be better covered and less troublesome because of identification with an admired role pattern. Each of the major traumata results, it would appear, in further oral fixations, and all of the psychosexual phases become fused with orality. A final psychological trauma of far-reaching consequences has been provided by confinement to reservation existence itself. The so-called paternalistic, but operationally lenient and inconsistently maternal, policies of the Bureau of Indian Affairs during the century or so during which the Apaches have been herded about have reinforced their dependent needs and irresponsibility.

There is no doubt that the female is the strong figure in the household and that the role of the woman is more consistent and respected in Apache society than is that of the male. Caudill has compared personality structure among two groups of Ojibwas in different stages of acculturation.[74] He found that women are able to make more satisfactory adjustments to conditions of acculturation than are men. It is biologically foreordained that in all societies the early identifications of children will be with the mothering figures. In Apache socialization, the male child is doomed to retain bisexual identification, partly because of faulty id-ego differentiation and partly because of the personal, familial, and societal weakness of the father.

As Peter Blos has commented in a personal communication about a previous paper,[75] today's Apache lack symbolic representations or derivatives that are detached from the original organ modes.[76] Rampant drunkenness and the flagrant male need to prove masculinity through promiscuity are cases in point. Blos wrote, "Other societies—like the Balinese—formalized in the trance and dance a psychotic transient state which permits a regression and simultaneously protects ego intactness."[77] Among the Apache, drunkenness may have similar functions, since alcoholic hallucinosis is frequent and sexual and hostile impulses can be discharged when the individual is intoxicated without meeting consistent societal disapproval. Drunkenness in itself, however, as employed by these Apache, constitutes a form of personal and societal suicide. R. M. Boyer has postulated that a societal safeguard against ethnosuicide is to be found in the widespread dependent tendencies combined with retention of individual rights of decision-making.[78] These characteristics provide positive relationships among the Apache, which make them feel relatively secure only when with one another on the reservation and help to preserve a sense of tribal identity.

Be that as it may, the cardinal point remains—that the nature of the Apache personality structure has its basis in the early abandonment of and failure to relate to infants by the narcissistic mother and available substitutes for her. The typical present-day Apache search for an adequate mother-infant relationship throughout their lives in all their activities. Even the universal seeking for a father figure constitutes, in the final analysis, a search for the mother, since the Apache conceptualization of the role of the father is, in general, maternal.

Hallowell[79] and Caudill[80] have concluded that major personality characteristics persist over time despite influences of acculturation. I suggest that the same is true even though deculturation[81] and inability or refusal to accept acculturation prevail, as in cases in which negative identity develops.[82] Among the Mescalero, a combination of partial acculturation and partial deculturation obtains; R. M. Boyer has suggested that Mescalero males have developed a type of negative identity.[83] It is my impression that the typical personality structure of the old-time Apache was very similar to that observed today, even though formerly the stable and internally flexible social structure provided means by which the conditions of abnormality stimulated and promoted by socialization processes could be consistently sanctioned and formalized, thus making individual functioning less conflictual than is the case today. This assumption appears to be borne out by an as yet incompletely studied series of about 250 Rorschach tests that I administered to Apache of all ages and the analysis of which is being supervised by Dr. Bruno Klopfer.

Let us now turn to the psychological meanings of Apache religion and shamanism.[84] In the past, all events influencing the lives of these Indians were ascribed to the actions of bosses, ghosts, and witches. The basic concept of religion consisted of animation of natural phenomena with supernatural power. The *diyin*, spirits, and sorcerers could be influenced by ceremonies, of which the major ones were the possessions solely of shamans. There were numerous food taboos. For example, Apache would not eat the meat of many animals, including members of the cat, bear, and dog families; batrachians; reptiles; some birds; fish; and insects. Ultimately, the common denominators among those various creatures resolve to only one: They were thought to be flesh-eaters. The bosses are logically, and in the minds of some Apaches actually, fused

with ghosts, obviously projections of individuals and their drive derivatives. Witches and shamans theoretically constitute aspects of the same
individuals, although people who have not been accorded the status of
shaman have been labeled witches. Witches exist because of their own
hostile personality components. Adult fears that plants and animals or
their *nantʔa* can retaliate for negligence in performance of gathering and
hunting rites constitute institutionalization of a trait that would probably
lose its adaptive purposes were the Apache not still strongly under the
influence of the oral phase and its utilization of the primary process. The
fear of retaliation by *diyin* for inadequate propitiation stems from employment of the *lex talionis* principle. All animation and anthropomorphization require projection. Power is conceived by the Apache largely
in oral and phallic terms, a phenomenon that can be traced to the emphasis on socialization stresses during the oral and phallic phases of
psychosexual and psychosocial development.

    The roles of the shaman and the witch are easily understood as dis-
placed representatives of the good and bad parents, in the final analysis
the mother, and of projections of portions of the individual. Kanzer
wrote of the scientific development of Freud's psychoanalytic thinking:

> The most primitive, or animistic system, which coincides with the stage of
> magic omnipotence of the ego, practices sorcery to control reality, "influ-
> encing spirits by treating them like people . . . The first theoretical accom-
> plishment of man was the creation of spirits" through which he delegated his
> freedom of the will to external powers, a stage in the development of reality
> testing. Religion, the next advance in thought, represents a systematized
> effort to restore to life the parricidally destroyed father in whom the magic
> of the spirits has become centrally vested—i.e., it is the mythology of a later
> stage of ego maturation in which the father serves as model for the organized
> and coercive nature of the forces in the external world (superego).[85]

He referred, of course, to Freud's now debunked *Totem and Taboo* formulation, which was developed before the concept of the superego was
introduced and its derivatives traced to a fusion of maternal and paternal
introjects.[86] Among the aboriginal Apache, supernatural power was apparently designated as asexual. This conceptualization can be understood
as deriving from projection of infantile portions of the self. It would seem
that the earliest formulation consisted of construction of the shamans and
witches as projections of the parents, with their protective and angry
aspects.

    With the influences of Western thinking, there have been changes in
the format. Many of the old taboos are losing their influence. Apache

religious philosophies have been altered by Christian influences. In the old days, treatment of psychogenic illnesses was the forte of the shaman. The same is true today; only the number of sicknesses that can be attributed to psychological forces has diminished. At present, as in the past, the success of shamanistic practices depends upon the degree of commitment by the patient to the philosophical system behind the shamanistic rituals and upon belief in the specific powers of the particular shaman. In turn, these beliefs depend upon the failure within patients and practitioners of id-ego differentiation and the pervasion of all levels of thinking with the influences of the primary process.

§ Some Points of Comparison
Between Apache Shamanism
and Western Psychiatry

Western psychiatry comprises in its philosophies and therapeutic techniques a vast continuum of points of view and methodologies, which vary between two opposite poles of approach: that of faith or magic healing, which utilizes primary-process thinking and exploitation of emotions as its *modus operandi,* and that of the scientist, which uses secondary-process thinking and objective investigation with the employment of rational remedies as its therapeutic method.

Let us examine these two therapeutic approaches in greater detail. Kubie has contrasted psychoanalysis and healing by faith or suggestion.[87] The psychoanalyst ideally maintains a scientific attitude and for him logic is not a substitute for evidence. His interpretations are offered as working hypotheses and are to be tested against further emergent data. He invites and expects his patient to preserve and utilize actively an observing segment of the ego and to co-operate in an investigative procedure.

> Nothing excites graver misgivings in him than the blind credulity and pious faith which some earnest patients struggle to maintain. Experience has taught the analyst that unless he can break down such attitudes they will make lasting therapeutic results impossible. He knows that the patient's effort to look upon him as omniscient and omnipotent is a symptom of the patient's neurosis, a direct carry-over from infancy; and he sets out not to exploit this uncritical worship but to analyze it away.[88]

All methods of faith healing share the basic premise that recovery depends upon supernatural forces that affect all illnesses equally. The construction of a differential diagnosis is thus ultimately superfluous. Healing based on magic and faith utilize exhortation and mobilize religious and personal emotional enthusiasms. The healer attempts to create altered moods and to induce changes in the levels of consciousness, regressed ego states.[89] Since his goal is to remove immediately a symptom or symptom complex and the duration of relief is not a crucial matter, he considers it legitimate both to introduce ideas that challenge the secondary-process logic of the patient and to exercise influence based upon his emotional hold over his client. "Thus the operation of suggestion in this sense is always dependent on the human relationship behind the ideas, a relationship which induces the patient to abrogate his right to judgment."[90] The analyst knows that abrupt symptom-removal frequently disguises the pathological condition that lies beneath, and his goal includes removal of that psychopathology itself. He does not expect to remove symptoms rapidly and is apprehensive at times when they disappear precipitously. In psychoanalysis, the relationship between the patient and the physician is used to facilitate the production of buried material that might otherwise remain inaccessible. Effort is made not to bind the analysand to the analyst or to his fantasies about the analyst but rather to clarify such fantasies and thus enable the subject to progress steadily toward greater freedom from the influences of his unconscious conflicts and the immature forms of logic used by his unconscious. Ultimately, the faith healer places himself and his supernatural powers in complete charge over the patient, who is expected to submit passively to his manipulations. Psychoanalysis demands conscious co-operative investigation. It demands willingness to accept in every detail the reality of the body, in a fashion that contrasts sharply with the faith healer's efforts to deny the existence of organic disease.

> Occasionally, however, an affiliation with a religious sect may be part of a more fundamental alteration in a distorted personality, a change sufficiently soond to place it on a sound basis so long as the faith persists.[91]

The psychoanalyst must strive to make the patient fundamentally different from what he once was and must expect to encounter the conscious and unconscious resistance to change that is inherent in all people.

Faith requires no evidence. Belief is the direct perception of a divinely revealed truth. Dependence on evidence is irreligious. The analyst must also trace the genesis of faith in the life of the individual to his ultimate dependence upon a belief in the omnipotence and omniscience of his parents, later displaced to other individuals and ultimately to the supernatural, which may be dehumanized or anthropomorphized.

Even in the most enlightened Western psychiatry, the utilization of physical therapies spans the two aforementioned poles. The rationale for use of drugs extends from the employment of the placebo for its purely suggestive properties to that of specific medicines like antiluetics that have been proved to counteract disorders. The employment of certain physical therapies has magical qualities, despite the fact that their efficacy has been demonstrated empirically; shock therapies provide a case in point.[92] The use of drugs and physical therapies by faith healers is ancillary to the ultimate philosophy of the therapeusis.

The aboriginal Apache philosophy was that all illnesses result ultimately from supernatural power and cure results from manipulation of agents of that power. The professional activities of the present-day shaman are, however, limited almost exclusively to the treatment of functional disorders. I observed a few instances in which individuals consulted shamans for treatment of obviously physical disorders—like gall-bladder disease and diabetes mellitus—but no curer, so far as I was able to determine, accepted such a case without insisting that the potential patient simultaneously consult white physicians. The majority of Apache now seek the services of shamans solely for pathological syndromes that they recognize to be psychogenic in nature. They call the pathogenic agent that has supposedly caused the functional disturbance "ghost," "witch, or "boss," but they are quite sure that the effective operative mechanisms through which such supernatural agents work is fear. Confronted with a psychogenic agent, the shaman makes a partially sincere attempt to formulate a differential diagnosis, but the labeling of a syndrome does not alter his therapeutic technique, which is reduced to a ritualistic, although somewhat individualistic, procedure. He demands complete faith in his system of thought and personal qualifications and total submission to his directives. He systematically exhorts and mobilizes religious and personal emotional enthusiasms. He induces altered, regressive ego states in his patients in his attempts to remove symptoms within a culturally set, magical time period. Although he prescribes drugs and physical therapies at times, their use is ancillary to the fundamental philosophy of his treatment. The aim underlying the administration of emetics, purgatives, and herbs that have been ethnocentrically and empirically determined to soothe mucosal and epidermal surfaces appears to be largely that of enhancing his own status. He tries to bind the patient to him and to strengthen the notion that he himself is omniscient and omnipotent. He never interprets transference reactions, although he appears at times to be well aware of their existence.[93] He makes no systematic effort to effect change in whatever underlying psychopathology may exist. To do so would be contrary to the Apache conceptualization of a man's nature as genetically or chemically determined and uninfluenceable. "Enlightened" persons who have read magazine articles that trace psychogenic disorders to childhood traumata pay lip service to such ideas and make pious pronouncements indicating they believe such ideas. When questioned, however, even the most acculturated attribute the "nature" of a person to his heredity and to the chemical effects of his parents' having used alcohol. When they are further pressed to explain why the parents have been drunkards, they ultimately resort to such statements as "Because such-and-such a person among his forebears was mean"; "They say he was witched"; or "I heard he started drinking right after that owl talked to him." The shaman generally uses treatment techniques that utilize suggestion, suppression, and reassurance. Sometimes his knowledge of the patient's life and current problems permits him to produce abreactions intentionally and an occasional shaman employes this technique. Opler wrote:

> Even if the shaman succeeds in establishing the nexus between the mental state of his patient and some terrifying experience with an evil animal, natural force or witch-suspect to which the patient was subjected, he gets no farther than this symbol and its attendant symptom. The animal or "witch" is, in keeping with the tenets of his culture, acceptable to the shaman as the final explanatory principle, and the personal or social situation which lurks behind the convenient symbol remains unexplored. If we were called upon to characterize the Apache shamanistic treatment of a mental disorder in a sentence, we could legitimately say that it entails dealing with symptoms alone by the method of suggestion.[94]

It is clear, then, that Apache psychiatry coincides with faith healing.

Since at least the beginning of reservation days, Mescalero and Lipan Apache have been nominally affiliated with the Roman Catholic religion. The Chiricahua were forcibly baptized as Catholics while held as prisoners of war in the Deep South. After their removal to Oklahoma, as a result of social-welfare activities by the Dutch Reform Church, they became formal members of that denomination. Some few years ago, the Assembly of God Church came to the reservation. Many Indians have renounced affiliation with the former two groups and joined the latter. Others remain nominally Catholics or "Protestants" but actually attend the Assembly of God services. A principal reason may be found in the utilization of faith healing and the denial of the existence of organic disease by the evangelists of the Assembly of God. Members who join that group can retain the essence of their old-time philosophies while accepting the Christian coloring of the Assembly of God.

Notes

1. An appendix to L. B. Boyer, "Remarks on the Personality of Shamans, with Special Reference to the Apaches of the Mescalero Indian Reservation," *The Psychoanalytic Study of Society*, 2 (New York: International Universities Press, 1962), 233-54, constitutes a representative breakdown of ethnic affiliations of tribal members and their offspring as of 1959.

2. Harry Hoijer, "The Southern Athabaskan Languages," *American Anthropologist*, 40 (1938), 75-87.

3. Franz Boaz, *Handbook of American Indian Languages* (Washington, D.C.: Government Printing Office, 1911) Part I; and Donald E. Worcester, *Early History of the Navajo Indians* (Unpublished Ph.D. dissertation, University of California, 1947).

4. Mary T. Shepardson, *Developing Political Process Among the Navaho Indians* (Unpublished Ph.D. dissertation, University of California, 1960).

5. Marvin H. Albert, *Apache Rising* (Greenwich: Fawcett World Library, 1957); J. Betzinez, with W. S. Nye, *I Fought with Geronimo* (Harrisburg: The Stackpole Co., 1959); James S. Calhoun, "Communication to the Commissioner of Indian Affairs, October 1, 1849," cited by William A. Kelleher, *Turmoil in New Mexico* (Santa Fe: The Rydal Press, 1952), p. 52; B. Davis, *The Truth about Geronimo* (Detroit: Burton Historical Collection, 1929); Logan A. Forster, *Proud Land* (New York: Bantam Books, Inc., 1958); Charles F. Lummis, *The Land of Poco Tiempo* (Albuquerque: University of New Mexico Press, 1952); Ross Santee, *Apache Land* (New York: Bantam Books, Inc., 1956); and C. L. Sonnichsen, *The Mescalero Apaches,* (Norman: University of Oklahoma Press, 1958).

6. J. C. Cremony, "The Apache Race," *Overland Monthly*, 1 (1868), 203.

7. Frederick Schwatka, "Among the Apaches," *The Century Magazine*, 12 (1887), 42.

8. Hiram M. Chittenden, *A History of the American Fur Trade of the Far West*, 2 (1902) (Stanford: Academic Reprints, 1954), 883.

9. Harry W. Basehart, *Chiricahua Apache Subsistence and Socio-Political Organization* (The University of New Mexico Mescalero-Chiricahua Land Claims Project, Contract Research, mimeographed, 1959); Basehart, *Mescalero Apache Subsistence Patterns and Socio-Political Organization* (The University of New Mexico Mescalero-Chiricahua Land Claims Project, mimeographed, 1960); Peter Kunstadter, *Culture Change, Social Structure and Health Behavior: A Quantitative Study of Clinic Use Among the Apaches of the Mescalero Indian Reservation* (Unpublished Ph.D. dissertation, The University of Michigan, 1960); Morris Edward Opler, *An Analysis of Mescalero and Chiricahua Apache Social Organization in the Light of Their Systems of Relationship* (1933) (Chicago: Private edition distributed by the University of Chicago Libraries, 1936); Opler, "An Outline of Chiricahua Apache Social Organization," Fred Eggan, ed., *Social Anthropology of North American Indian Tribes* (enlarged ed.; Chicago: University of Chicago Press, 1955); Opler and Catherine H. Opler, "Mescalero Apache History in the Southwest," *New Mexico Historical Review*, 25 (1950), 1-36; Alfred B. Thomas, *The Chiricahua Apache: 1695-1876* (The University of New Mexico Mescalero-Chiricahua Land Claims Project, Contract Research, mimeographed, 1959); Thomas, *The Lipan Apache: 1718-1856* (The University of New Mexico Mescalero-Chiricahua Land Claims Project, Contract Research, mimeographed, 1959); and Thomas, *The Mescalero Apache: 1653-1874* (The University of New Mexico Mescalero-Chiricahua Land Claims Project, Contract Research, mimeographed, 1959).

10. Basehart, *Chiricahua;* and Basehart, *Mescalero.* Basehart and I have observed that, while elderly Chiricahua are able to answer in generalizations to inquiries, the answers of old Mescalero deal only with specific situations and incidents. I have ad-

ministered Rorschach tests to almost all living Chiricahua and Mescalero sixty years old and older. Dr. Bruno Klopfer, who evaluated the protocols, found clear, consistent, statistically significant differences in perception and cognition. It seems likely that the comparatively rapid, enforced acculturation of the Chiricahua accounts for their responses' being so much more like those of whites (Bruno Klopfer and Boyer, unpublished data).

11. Margot Astrov, *The Winged Serpent* (New York: The John Day Company, Inc., 1946); John G. Bourke, "Notes on Apache Mythology," *Journal of American Folk-Lore*, 3 (1890), 209-12; Evelyn P. Breuninger, "Debut of Mescalero Maidens," *The Apache Scout*, II (Mescalero, New Mexico: 1959), No. 8, 5-6; Ann Pence Davis, "Apache Debs," *New Mexico*, 15 (1937), 10-1; Hoijer, *Chiricahua and Mescalero Texts* (Chicago: University of Chicago Press, 1938), pp. 48-65; Dan Nicholas, "Mescalero Apache Girls' Puberty Ceremony," *El Palacio*, 15 (1939), 110-5; M. E. Opler, *An Apache Life-Way* (Chicago: University of Chicago Press, 1941) pp. 82-134; Evelyn Pellman, "Debut of Apache Maidens," Mescalero Indian Agency brochure, 1950; and Sonnichsen, *op. cit.*, pp. 25-7.

12. Basehart, *Mescalero*, p. 105.

13. Regina Flannery, "The Position of Women Among the Mescalero Apache," *Primitive Man*, 5 (1932), 26-32.

14. Basehart, *Mescalero*, p. 58; Edward F. Castetter and M. E. Opler, *The Ethnobiology of the Chiricahua and Mescalero Apache. A. The Use of Planting for Foods, Beverages and Narcotics* (The University of New Mexico Bulletin No. 507 [1937]); and Kunstadter, *op. cit.*, pp. 97-100.

15. Betzinez, *op. cit.*

16. Bruce B. MacLachlan, *Contemporary Mescalero Apache Legal System*. Paper presented before the 59th Annual Meeting of the American Anthropological Association, Minneapolis, November 17-20, 1960, pp. 1-2.

17. Kunstadter, *op. cit.*, p. 270.

18. M. E. Opler, *An Apache Life-Way*, pp. 5-139.

19. *Ibid.*, p. 25.

20. The modern socialization data presented here so scantily were collected primarily by R. M. Boyer. Incomplete reports have been written (L. B. Boyer, *Identity Problems of the Eastern Apache: Alcoholic Hallucinosis and Latent Homosexuality Among Typical Men* [Unpublished ms., 1962]; and R. M. Boyer, *Social Structure and Socialization Among the Apache of the Mescalero Indian Reservation* (Unpublished Ph.D. dissertation, University of California, 1962). See also Kunstadter, *op. cit.*

21. M. E. Opler, *An Apache Life-Way*, pp. 5-76.

22. *Ibid.*, pp. 54-65.

23. Cremony, *op. cit.*

24. M. E. Opler and Hoijer, "The Raid and Warpath Language of the Chiricahua Apache," *American Anthropologist*, 42 (1940), 617-34.

25. William W. Clements and Duane V. Mohr, *Chronic Subdural Hematomas in Infants*. Paper presented at the Annual United States Public Health Service National Clinical Society Meeting, Lexington, Kentucky, April 5, 1961.

26. Bourke, "The Medicine-Men of the Apache," *Ninth Annual Report, Bureau of Ethnology* (Washington, D.C.: Government Printing Office, 1892); Breuninger, *op. cit.*; Pliny E. Goddard, "The Masked Dancers of the Apache," *The Holmes Anniversary Issue* (Washington, D.C.: 1916), pp. 132-6; M. R. Harrington, "The Devil Dance of the Apaches," *Museum Journal*, 8 (Philadelphia: 1912), 6-9; Hoijer, *Texts*, pp. 27-36, 53-65, 143-5; M. E. Opler, "The Sacred Clowns of the Chiricahua and Mescalero Indians," *El Palacio*, 14 (1938) 75-9; M. E. Opler, pp. 100-15, 267-80; and M. E. Opler, "Chiricahua Apache Material Relating to Sorcery," *Primitive Man*, 19 (1946), 81-92.

27. Hoijer, *Texts;* and M. E. Opler, *Myths and Tales of the Chiracahua Indians* (Memoirs of the American Folk-Lore Society, Vol. 37 [New York: J. J. Augustin, 1942]).

28. Bourke, *Skatological Rites of All Nations* (Washington, D.C.: Lowdermilk & Co., 1891).

29. M. E. Opler, "The Influence of Aboriginal Pattern and White Contact on a Recently Introduced Ceremony, the Mescalero Peyote Rite," *Journal of American Folk-Lore*, 49 (1936), 143-66.

30. Edith Jacobsen, "The Wish for a Child in Boys," *The Psychoanalytic Study of the Child*, 5 (New York: International Universities Press, 1950), 141.

31. Judith Kestenberg, "Vicissitudes of Female Sexuality," *Journal of the American Psychoanalytic Association*, 4 (1956), 453-76; Kestenberg, "On the Development of Maternal Feelings in Early Childhood," R. S. Eissler, A. Freud, H. Hartmann, E. Kris, Eds., *The Psychoanalytic Study of the Child*, 11 (1956), 257-91; and Noel Bradley, "The Doll," *International Journal of Psychoanalysis*, 42 (1961), 550-5.

32. *Ibid.*, p. 551.

33. Anna Freud, "Observation on Child Development," R. S. Eissler, A. Freud, H. Hartmann, E. Kris, eds., *The Psychoanalytic Study of the Child*, 6 (New York: International Universities Press, 1951), 18-30.

34. Robert Fleiss, *Erotogeneity and Libido* (New York: International Universities Press, 1956), p. xvii.

35. Edward A. Marinsek, *The Effect of Cultural Difference in the Education of Apache Indians* (The University of New Mexico Research Study, The College of Education, mimeographed, 1960); and Miles V. Zintz, *The Indian Research Study* (University of New Mexico, College of Education, mimeographed, 1957-1960). See also Robert J. Havighurst and Bernice L. Neugarten, *American Indian and White Children: A Sociopsychological Investigation* (Chicago: University of Chicago Press, 1955).

36. Thomas Gladwin and Seymour B. Sarason, *Truk: Man in Paradise* (New York: Wenner-Gren Foundation for Anthropological Research, 1953); Abram Kardiner, *The Individual and His Society* (New York: Columbia University Press, 1939); and Kardiner, *The Psychological Frontiers of Society* (New York: Columbia University Press, 1945).

37. L. B. Boyer, "Remarks,"; L. B. Boyer, "Identity Problems"; and Klopfer and L. B. Boyer, "Notes on the Personality Structure of a North American Indian Shaman: Rorschach Interpretation," *Journal of Projective Techniques*, 25 (1961), 169-78.

38. Eugen Bleuler, *Dementia Praecox or the Group of Schizophrenias* (New York: International Universities Press, 1950).

39. Edward Glover, "A Note On Idealization," *International Journal of Psychoanalysis*, 19 (1938), 91-6.

40. Heinz Hartmann, Ernst Kris, and Rudolph M. Lowenstein, "Notes on the Theory of Aggression," *The Psychoanalytic Study of the Child*, 3-4 (New York: International Universities Press, 1949), 9-35.

41. Hartmann, *Ego Psychology and the Problem of Adaptation* (1939) (New York: International Universities Press, 1958).

42. Daniel G. Brinton, *Myths of the New World* (New York: 1868), cited in Bourke, "The Medicine-Men," pp. 593-4.

43. M. E. Opler, "The Concept of Supernatural Power among Chiricahua and Mescalero Apaches," *American Anthropologist*, 37 (1935), 65-70. Opler (In Hoijer, *Texts*, p. 141) has explained that the conception of a Creator is not sharply defined for the Chiricahua and appears to have little relation to other phases of their religious thinking. Support for this view seems to be implicit in the following quotations from Asa Daklugie ("Coyote and the Flies," *New Mexico Folklore Record*, 11 [1955-1956], 12-3): "In the beginning, the Chiricahuas were born from a cloud. It was hanging

in the sky when Lightning struck it. The Apache came to earth like a flock of birds,"
"Fire came from lightning, too . . . It belong to Yussen, Creator of Life." *Yussen* is
an Apache word that derives from contact with Mexicans and is a distortion of *dios*.

44. M. E. Opler, "Notes on Chiricahua Apache Culture. 1. Supernatural Power
and the Shaman," *Primitive Man*, 20 (1947), 1.

45. M. E. Opler, "Influence," pp. 144-5.

46. M. E. Opler, "Notes," p. 1.

47. M. E. Opler, "Influence," p. 145.

48. M. E. Opler, "Notes," p. 5.

49. M. E. Opler, "Supernatural Power," p. 70.

50. Bourke, "Medicine-Men," p. 412.

51. L. B. Boyer, "Fantasies."

52. M. E. Opler, *An Apache Life-Way*, p. 200.

53. A basic problem in the presentation of data dealing with attitudes and beliefs
about the supernatural in the modern reservation community is how to convey the
absence of clarity about them among individual Indians in a single short essay. The
discussion of contemporary empirical materials in this section has thus been oversimplified; it is important, however, to note that this reduction of a range of quite variable
data to a common element is consistent with the generalized formulations provided
by a few informants.

54. Jules Henry, "The Cult of Silas John," (Unpublished ms., n.d.).

55. L. B. Boyer, "Remarks," Appendix II.

56. Hoijer, *Texts*, pp. 143-4.

57. *Ibid.*, p. 144.

58. M. E. Opler, *An Apache Life-Way*, pp. 229-37; M. E. Opler, "Chiricahua
Apache Material"; and M. E. Opler, "Mountain Spirits of the Chiricahua Apache,"
The Masterkey, 20 (1946), 125-31.

59. M. E. Opler, *An Apache Life-Way*, pp. 248-53.

60. Schwatka, *op. cit.*

61. L. B. Boyer, "Remarks."

62. M. E. Opler, "An Interpretation"; and M. E. Opler, "Further Comparative
Anthropological Data Bearing on the Solution of a Psychological Problem," *The Journal of Social Psychology*, 9 (1938), 477-83.

63. M. E. Opler, "Influence," p. 1372.

64. *Ibid.*, p. 1373.

65. *Ibid.*, pp. 1375-6.

66. *Ibid.*, p. 1377.

67. *Ibid.*, p. 1379.

68. *Ibid.*, p. 1383.

69. Wolfgang Born, "The Dream," *Ciba Symposia*, 10 (1948), No. 2; Joseph
Campbell, *The Masks of God: Primitive Mythology* (New York: The Viking Press,
Inc., 1959); Sigmund Freud, *The Interpretation of Dreams*, 4, 5 (1900) (Standard
ed.; London: Hogarth Press, Ltd., 1953); and A. Leo Oppenheim, *The Interpretation
of Dreams in the Ancient Near East* (Transactions of the American Philosophical Society, New Series, Vol. 46 [1956], Part 3).

70. A. Irving Hallowell, "Psychic Stresses and Culture Patterns," *American Journal of Psychiatry*, 92 (1936), 1291-1310; M. K. Opler, "Dream Analysis in Ute Indian Therapy," *Culture and Mental Health* (New York: The Macmillan Company,
1959), pp. 97-117; Geza Roheim, *The Gates of the Dream* (New York: International
Universities Press, 1952); and Anthony F. C. Wallace, "Dreams and the Wishes of the
Soul: A Type of Psychoanalytic Theory Among the Seventeenth Century Iroquois,"
American Anthropologist, 60 (1958), 234-48.

71. L. B. Boyer, "Remarks"; and M. E. Opler, *An Apache Life-Way*, pp. 190-3,
233-4.

72. *Ibid.*, p. 190.
73. *Ibid.*
74. William Caudill, "Psychological Characteristics of Acculturated Wisconsin Ojibwa Children," *American Anthropologist,* 51 (1949), 409-27.
75. L. B. Boyer, "Identity Problems."
76. Erik H. Erikson, *Childhood and Society* (New York: W. W. Norton & Company, Inc., 1950); and Erikson, *Identity and the Life Cycle* (Psychological Issues, Vol. I [New York: International Universities Press, 1959], Monograph I).
77. Merton M. Gill and Margaret Brenman, *Hypnosis and Related States* (New York: International Universities Press, 1959), pp. 294-320.
78. R. M. Boyer, *op. cit.,* Chap. 14.
79. Hallowell, "Some Psychological Characteristics of the Northeastern Indians," *Culture and Experience* (Philadelphia: University of Pennsylvania Press, 1955), pp. 125-50.
80. Caudill, *op. cit.*
81. Bernard J. James, "Some Critical Observations Concerning Analyses of Chippewa 'Atomism' and Chippewa Personality," *American Anthropologist,* 56 (1954), 283-6.
82. Erikson, *Identity,* pp. 131-2.
83. R. M. Boyer, *op. cit.,* pp. 335-41.
84. L. B. Boyer, "Remarks."
85. Mark Kanzer, "Freud and the Demon," *Journal of the Hillside Hospital,* 10 (1961), 198.
86. S. Freud, *Totem and Taboo,* 13 (1913) (Standard ed.; London: Hogarth Press, Ltd., 1955).
87. Lawrence S. Kubie, *Practical and Theoretical Aspects of Psychoanalysis* (New York: International Universities Press, 1950), pp. 145-54.
88. *Ibid.,* p. 145.
89. Gill and Brenman, *op. cit.,*
90. Kubie, *op. cit.,* p. 147.
91. *Ibid.,* p. 149 .
92. L. B. Boyer, "Fantasies"; and Max Rinkel and Harold E. Himwich, eds., *Insulin Treatment in Psychiatry* (New York: Philosophical Library, Inc., 1959).
93. L. B. Boyer, "Remarks."
94. M. E. Opler, "Influence," p. 1385.

William Madsen

Value Conflicts and Folk Psychotherapy in South Texas*

MUCH HAS BEEN WRITTEN about primitive ethnocentricity but remarkably little about our own, in regard to the sanctity of modern science. This paper attempts to demonstrate how the ethnocentric orientation of modern medicine and psychiatry has braked the acculturation of the Mexican-American population in South Texas. The intolerance of medical science toward other curing traditions has hindered its acceptance in folk societies. It has also blocked medical recognition of the actual therapeutic value of many folk curing techniques.

More than 75% of the population of Hidalgo County, Texas, is of Mexican descent. Most of these Mexican-Americans belong to the lower class. Today this population is characterized by an increased rate of acculturation to many aspects of the Anglo-American pattern of behavior. The resulting threat to social and cultural traditions is producing psychological stress and high levels of anxiety. In such a situation some might expect to find a heavy reliance by the Mexican-Americans on medical and psychiatric resources. That is not the case. Rather, most Mexican-Americans in need of help for psychological or social maladjustment seek the services of the *curandero* or folk curer. One reason for preferring the *curandero* over the psychiatrist or physician is the widespread inability of the latter to communicate linguistically or culturally with this pre-

* This paper is one of the reports of the Hidalgo Project on Differential Culture Change and Mental Health, which conducted field research in southern Texas and northern Mexico from 1957 to 1962. This work was supported by the Hogg Foundation for Mental Health at the University of Texas. Personnel of the project include William Madsen (director), Antonieta Espejo, Albino Fantini, Octavio Romano, and Arthur Rubel.

dominantly Spanish-speaking group. Another reason is the high degree of success the *curandero* has demonstrated in treating patients. An understanding of the factors favoring the *curandero* over medical practitioners can be gained from an examination of the history and culture of this area.

Except for the descendants of the early settlers from Mexico, the bulk of the modern population of this area came in two waves of migration beginning in the second decade of this century. At that time, several investment companies began clearing and irrigating the land that today supports the thriving vegetable and citrus farms of the lower Rio Grande Valley. The purchasers of these improved lands were mainly Anglos from the midwestern and northeastern parts of the United States. The men who cut the brush and dug the irrigation ditches were laborers from Mexico. Many remained as field hands. Migration from Mexico was further increased by refugees from the Mexican Revolution of 1910 and included some members of the middle and upper classes.[1]

The towns that grew up in the area were carefully planned to separate the residential areas of the Anglo and Latin peoples. Each town is divided by a railroad line or a highway, which marks the boundary between the homes of the predominantly Spanish-speaking and English-speaking groups. Originally each half of each town was a relatively self-contained community with its own schools, stores, and churches. The absolute rigidity of this system is breaking down today. Many of the schools are integrated, and an increasing number of Mexican-Americans are moving into homes on the Anglo side of town.

The predominantly middle-class Anglos have borrowed little from Mexican-American culture aside from occasional visits to Mexican restaurants. Their speech and culture conform closely to those of greater middle-class America. The Mexican-Americans are generally bilingual, and the traditional Mexican patterns of behavior have been modified among them by the acceptance of many Anglo ways and ideas. Most of these modifications and additions are in the sphere of technical culture. The basic social structure and the core values are largely drawn from Mexico.

Despite increasing intercourse between these two groups, each lacks understanding of the other and feels threatened by it. The Anglo frequently regards the Latin as unreliable, childlike, and in need of supervision and guidance. Latins are also characterized by the Anglos as superstitious, morally lax, and dirty. On the other hand, the Latin often views the Anglo as grossly materialistic, self-centered, untrustworthy, and clownish. The Mexican-American believes that desire for economic advancement is the prime motivation in Anglo behavior. In the usual Anglo employer and Latin employee relationship, the Mexican-American is liable to believe himself exploited and underpaid. This idea is frequently based on fact. In turn, as increasing use is made of Mexican-American white-collar workers, their Anglo equivalents feel their jobs threatened because Spanish-speaking employees often work for lower wages. Latin upper mobility and the increasing rate of anglicization is not reducing the mutual suspicion and distrust between these two ethnic groups.

Because of the cultural changes taking place in Hidalgo County, it would be a gross oversimplification to picture two ethnic groups separated by a sharp line of cultural difference. In individual Latin behavior, many degrees of acculturation can be observed, ranging from almost total conformity to Mexican folk culture to integration of Mexican-American professionals into the Anglo upper class. Generally speaking, one finds increasing anglicization as one moves from the lower to the upper class and from the older to the younger generation.

Those Mexican-Americans who are actively attempting to anglicize themselves are often contemptuously called *Inglesados* (the anglicized) or more commonly *agringados* (the "gringoized") by the more conservative Latins. Overt attempts at cultural transfer are slowed by fear of such ridicule from conservative friends. The Mexican value of submission to the will of one's parents, who are usually conservative, also prevents many members of the younger generation from freely following Anglo patterns. Anglo resistance to purely social relations with Mexican-Americans also slows the process of anglicization. The Latin wants to benefit from the material advantages of Anglo society but is dubious about overtly declaring affiliation with a group that rejects him and is contemptuous of his origins. Easy identification of their background by physical appearance and often language prevents most Mexican-Americans from "passing" in Anglo society.

The conservative Mexican-American culture is basically derived from that of rural Mexico although it is modified by the sociocultural setting in Texas. The people have mixed attitudes toward Mexico. The mother country south of Texas is regarded as the fountainhead of philosophical truth, religious devotion, and beauty in literature and the arts. At the same time, Mexicans are regarded as unreliable, impractical, and inefficient. These attitudes toward Mexico are in part a reflection of the Mexican-Americans' acceptance of the Anglo value of technical proficiency and the rejection of many of the nonmaterial values associated with English-speaking society.

The conservative Latin world-view follows the common folk pattern of blending the supernatural and the natural in one integrated system.

Although the Anglo may be a devout church member, he usually distinguishes clearly between supernatural and natural phenomena. The scientific isolation of the natural world is incomprehensible to the conservative Mexican-American. Usually a Roman Catholic, he tends to view the Anglo belief as a part of the "Protestant heresy." Even continuous attempts by the Catholic clergy to educate the lower-class Latins to the basic concepts of modern medicine usually fail.

As in much of rural Mexico, the Texas Latins see normality as a balance of elements. As long as a proper relationship among beings and things is maintained, all is well. Disease, social strife, and misfortune in general are due to planned or accidental contradictions of the normal balance. An elaborate example of the theory of balance is seen in the hot-and-cold concept of disease and curing. This system came to Mexico from the classical Mediterranean world by way of colonial Spain. In brief, it holds that health is a "temperate" condition in which there is no excess of "hot" or "cold" elements. These classifications often have no real relationship to actual temperature. An excessive exposure to or intake of things classified in one or the other of the temperature extremes can produce illness. Treatment, in part, consists of feeding "hot" foods for "cold" diseases and the reverse.

Man's violation of the moral and ethical code can cause supernatural beings to upset the balance further by sending accident or illness as punishment. These saints and spirits are borrowed from the folk-Catholic hierarchy of Mexico. Even in the supernatural sphere, balance is essential to being. God is opposed by Satan and angels by imps. Like humans, saints are balanced between male and female. Existence itself is a balance of the natural and supernatural. Each human body contains a divine soul.

The Mexican-American considers himself a member of *la raza*, the "race" of native Spanish-speakers in the Americas. The term "race," in this sense, is not restricted to its biological meaning but includes the concepts of shared culture and common spiritual heritage. It is believed that God intended a glorious destiny for the members of *la raza*. This destiny, the Mexican-American says, is one that the Texas Latins will probably never achieve. The spiritual potential of *la raza* is continually weakened by the immoral and destructive behavior of a few. It is stated that, if the drunks would dry up, the thieves reform, and the irresponsible meet their obligations, *la raza* in Texas would again return to the path of greatness. Universal conformity among its members to the values of *la raza* could restore it to its rightful place in the balance of the universe, according to conservative Mexican-Americans.

Some believe that the ideal family should be based on divine example. The mother is frequently equated to the Virgin of Guadalupe,[2] and the father's role is the human equivalent of God, the authoritarian. The pure mother is the source of comfort and affection, and the aloof father is the protector and the administrator of justice.

As *la raza* as a whole has failed to achieve God's plan for the group, individual members never conform perfectly to the divine models of male and female. Although ideally all women should be sexually pure, it is believed that they are weak-willed. Familial supervision and protection are therefore necessary to protect them from sexually aggressive males. No woman, it is believed, can protect herself against the superior intelligence of the male.

Unlike God, the Mexican-American male must constantly prove his worth. Male values are encompassed by the concept of *machismo or* manliness. A true man is proud, dignified, and reliable. Such a man will remain aloof from petty argument and intrigue. When his honor is challenged, he will seek vengeance. Vengeance may not be immediate, but it is certain. The respected man is in control of himself in any social situation because of his experience in life and his ability to defend himself socially and physically. In time he will be addressed with the honorific *don* and his first name.[3]

These qualities of manliness are associated with sexual prowess and ability. While monogamy is a virtue, extramarital affairs are expected as the mark of a successful man. If he has the financial means, he may maintain a second household, or *casa chica*, without fear of losing respect in the conservative Latin-American community. At no time, however, must he allow his attentions to endanger the security and well-being of his wife and family.

Homosexuality is an indication of individual inadequacy. To be labeled "homosexual" is the ultimate debasement in the sphere of male behavior. The only occasion on which accusations of effeminacy in males is tolerated is during the ritual of verbal dueling among younger men who are together.[4] Such dueling may be partly an anxiety release from fear of latent homosexual tendencies.

As female purity is threatened by the male sex drive, so manliness is threatened by homosexuality. These beliefs are only two manifestations of the hostility that the Mexican-American sees in his environment. It is believed that no individual outside the family can be fully trusted. This distrust applies to Anglo and Latin alike. Children learn early to be suspicious of the motives of others and to acquire the art of social self-defense.

In contrast to the outside world, the family is ideally the haven from threat and trouble. Here the maximum co-operation in Mexican-American activity is seen. Familial roles are well defined, with the female sub-servient to the male and the young to the old. The family is extended beyond the nuclear unit to include both ascending and descending gen-erations. Before marriage, the primary authority is the father. Following marriage, a woman should respect her husband's wishes over those of her parents. A man, ideally, never allows the ultimate authority of his own father to be compromised.

As the individual owes allegiance to the family, so the family owes protection to its members. Because of strict definition of familial relations, however, certain types of problem are usually solved without family help. For example, serious sexual difficulties are rarely taken up with the parents. Knowledge of them would offend the purity of the mother and be a confession of inadequacy to the father. Children from conservative families learn early of their parents' disapproval of many Anglo customs. If the children imitate the Anglos in any of these areas of behavior, they usually conceal their behavior from their elders. The conflicts between the conservative Latin culture and values acquired at school are rarely discussed or resolved at home. The parents regard many Anglo values as silly, irresponsible, and dangerous. Children who express them orally are silenced. Many Latin interpretations of reality, on the other hand, are dismissed by school teachers as "superstitions" and may bring ridicule from classmates. The child in an integrated school frequently develops agility in shifting values in his everyday behavior. He will conform to conservative Latin values in the family environment and may seek ap-proval at school by attempting to conform to Anglo ways of life as he perceives them. Another possibility is that he may rebel against one or both of these systems.

The Mexican-American godparent system is structured to reinforce conservative values. There is reluctance to mar the traditionally formal relationship with familial value conflicts. Although these *compadres* (coparents) are expected to co-operate in time of need, such aid is usually expected only within the sphere of traditional behavior. With increased acculturation and geographical mobility, the bonds of the *compadre* re-lationship are weakening in the Mexican-American population.

The growing child or young adult, then, is forced to seek advice out-side the home in many fields of activity. The maturing female turns to one of her few close friends. The male may rely on fellow members of an informal association called the *palomilla*. The word *palomilla* means moth and refers to the tendency of these insects—and of youths—to cluster around street lamps after dark. A young man's need to maintain his dignity and self-respect, however, rules out exposing many of his problems to his friends in the *palomilla*. His final hope for guidance in these problem areas is his *amigo de confianza*, his "trusted friend." Each male has such a relationship with another his age, and it constitutes his closest social relationship outside the family. Even here, however, complete frankness is not always possible. Since the fellowship and trust of the *amigo de confianza* are valued, the male will not risk breaking the relationship by admitting to problems or behavior that might lower his friend's esteem for him. There is also the fear that even a close friend may become an enemy.

As personal shortcomings or failures are not easily admitted, so personal gains or advancements may be concealed. Such concealment prevents *envidia* or envy in others. A person should not experience envy of the success of a friend or neighbor. Nevertheless, the Mexican-American regards envy as a powerful emotion and one difficult to control. Because of his suspicion of others, the Latin who has experienced any self-satisfaction may think he detects envy among them.

One of the most frequent manifestations of envy is *mal ojo* or evil eye. It is believed that some people are born with "strong vision," which can harmfully project their admiration or desire of possession into a person or thing. Children are especially susceptible to this misfortune for they lack the spiritual strength and defenses of the adult. Their purity is also a quality that solicits admiration. To suffer from the evil eye is a proof to all of the child's appeal. Following the diagnosis of evil eye sickness in a child, the cure is standard. The parents review the list of those who may have admired the child during the day and decide which one sent the affliction. That person is then sought out and asked to touch the child on the head. This action removes the foreign force that the admiring look sent into the child and returns the patient's body to its normal balance. If the touch of the first person does not produce a cure, another who has seen the child recently is approached. If the person who is responsible for the disease cannot be located, the patient's body is "cleaned" with a raw egg in the shell and brushed with certain herbs that remove the condition.

If a person knows that he has the power of the evil eye, he should always touch a child he has admired on the head. This prophylactic gesture protects the child. In admiring any fragile object, he should handle or caress it for the same reason. If he fails to do so, it may later crack or break.

Theoretically, if a person with "strong vision" takes these precautions systematically, he is in no way feared or avoided. In fact, he quite often is feared. A person responsible for inflicting the evil-eye disease unintentionally may detect strains in certain areas of his interpersonal relations. He or she may not be invited into homes where there are young children or objects subject to damage by strong vision. If a person suspected of having the evil eye takes no precautions with children after addressing them, the avoidance pattern is even more marked. One Anglo public-health nurse was under a severe handicap for years until she was finally informed that she had "very strong vision." Although having strong vision is a matter of fate, the evil-eye complex is sometimes loosely associated with the whole feared complex of black magic and witchcraft. A person with the evil eye is more likely to be suspected of witchcraft than one without it. One staff member of the Hidalgo Project was once suspected of having the evil eye. A few weeks later, this person was accused of being a witch. Such associations of evil eye and witchcraft, however, are not common.

While possessing the evil eye is in itself not a matter for condemnation, being a witch always is. Witches are greatly feared and are believed to obtain their power from the devil. Those who believe that they are arousing envy or jealousy in others frequently fear that a witch will be hired to harm them. So dangerous is the subject of witchcraft that most Mexican-Americans are hesitant to discuss the subject except within the family or with a close friend. It is believed that witches can transform themselves into animals, fly disguised as owls, and become invisible. Their evil is frequently worked by sympathetic image magic although other techniques are known. Some witches force an evil wind (*mal aire*) to enter the patient's body and cause acute pain. One witch, who was later driven out of town, was said to keep magical worms in a bottle of human milk and to send them to cause illnesses. Another witch is believed to be a satanist who controls demons that possess their master's victims. Such naming of particular witches is unusual. While belief in witchcraft is widespread, few Mexican-Americans will name particular persons as witches. Most of those so identified are transients.

Another ailment of supernatural origin is *espanto* (fright), which is caused by seeing a ghost or demon. *Susto* (fright) is a similar complaint caused by such a natural fright as being nearly run over by an automobile. Many Mexican-Americans do not distinguish between the two but lump them together as *susto*, especially among the more acculturated individuals.

Bilis (bile), like *susto* and *espanto,* is a disease caused by an emotional upset. *Bilis* is quite often the result of anger (*coraje*), which stimulates yellow-bile production and causes an imbalance of the humors. Like the hot and cold complex, *bilis* derives from the Hippocratic system of medicine.

Though emotional in origin, both *susto* and *bilis* are classified as "natural diseases." They are believed to be due to natural imbalances, as opposed to those ailments like *mal ojo,* which are said to be caused by supernatural forces. Other examples of natural illnesses are *empacho* (impediment or blockage) and *caida de la mollera* (fallen fontanelle). In cases of *empacho,* certain foods cling to the digestive tract causing constipation and pain. *Caida de la mollera* is an infant's disease caused by the collapse of the loose fontanelle.

The older conservative Mexican-Americans believe that all natural diseases are the result of physical imbalance. Even many of the younger conservatives reject the theory of germ causation of illness. An ever-increasing number do, however, admit the role of the bacterium and the virus in such contagious diseases as measles and chicken pox. Infectious diseases are the ones most frequently referred to physicians. Other "natural diseases" are often said to be beyond the scope of modern medicine. They include *empacho* and *caida de la mollera.*[5] Patients suffering from diseases of supernatural origin are seldom taken to physicians by the conservative Mexican-Americans.

The physician is regarded as an unreliable curer for many reasons beside his ignorance of the folk diseases. His intolerance of Latin "superstitions" is frequently noted as is his inability to speak Spanish. The conservative Mexican-American regards the physician-patient relationship as cold and impersonal, reflecting absence of concern on the part of the physician. Above all, the Latin cannot understand why the medical profession chooses to "forget God." It is believed that no cure is possible without His will. Whenever modern medical help is solicited, facilities and persons with some overt religious identification are preferred. For this reason, a Seventh-Day Adventist hospital in northern Mexico receives a number of Latin patients from South Texas.

Hospitalization is usually dreaded and resisted in the lower Rio Grande Valley. Families are regarded as morally delinquent for surrendering their members to Anglo institutions for care and treatment. Patients are uncomfortable in a system they do not fully understand, dislike the food, and long for the affective relationships of the home. An increasing exception is the case of childbirth. Pregnancy and delivery, however, are regarded as normal functions, not as diseases. Referral of maternity cases to a hospital by midwives when complications develop has allowed demonstration of medical proficiency in delivery.

Curanderos also refer critical cases to hospitals on occasion. Such cases usually involve seriously advanced illnesses that the *curanderos* believe are in the terminal stages. The curer thus avoids a reputation for losing cases and possible legal action. When such cases do die in the hospital, the deaths reinforce the belief that "hospitals are where people die." Even patients who know they have fatal diseases resist hospitalization. It is far preferable to die at home surrounded by one's family and "at peace with God."

A few Mexican-Americans argue that death is perhaps preferable to a successful operation, especially if one of the organs is to be removed. A person who has recovered from such an operation is going to suffer for the rest of his life. The normal balance of his body has been disturbed, and this imbalance will affect his relations with the world and humanity. He is no longer whole.[6]

While the conservative Mexican-American looks with disapproval on the philosophy and techniques of the physician, he sees the *curandero* as an enlightened individual with a divine gift for returning ailing souls and bodies to normal condition. In part, preference for the *curandero* is owing to the attitude toward his role in healing. While the physician claims to cure merely through acquired knowledge, the *curandero* operates through the grace of God.

The *curandero* may be either male or female (*curandera*). The conservative Latin distinguishes sharply between the witch and the curer. The witch's power comes from Satan and the *curandero's* from God. The witch is feared and despised, while the successful curer receives the honorific *Don* (or *Doña* for a female) before his first name. The more acculturated Mexican-Americans, however, may follow the Anglo pattern of lumping witchcraft and folk curing together into one system and labeling both types of practitioner as "witches."

Both professional and part-time *curanderos* are found in Mexican-American society. Some curers are equivalent to the Anglo general practitioners, while others are specialists. Most practice in their homes, although a few have regular offices.

Despite these differences, certain characteristics are common to all *curanderos*. Their power to heal is a gift (*don*) from God, and all treatments are accompanied by appeals to Him or to one of the saints. The holy nature of their office is reflected in the altar maintained in the consulting room. *Curandero* and patient frequently pray together before this table, which is laden with statues of saints, holy pictures, containers of blessed water, and flowers. The patient's payment is ritualized to show his awareness that the curer has merely served as a mechanism for God during the treatment. Rather than paying a small fee to the *curandero,* he leaves an offering before one of the saints. This system also relieves the *curandero* from the fear of conviction for receiving payment for practicing medicine without a license. The convicting evidence usually shows that the curer uses medicines obtained from Mexico, which are frequently administered by hypodermic injection.

Beside the preparations borrowed from modern medicine, Mexican-American folk curers rely heavily on herbs, eggs, earth, holy water or water blessed by themselves, printed prayers, and holy objects. Some curers rely entirely on one of these elements. Water is especially favored, probably because of the ancient Mexican tradition that water is a holy and purifying element.[7]

The method by which the curer realizes the will of God or the saints during treatment varies. Some curers claim that they can hear the commands from beyond. Others are possessed. One famous curer in Hidalgo County today is a nine-year-old girl who becomes possessed by the spirit of a deceased *curandero.* While she is in a state of possession, the soul of the dead *curandero* speaks through the child's mouth, and its orders are carried out by an adult assistant. A few curers are members of one of the spiritualist churches.

The techniques utilized by the *curandero* usually depend on the way he entered the profession. Most *curanderos* claim that they were ordered or inspired by God to become curers. This divine election is most frequent among those who have parents in the profession. Training is usually under the guidance of practicing *curanderos.* Some are instructed in one of the centers of folk curing in northern Mexico. Others train by means of correspondence courses from one of the spiritualist temples in Mexico City.

Simplified forms of the *curandero's* techniques are utilized in home curing. A mother may treat what she has diagnosed as a simple case of *susto* in her child. Accompanied by the usual prayers for recovery, the child's body may be swept with a palm frond, preferably one that was used in Easter church ceremonies. When home treatment fails, a *curandero* is sought.

Treatment by folk techniques at home or by a *curandero* is meaningful in the context of the conservative Mexican-American culture. The patient and the family are interested in and are informed of the reasoning behind the diagnosis and each step of the treatment. Illness is never a matter of mere individual concern. The diseases recognized and treated are real to the Mexican-American and do in fact fulfill important social functions. Rubel, for example, has pointed out that three of these "illnesses function to sustain some of the dominant values of the Mexican-American culture."[8]

As most of these diseases are not recognized by modern medicine and do indeed make people ill, it seems proper to inquire into their exact nature. The symptoms characteristic of each, as listed by Mexican-Americans, are vague and insufficient for medical diagnosis. For example, a pain in any part of the body may be attributed to *aire* or air, a supernatural concept. *Empacho* may be characterized by abdominal pains and nervousness. *Espanto* may produce feebleness, musular aches, insomnia, nervousness, or burning eyes. *Mal ojo* may be signaled by insomnia, crying, lassitude, temperature, rashes, or sores. The symptoms of *susto* may be general aches and pains, feebleness, mild paralysis, nightmares or insomnia, rapid palpitations of the heart, and difficulty in breathing. Variation in these symptoms for any one ailment is impressive and argues against any claim that a direct relationship necessarily exists between the complaints and the diagnoses. Most of these symptoms could be caused by any of the commoner virus diseases. They might also be the psychosomatic manifestations of anxiety or fear resulting from value conflicts and strained social relations. Examination of a number of cases of Mexican-American folk diseases tends to confirm the impression that they are associated with sociocultural crises. Illness frequently enables a patient to avoid a crisis. If the ailment follows the crisis, it may be partially a mechanism for relief from individual guilt and social disapproval. A few examples will clarify this point.

Miguel had bragged to members of his *palomilla* that he would "win over" the affections of Margarita at a Friday dance. He later discovered that his elder brother was interested in the same girl. To retreat from this amatory challenge would be an admission of shortcomings in manhood to his friends. To attempt to take the girl from his brother would be a threat to family solidarity and authority. On the day before the dance, he developed a painful and stiff leg. Within the family, it was diagnosed as *aire*. Miguel had to remain in bed while his brother danced with Margarita.

Memo was fired by his boss and consoled himself that night at a bar with friends. He told the group that no reason had been given for his dismissal, although weeks later he admitted that he had been guilty of consistent absenteeism. His close friend Alejandro said that Memo should have demanded a reason for the action or the continuation of his job. Memo agreed and, as the evening passed and beer was consumed, repeated expressions of increasing hostility against his ex-boss. Finally, he announced that the following day he would see his former employer and have a showdown. Alejandro, who worked at the same canning plant, said he would watch for the encounter, wished Memo luck, and urged him to be firm. Walking home from the bar, Memo fell in the street and was nearly struck by a truck. The next day he awoke with a headache, an uneasiness in his stomach, vague body pains, and a shaky hand—symptoms of the *susto* resulting from his frightening experience with the truck. A neighbor made the diagnosis, treated him, and ordered him to bed for a few days. Confrontation of his ex-boss was postponed and finally forgotten. Alejandro was extremely sympathetic about his friend's illness.

Enrique borrowed a truck from his cousin to transport some furniture for his father. While returning home with the load, he stopped to chat by the roadside with Berta, a young woman with a reputation for promiscuity. At her request, he drove her to another town considerably out of his way and there drank some beer with her. On parting, Enrique realized the lateness of the hour and accelerated to reach home before arousing his father's wrath. In turning a corner, the truck jumped the curb and tipped over. Enrique was badly cut, the truck dented, and much of the furniture broken. Enrique was taken by the police to the hospital where his wounds were dressed. The cousin was dismayed at the damage to his truck, and Enrique's father was angered by his son's irresponsibility. Enrique retired to his room shaken with guilt and anxiety. His mother took his torn clothing to mend. Pinned to his shirt she "found" a tiny envelope of cloth containing some hair and threads adhering to a small piece of greasy clay. This indication of bewitchment by Berta lessened Enrique's guilt and tended to mollify somewhat the strong feelings of his father and his cousin. The magical love charm was burned with lime by the father, and the mother sprinkled Enrique with water containing pieces of palm leaf. Enrique promised his father to avoid women like Berta and the next day helped to repair the truck and the furniture.

The first two cases illustrate the manner in which the diagnosis of illness can avert a social situation in which conflicts internal to the Mexican-American complex would have resulted in the compromise of one or the other of two basic values. Miguel's image as a man would have conflicted with the expected role he should play toward an elder brother. Had Memo confronted his ex-boss, his friend would have heard the charge of Memo's absenteeism. This charge would seriously reflect on Memo's image as a man of honor and integrity. To contradict the older employer's charge would be a violation of respect and subordination toward one's elders. Deliberately to avoid the encounter would weaken Memo's self-and public image as a true man. The incident was avoided by the diagnosis of hangover symptoms as an illness. I doubt that deceit was present in either case. The desire to withdraw into the role of a patient tends unconsciously to increase the awareness of any bodily complaints that are present. The concepts of disease present an explanation of the symptoms and provide an escape from a seemingly hopeless social situation. In the third case, the fortunate "discovery" of the magical packet by Enrique's mother explained the son's behavior as beyond his control rather than as a reflection of irresponsibility and disrespect toward the family. The purification rites of burning the magical packet and sprinkling Enrique ritualized the submission of the son to the dominant and protective roles of the parents. By working with the father and cousin to repair the truck and furniture, Enrique was reinstated as a co-operative and dutiful family member.

One function then of folk diseases in South Texas is to provide a mechanism to avoid or relieve situations involving a conflict of Mexican-American values. With increasing acculturation and personal interaction between Anglo and Latin since World War II, value conflicts are increasing. These conflicts are especially marked in those individuals who attempt cultural transfer, the *Inglesados*. The individual who has internalized values from both subcultures usually at some point becomes aware of painful cognitive dissonance.[9] The individual's self-image loses its focus, and decision-making becomes a matter of profound anxiety. The partly acculturated *Inglesado* finds identity with any recognized role in either subgroup almost impossible. He is scorned by the conservative Mexican-Americans and refused admission to Anglo society. Some *Inglesados* in this situation seek closer identity with Anglo culture through such means as conspicuous display of Anglo mannerisms or conversion to a Protestant church. Others seek to escape geographically and move to another state or to one of the larger cities in Texas. Others attempt to retreat into the conservative Mexican-American culture. Those who retreat are usually afflicted with a series of folk diseases. As Anglos are believed to be immune to such ailments, merely being afflicted by one is a means of cultural identification with *la raza*. To accept the diagnosis and to co-operate in the treatment are a declaration of acceptance of the conservative Mexican-American world-view. The treatment involves the re-establishment of traditional roles and frequently some form of penance. Such treatments are nearly always conducted by *curanderos*.

María is an example of an *Inglesada* who was successfully reintegrated into conservative Mexican-American society. She is an attractive girl and is married to José Romero. Her best friend and confidante, Emilia, became the godmother of her first child and thus her *comadre*. Shortly afterward Emilia's husband obtained a job as foreman, and their increased income was soon visible in a new automobile and wardrobe. Although inconspicuous consumption outside of religious duties was once the only accepted means of utilizing sudden increases in wealth, such conspicuous displays in the Anglo pattern are increasing. María's envy soon became a poorly suppressed hostility. Her husband ridiculed her hints that they should improve their financial status and denied her permission to take a job. As a good wife, María did not mention the deeper resentment she felt at his spending money on another woman. During the next harvest season, José went north as a migratory laborer. He wanted María to accompany him as she had in the past. On her plea that their child was sickly and should not travel, however, he allowed her to remain at home. His eldest sister moved in with her before he left.

Free of her husband's authority, María obtained a job as a clerk in a neighboring town. Her small weekly salary at first went to buy household decorations and clothing to equal those of her *comadre*. Soon, under the influence of a fellow clerk, she was paying for night courses at a secretarial school. José's sister, who now had the responsibility of María's child, most of the time objected strongly to María's behavior but to no avail. Emilia, the *comadre*, tried gently to convince María that disobeying José's orders not to take employment would only end in trouble. María retorted that if José objected she would leave him and become a success on her own as a secretary. In defiance of growing community disapproval, María began to flaunt her rebellion in accentuated Anglo mannerisms and dress. Her own family expressed disapproval of her behavior and withheld the close affection usually displayed when she visited them. Her reputation as a rebel spread and was enlarged by gossip. As her alienation from the community continued, she received word that her husband was returning early from his harvesting trip. That evening at school she accepted the invitation of an anglicized girl friend to attend a mixed beer party the following night.

The next morning, a Saturday, María was in menstruation and felt as though her bones "were pliable." Her bleeding was exceptionally heavy, and she suffered nausea and dizziness. By noon she was sweating and experiencing periods of hysterical weeping. Her sister-in-law gave her aspirin and herbal teas and massaged her. When these aids brought no relief, she summoned María's mother. Shortly thereafter José's mother joined them. María moaned that she was bewitched, and the attendant women agreed that bewitchment was indicated by the symptoms. The mother and mother-in-law left, ostensibly to obtain some medicines but in fact to consult with their husbands. They returned in a couple of hours with some herbs and the sanction for taking María to a *curandero*. Her illness had returned her to her family and family-in-law. The *curandero* would be expected to return her to health and society.

It was decided to consult Doña Inés, a respected and pious *curandera*. Supported by the two mothers, María was taken to the curer's home. The patient's hysterical self-diagnosis of bewitchment or *mal puesto* was politely heard but not commented on. The *curandera*, who knew the gossip about María, passed a glass of blessed water over the patient's head and observed that ripples formed on the surface as though it was rejecting María. Doña Inés then examined María's tear-laden eyes and felt her face. After closely questioning María and the attendant mothers, the *curandera* retired to pray and "commune with God." She returned later and, with bowed head, gave her diagnosis: *castigo de Dios* or punishment from God.

Due to the seriousness of this condition, Doña Inés requested that María remain in her house during treatment. María's mother and sister-in-law would care for her child. María remained for nearly two weeks. The treatment consisted primarily of prayers, although the patient was also given teas and massages. During this period, Doña Inés, by analogy and later by direct statements, pointed out to María the sin involved in her actions. María became convinced that her suffering would not end until she had paid to God and to those she had injured for her transgressions. Far from relieving her condition, the treatment heightened her anxiety and increased the periods of convulsive sobbing. She also suffered insomnia, loss of appetite, and bodily pains. These symptoms increased when she learned that her husband José had returned and was regularly conferring with Doña Inés. Despite the patient's continual pleas, the *curandera* gently refused to tell her how José was reacting to the news of her behavior and condition.

In her meetings with José, Doña Inés freely stated that María had been behaving very badly and that the divine punishment was deserved. She also, however, instilled a sense of guilt in the husband. By indirection she made him aware that he too had sinned. She led him to believe that he had failed to supply María with "those things a woman needs to be fully a woman." These talks also convinced him that parting with his wife when she was experiencing envy of her *comadre* and anxiety over her sick child signified failure in his role as a husband and father. His mother attended these conferences with him, and her knowledge of his own failings diluted his overt expressions of anger at María.

When Doña Inés finally permitted the meeting of husband and wife, the encounter took place in her presence before her altar. Before allowing them to speak, she made them kneel together before the altar, sprinkled them with blessed water, and prayed aloud over them. The prayer asked forgiveness for mortal weakness and praised the wisdom of God. The prayer included the sentiment that no person can be whole in isolation. It stated that "a man is because of woman and a woman is because of her man." Following the prayer, the *curandera* ordered the patient to welcome her husband and beg his forgiveness. Although José's reaction was silence, he made no protest when María followed him home. Later, he accompanied her on a pilgrimage to a holy shrine to beg God's forgiveness. María still wears clothing of the dark shades of humility and penance, and José has accelerated his extramarital demonstrations of manliness. Although their relationship is strained, both husband and wife are filling their roles in conformity with the expectations of conservative Mexican-American society.

In cases like María's, folk disease represents the means for retreat to the conservative roles of Latin society. The utilization of this mechanism is probably rarely conscious. The anxieties and threats of cultural transfer combined with the desire for relief may provide the psychosomatic genesis of disease symptoms. Successful reinstatement in society and resulting relief from physical complaint reinforce the cultural acceptance of folk illnesses. Belief in the reality of these diseases frequently results in the diagnosis of completely physical ailments as *susto, mal ojo,* or one of the other afflictions in the folk system. Even then, traditional treatments may be of value. The teas and massages probably relieve some of the patients' pain, and close affective relationships during treatment are conducive to psychological comfort. Each case of illness, moreover, reinforces family solidarity and patterns of co-operation. From the point of view of public health, the main dangers of folk medicine are the cases of communicable diseases that go unrecognized and receive improper treatment.

Although the *curandero* may not be able to cure such diseases as smallpox and measles, he often successfully cures psychiatric disorders that are generally regarded as being unlinked to cultural variation. This success indicates that, although the generic manifestations of these diseases are similar, the factors contributing to their development and cure vary within different cultures. This point is demonstrated in the case of Catalina.

Catalina was committed in her early twenties to a state mental institution over the protests of her parents. She was classified as paranoid and was under treatment for more than two years. During this period, no improvement in her condition was noted. Her family finally succeeded in obtaining her release in their custody. They placed her under the care of a *curandera,* and six months later she had been relieved of all her gross symptoms.

The folk treatment that Catalina received differed markedly from treatment in the mental hospital. After a few sessions with the *curandera,* Catalina made it clear that she believed that all who knew her hated her. The curer asked her why. Slowly and painfully, the *curandera* extracted from Catalina a confession of sexual perversion with an Anglo male that had produced an unbearable feeling of guilt and self-condemnation. Rather than expressing understanding and sympathy, the *curandera* threw up her hands in horror and drew back from the girl. The *curandera* said, "For this I, too, hate you as does God." Due to her divine appointment to relieve human suffering, however, the *curandera* agreed to help Catalina atone for her sin.

The healer prescribed an intensive program of self-debasement and punishment for her patient. She learned that Catalina loved the rabbits that her family raised. Every other day, Catalina was ordered to rise before dawn and strike open the skull of a live rabbit. She was then to eat the brains from the carcass. Periodically Catalina was to come to the *curandera* to be flogged. The girl's diet was restricted to drab and taste-less food, and she was denied all pleasurable activity. For hours daily she was to kneel in prayer. Catalina's family was led to believe that their daughter was paying for a mental transgression of God's commandments. A successful social rehabilitation would have been impossible had they been informed of the true nature of the wrongdoing that had brought the punishment from God. The *curandera's* respect for her need to conceal the truth increased Catalina's faith and reliance on her.

Although Catalina's physical suffering and anxiety were heightened, she endured the treatment with the vision of possible divine and social forgiveness and reacceptance. Various curing rites upheld her hope that she was being purged of sin. Several of the rituals that she underwent with the *curandera* were explained as serving "to remove the evil and replace the purity" that she had lost through sin.

Nearly six months later, when Catalina appeared for her flogging, the *curandera* informed her that this punishment was no longer necessary. God's voice forgiving Catalina and sanctioning her return to a normal life had been heard by the curer. And she returned. In honor of the miracle, her family invited friends to a party marking Catalina's re-entry into her proper role in Mexican-American society.

Catalina's rehabilitation must be regarded as a successful cure despite the fact that "paranoia" is an unknown term to most *curanderos*. Another Anglo disease classification rarely accepted by folk curers is alcoholism. This affliction is sometimes believed to be a consequence of *mal ojo*[10] or *susto*. Although compulsive drinkers are occasionally treated by *curanderos*, success in this area is as rare as with Anglos undergoing standard psychiatric treatment. As alcoholic rehabilitation is impossible without total abstinence, the recovery of a compulsive drinker in Mexican-American society is probably more difficult than for many Anglos. Drinking is tightly integrated into the concept of *machismo* and plays an important role in the accepted patterns of male social intercourse. One of the strongest insults to a Latin male is a refusal to drink with him.

The most successful institution for alcoholic rehabilitation in Anglo society is Alcoholics Anonymous. Association with this group is almost impossible for the conservative Mexican-American. The required abstinence denies his manliness and disrupts his interpersonal relations. Reliance for aid on institutions alien to Latin culture is regarded as a threat to the family and society. Furthermore, the philosophy and integrated nature of A.A. tend to categorize any Latin member as an *Inglesado* in Mexican-American opinion. One Spanish-speaking member of Alcoholics Anonymous admitted that successful dryness compromised most of his traditional values and his social identity. The possibility of an alcoholic death had so frightened this man that he accepted these consequences. As he put it, "It is better to be a live chicken than a dead rooster."

Occasionally, however, a *curandero* can obtain individual and social acceptance for the nondrinking alcoholic undergoing treatment. The example of Raul is such a case. This young man was a compulsive drinker with a history of repeated arrests. Despite the pleas of his wife and family, he was unable to control his drinking. One night while drunk, he knocked over a large cupboard while staggering across the room. The furniture fell, knocking his wife to the floor and severely injuring her. Neighbors took her to a hospital. The following day Raul sought to enlist the services of a *curandero* to effect his wife's recovery. The curer informed Raul that, as the accident was his fault, the wife's recovery depended on his humility and penance. At the curer's suggestion, Raul took candles to the church and made a pledge of abstinence if his wife recovered. A week later, she was home and apparently suffers no permanent injury. Raul appears to be remaining sober. No individual would urge a man to break a vow (*promesa*) in order to conform to a nonreligious behavior pattern. Raul's sacrifice is regarded as a proof of his strength rather than as a reflection on his manhood.

The cited cases demonstrate that many *curanderos* are knowledgeable about the nature of the value conflicts inherent in the structure of Mexican-American society and those arising from contact with Anglo culture. Folk treatment involves a return to the ideal values and social relationships of the conservative Latin way of life.

It is probable that many psychiatrists treating Mexican-Americans fail to recognize the core values involved in their patients' complaints. These values are primarily assimilated during childhood and within the family. They represent the pivot for the secondary Mexican-American values acquired later in life. These core values can be equated to Hall's "formal level of culture,"[11] except for the value of *machismo*. Though formation of this value begins in childhood, its crystallization is one function of adolescent experience.

Secondary values derived purely from Mexican culture are rarely in direct conflict with the core values. Those modified or derived from Anglo culture frequently represent contradictions or involve compromises of the more basic values. In the pursuit of immediate goals, secondary Anglo-derived values may seem to override the core values. Such was the case in María's temporary pursuit of economic independence in defiance of tradition. When such endeavors threaten all community identification of the individual, however, the usual response is retreat into the core value system of Mexican-American culture. In treating an *Inglesado,* there is danger that a psychiatrist, who is not conversant with Mexican-American culture, may identify Anglo-derived values as primary motivational factors rather than as secondary alternatives.

It is not surprising, therefore, to find folk psychiatry frequently successful where established psychotherapeutic techniques fail. Each success of a *curandero* and of home treatment reinforces faith in this complex of beliefs known as *curanderismo.*

Curanderismo seems assured of continued adherence despite multiple attempts to accelerate anglicization of Mexican-Americans in South Texas. Its persistence is due to its meaningfulness in the Latin world-view, its social functions, and its actual medical effectiveness in the area of psychotherapy. Acceptance of Anglo medical philosophy is slow because of its practitioners' attitudes toward Latin belief and their failure to comprehend the nature of Mexican-American culture and personality. The inconsistencies of Anglo intolerance in the area of curing confuse the Latins. As one Mexican-American put it, "Why do Anglos assume that Oral Roberts has a monopoly on the healing powers of Christ?"

Notes

1. William Madsen, *Society and Health in the Lower Rio Grande Valley* (Austin: The Hogg Foundation for Mental Health, 1961), pp. 5-6.

2. J. Bushnell, "La Virgen de Guadalupe as Surrogate Mother in San Juan Atzingo," *American Anthropologist*, 60 (1958), 261-5.

3. Octavio Romano, "Donship in a Mexican-American Community in Texas," *American Anthropologist*, 62 (1960), 966-76.

4. *Ibid.*, p. 972.

5. Arthur J. Rubel, "Concepts of Disease in Mexican-American Culture," *American Anthropologist*, 62 (1960), 797.

6. Albino E. Fantini, *Illness and Curing Among the Mexican Americans of Mission Texas* (Unpublished M.A. thesis, University of Texas, 1962), p. 44.

7. Madsen, *The Virgin's Children: Life in an Aztec Village Today* (Austin: University of Texas Press, 1960), pp. 11-2.

8. Rubel, *op. cit.*, p. 813.

9. Leon Festinger, *A Theory of Cognitive Dissonance* (Stanford: Stanford University Press, 1957).

10. Fred R. Crawford, *The Forgotten Egg* (Austin: Texas State Department of Health, 1961), p. 13.

11. Edward T. Hall, *The Silent Language* (Garden City: Doubleday & Company, Inc.), pp. 87-92.

Part Four

Western psychiatry must learn to make
more creative use of native culture if it is to increase
its effectiveness in dealing with mental illness
and to hasten the acceptance of modern medicine
among primitive peoples.

T. Adeoye Lambo

Patterns of Psychiatric Care
in Developing African Countries

MANY AFRICAN societies are today in a state of rapid change—
social, economic, and cultural. By the very nature of their economic and
manpower positions, developing countries in Africa cannot afford, at
this time, the building and administration of huge medical institutions.
Necessity therefore forces us not only to compromise but also to explore
all possible avenues for the most effective, economical, and socially acceptable ways of treating the mentally ill in Africa. Because of the essential nature of the societies and their dynamic characteristics, an
independent diagnosis of our position, followed by formulation of patterns
of care in tune with our social structure, would be the most realistic approach. In order to find the most practical way of treating the mentally
ill in Africa, a special study was made of traditional social institutions
among various African peoples. This paper first describes certain general
aspects of African traditional beliefs and customs and then examines in
detail experiences in Nigeria that have involved the integration of modern
and traditional methods of psychiatric treatment in the village communities of Aro, Nigeria.

§ Traditional Beliefs and Customs

The subject of African traditional beliefs, concepts of health, and
medical practice has certain paradoxical and complex features that do
not readily lend themselves to finer analysis and exotic interpretation. The
function of traditional beliefs as natural carriers of a culture and, therefore as a cluster of socially determined attitudes and behavior patterns,
grouped and elaborated around operationally determined roles and re-

lationships, is well known. African culture,* in common with most non-literate cultures, manifests an intensely realized perception of super-natural presence but with a kind of adolescent impetuousness and a fatuous, almost fanatical, faith in the magic of certain symbols to produce certain results. Most nonliterate cultures are thus especially conducive to states of morbid fear and anxiety. Rituals, involving sacrifice that may connote life-taking (actual or symbolic), are a logical outcome. Sacrifice, which is among the earliest popular traditions of man, is the crucial psychological point of all cults, the essential bond between man and deity. In the past, the African peoples, addicted to the cult of animals, have indulged in peculiar types of sacrifice. In times of tribal distress—famine, drought, or epidemic, for example—the tribe may offer an ex-piatory sacrifice to its tutelar animal. In many instances, the method is more complex. For example, a grand synod of tribal chiefs is called, an animal is caught and killed, and finally every man present eats a portion of the flesh. This ritual is a form of sacrament, since it is argued that it is a sort of self-deification. The animal killed and eaten represents the tribal mascot, which has withdrawn its protection, thus exposing the tribe to the current catastrophe of epidemic or famine.

In more recent times, there have been some malignant forms of ritualistic observances. In 1960, I coined a clinical term, "malignant anxiety," to describe the essential features of an abnormal psychosocial condition after a close study of twenty-nine subjects and a careful an-alysis of three major epidemics in Kenya, Nigeria, and the Congo.[1] The cults or subcultural societies studied were Odozi Obodo in Nigeria, Leopard Men Society also in Nigeria, Boro Society of Sierra Leone, and Mau Mau of Kenya. These societies, even in the middle of the twentieth century, appeared determined to assert and vindicate their ancient rights and privileges.

The Leopard Men of Nigeria were a secret and subhuman society, involved in savage sacrament, about which an observer has written: "The witnesses—there were witnesses on some occasions—said they had never seen a man. They had seen a leopard, or 'a thing on two legs' and they had run away to call for help. Even if they knew the murderer they would not say, not merely because of their fear of reprisals, but because,

---

* We know that this culture is far from homogeneous and that there are distinct and characteristic configurations of culture in Africa. The great diversity of tribes and cultures makes any examination of their social institutions peculiarly difficult, and the task is not rendered easier by almost complete ignorance of some of the customs in the smaller tribes.

to an African, a man becomes the thing he says he is, even if he isn't, by an act of faith . . ."[2]

We have found that malignant anxiety has developed under the impact of social and emotional difficulties encountered by personalities psychologically ill equipped to meet them. When adaptation to new and stressful life situations becomes difficult for the African, anxiety, expressed in aggressive behavior, is apt to occur, leading, in some instances, to crimes akin to ritual murder. The psychological attitudes and phantasies underlying these ritual murders and other criminal acts have the same etiological basis as those of the more benign tribal rituals of old.

Related to this phenomenon is the phenomenon of *le mythe du mpaka-fo,* vividly described by Dr. Louise Marx from observation in Madagascar. It is associated with an acute castration anxiety state, which can only be relieved, warded off, or expiated by tearing out the heart of a young child and offering it to Mpaka-Fo. Thus a sporadic psychosocial condition has led to a new form of ritual murder. The source of this myth is not known.

One of the essential elements of the African's traditional beliefs is his awareness of man. He is fundamentally concerned with establishing good relations with man, not only man here and now (empirical man) but also man who has vanished from mortal sight (transcendental man, the basis of ancestor worship). This psychological and philosophical attitude expresses the profoundly human motives underlying the institutions of "ancestor worship" and certain secret societies. The African tribal names are other evidences of the basic concept underlying the consecration of ancestor worship, which strengthens all family relations, enabling the departed father to retain his role as powerful leader of the group (a spiritual force) and at the same time to become a being of far more than human excellence.

That these traditional beliefs, basic concepts, and attitudes of life are deeply ingrained irrespective of degree of sophistication is suggested by a number of studies.

In a study of a group of Nigerian students who broke down during their courses of university study in Great Britain in 1957, it was found that the symptoms in more than 90% of the patients offered clear-cut evidence of African traditional beliefs in bewitchment and machinations of the enemy.[3] The students tended to regard their dream-lives as objective reality. The appearance of dead persons in dreams thus took on a quality of reality with deep psychological significance.

In 1960, I described the case of an English-university-trained West

African patient who had been promoted to the Administrative Service, superseding quite a number of able West African contemporaries by virtue, it was alleged, of his high social position and contacts. A few weeks after his promotion, he had an accident in unusual circumstances and became terrified that his colleagues were trying to get at him in a mysterious way.

During this period, his grandfather appeared in a dream, assured him of long life, and asked that a goat be sacrificed. He bought a goat the following day, carried out his "instruction" and quickly recovered from his severe anxiety state. Even though he did not like to discuss the matter, the patient conceded that he believed there was something in this "native thing." This case is not an isolated one. I found innumerable examples among Westernized professional Africans and also among our students in England at the university level. I found in 1950 that more than 60% of the patient population of a large general hospital in Western Nigeria received "native treatment" in one form or another during the time they were in the hospital. In psychiatry, the percentage would probably be much higher.

It would seem, therefore, that under stress, emotional or otherwise, newly acquired and highly differentiated social attitudes and ideologies are more susceptible to "damage," leaving the basic traditional beliefs and indigenous moral philosophy functionally overactive. The realization of this fact has led me (and my Sudanese colleague, Dr. Tigani El Mahi) to recognize the part played by indigenous psychotherapeutic approaches in the total management of the patient, without any lowering of standards of medical practice. Although by Western standards this approach is indefensible and although some of these indigenous cultural factors may be caricatured as primitive and antediluvian, they are nevertheless emotionally reinforced. They are an historical and traditional legacy, and the behavioral scientist working in an African cultural setting must be sensitive to their implications.

Concepts of health within the framework of African culture are far more social than biological. In the mind of the African, there is a more unitary concept of psychosomatic interrelationship, that is, an apparent reciprocity between mind and matter. Health is not an isolated phenomenon but part of the entire magico-religious fabric; it is more than the absence of disease. Since disease is viewed as one of the most important social sanctions, "peaceful living with neighbors, abstention from adultery, keeping the laws of gods and men, are essentials in order to protect oneself and one's family from disease."

When analyzed closely, the concepts of health and disease in African culture can be regarded as constituting a continuum with almost imperceptible gradations. Burstein, writing on public health and prevention of disease in primitive communities, notes: "Medicine in our sense, at primitive culture levels, is only one phase of a set of processes to promote human well-being; averting the wrath of gods or spirits, making rain, purifying streams or habitations, improving sex potency or fecundity or the fertility of fields and crops—in short, it is bound up with the whole interpretation of life."[4]

The African within his indigenous culture constantly asks the same existential questions posed by Heidegger: "Who am I?" "What am I doing here?" The richness of his culture provides him with adequate answers, thereby averting a breakdown of normal psychological mechanisms. The whole question of traditional beliefs, concepts of health, and medical practice in African cultures is manifestly one question, and every attempt in the past to classify various solutions as essentially "social," "religious," "personal," or "utilitarian" has proved too arbitrary and has not advanced our understanding of the question.

§ The Nigerian Experience

With these kinds of cultural consideration in mind, a pilot experiment in community psychiatry was started in Aro, Abeokuta, Western Nigeria, in 1954. It has now become a model for other developing African countries.* The original experiment took the form of a "village system," which permitted full treatment of the mentally ill by utilization of inherent dynamic resources of the social environment as the principal therapeutic technique.

In October, 1954, two projects were started at Aro, a rural suburb of the ancient town of Abeokuta, sixty miles from the federal capital. The first phase was the adoption of a day-hospital scheme. This and other projects dealing with community psychiatry were undertaken in full recognition that the African patient must ideally be treated within his social environment. The scheme of treatment within the framework of the community was based on the use of four large traditional villages. On to these four villages, we grafted our therapeutic unit, which could accommodate 200 to 300 patients. The normal population comprised Yoruba tribesmen and their extended families, the majority of whom were

* A modified version is now used in Ghana, and various adaptations are being contemplated in East African countries.

peasant farmers, fishermen, and local craftsmen. The four villages sur-
round a central institution—Aro Hospital—a most modern 200-bed mental
hospital with all the modern facilities for treatment and research.

It was part of the regulation leading to admission to the treatment program that each patient should be accompanied by at least one member
of the family—mother, sister, brother, or aunt, who should be able to
cook for him, wash his clothes, take him to the hospital for treatment
in the morning, and collect him in the afternoon. This regulation was
easily enforced, and the relatives of the sick people came forward readily.
This approach was due to our appreciation, gained during our preliminary study of the African community, of the important fact that there was
still in many places a strong sense of social security in this closely knit
society—of well organized and well defined kin groups with definite traditional roles and culturally prescribed mutual obligations.

This first phase went on for two years.[5] Patients and their families, as
well as the ordinary villagers, were regularly invited to attend church
services, films, traditional plays, dances, and social functions in the hospital itself. One of the most important lessons learned during the first
phase of the experiment was that this form of treatment provided the
best and the most effective way of dealing with family attitudes toward
patients from the beginning of treatment. Personal experience and insight
gained by members of the family accompanying their sick relatives to,
and fully participating in, therapy proved to have a great deal of influence on the rehabilitation of the patient, since this unique experience
gained by the families considerably influenced social attitudes within the
family and within the community. It also made it easier for the relatives,
who were in constant contact with the patients, to adjust smoothly to the
latter and their future emotional needs. In view of this design, we therefore regard village admission and therapy for the patient (in the company
of his relatives) as only one point in the therapeutic continuum.

The second phase of our experiment took the form of comprehensive
village-care services through gradual extending of the first phase. All
treatment facilities are now provided in two smaller villages, and, in
addition, we have now taken full responsibility for health administration,
management, planning, and public health of these villages, in full collaboration with the village elders, who serve on the health planning
council. Regular monthly meetings are held between the staff of the
Department of Psychiatry of the University of Ibadan (which has now
assumed full responsibility for teaching, research, and clinical work in
these villages) and the village chiefs and their councils.

Clinics have now been built in two villages, where all forms of modern therapy are provided; the doctors and nurses also use these clinics as their administrative centers. Each clinic is equipped with a small laboratory sufficient to carry out routine laboratory investigation. In addition, a mobile clinic is used to penetrate other distant villages in the area in which epidemiological research has been going on for some time.[6]

Loans are made available to the people in the two central villages to enable them to expand or build new homes to accommodate the influx of new patients from distant villages and towns. Care is taken, however, that the ratio of normal villagers to patient population is constantly maintained at six villagers to four patients. To this end, small villages in the immediate vicinity of our mental health clinics have been encouraged to take new patients into their homes. There have been no difficulties, since the rewards accorded to the original villages participating in this unique scheme are obvious. Among other things, we have paid for the installation of water pipes, which bring scientifically purified water from the water works of the town of Abeokuta a few miles away; pit latrines; and a mosquito eradication squad. Men and women from the villages are employed in the clinics and the hospital (as gardeners, porters, cooks, and so forth), and they are in turn the landlords and landladies of the patients. Efforts are thus made to raise the public-health standards and subsistence economy of the village population without interfering in any significant measure with the social structure and traditional atmosphere of village society.

Facilities available at the clinics include EST, modified insulin therapy (because of the resulting cachectic states of most African patients), abreactive techniques, various group psychotherapies of the most diversified nature, and drug medication. Emphasis is laid on utilizing every conceivable sociopsychological concept and method.[7]

One of the most unusual features of our pattern of care for the mentally ill in Nigeria is our unorthodox collaboration with the traditional healers. We have discovered through our long practice in Africa that it is essential to the scientific understanding of man and his social environment to work in close collaboration with other disciplines and even to establish some form of interprofessional relationship on a fairly continuing basis—even with those who, by Western standards, are not strictly regarded as "professional." For example, Dr. El Mahi and I have for a number of years made use of the services of African "witch doctors," especially selected for epidemiological work and other aspects of social psychiatry (for example, a community attitude survey), a procedure that is indefensible by Western standards. Through their participation we have enriched our scientific knowledge of the psychopathology and psychodynamics of the major psychiatric disorders occurring in these exotic societies. We have also been able to accumulate a mass of data on the natural history and prevalence of many psychiatric disorders, in terms of cultural and social variables (variables that are ill defined and remain resistant to Western forms of categorization). Without the help of the "witch doctors," we would not have known how and where to look and what obstacles to skirt in searching for simple disorders like obsessional neurosis in the indigenous population of Africa. Most of these traditional healers who are employed by us and are participating in this scheme have considerable experience in the management of African patients. They supervise and direct the social and group activities of our patients in the villages under our guidance.

During the first phase of this community psychiatry, the patients who were boarded out in the villages were especially chosen, hand picked as it were, but now no selection of patients is made. We admit, among others, catatonics and other schizophrenics with symptoms. Even patients who have exhibited aggressive and antisocial tendencies in their homes and have to be heavily restrained mechanically have become quite manageable under the village conditions.

In the second phase, we emphasize the fact that a patient can be admitted into the village, treated within the village community, and discharged from the village without having entered any kind of formal institution like a hospital.

Before turning to a brief description of the third and final phase of our experiment, let me summarize and, perhaps for the first time, highlight our therapeutic rationale, including our major therapeutic techniques, and dilate on the advantages and limitations of our approach.

Our approach is fundamentally based upon our discovery that certain practices with an obvious therapeutic tinge were opportunely present in the indigenous culture and that certain factors in the traditional environment and the village in particular act as powerful buffers against social pressures and conflicts and consequently promote good mental health. Confession, dancing, rituals, suggestions inherent in traditional cults, flexibility, and tolerance of the environment, to mention a few, could be mobilized and utilized as powerful psychotherapeutic armament, especially in psychoneurosis. Anxiety, which is the most common and crippling psychiatric disorder in Africa, also forms the central core of other neurotic reactions in the African.

In any group situation (normal or therapeutic) in Africa, transference is a vital problem. We have found that, where recovery is probable, the success of all other measures depends upon an adequate affective transfer. Even when the prognosis is unfavorable, a positive transfer of affect under the empathic conditions of the village and within the context of a warm, sympathetic, and tolerant therapeutic relationship, may be used to prevent patients from deteriorating (secondary prevention). By permitting the ego of the patient to gain sufficient strength to function without overwhelming anxiety through reality testing wihout any fear of being further traumatized, the village community disinhibits and desensitizes the sensitive ego. Multiple therapy techniques are applied through the participation of two or more therapists (the traditional healers and one psychiatrist) with one patient. The permissiveness of the group in the traditional village facilitates the effective use of learning situations, which bring about desirable effects in certain individual patients; it is also through the atmosphere of the group that frequently latent behavior becomes manifest in some patients and that this behavior is dealt with without fuss.

Constant evaluation of the effects of therapy goes on and forms a major part of our operational research. As a result, comparison of the patient before and after therapy in terms of his described and observed behavior and feelings in his relationships with others is always fully explored and recorded. Such comparison is based upon reports from the patients and their families, and these reports are frequently supplemented by reports from the village heads, friends, and workmates on the farm, especially in terms of modification and alteration in social roles.

After nine years of continuous experiment in this pattern of community psychiatry in Nigeria, a pattern that would seem to be acceptable to the African populations and that has proved to be the most economical and practical way of providing therapy for a large group of people in need of help, what then are its advantages and limitations?

The advantages are threefold—social, medical (therapeutic), and economic.

SOCIAL ADVANTAGES

1. It makes psychiatric care an integral part of the community and therefore part of the culture, to which it is highly sensitive.

2. It promotes a measurable degree of relaxation in community attitudes.

3. It creates a positive and more natural environment for measuring

the degree of social competence or impairment in patients, in contrast to the very often artificially structured social environment of the institution (hospital).

4. It makes it easier for psychiatric personnel to communicate freely with one another and with the community.

5. It lessens the risk of social stigma and promotes better social adaptation and integration of the patients.

MEDICAL (INCLUDING THERAPEUTIC AND RESEARCH) ADVANTAGES

1. It provides an optimal therapeutic environment for the treatment of certain psychiatric disorders, such as character disorders, sociopathy, alcoholism, and neurosis, especially nonrational malignant forms of anxiety. It creates the opportunity, through utilization of environmental factors, to conduct treatment and rehabilitation at almost the same time. It is our finding, through follow-up studies, that it promotes quick recovery, lessens the risk of social and other disabilities, and reduces the problem of rehabilitation or after-care.

2. It promotes a spirit of collaboration with behavioral scientists (anthropologists, sociologists, social psychologists), thus creating opportunities for an interdisciplinary approach allowing major variables to be measured multidimensionally.

3. It allows for built-in research. Community psychiatry of this type offers a "laboratory" in which certain variables can be observed to operate without contamination. It affords full opportunity for empirical researches in the general area of group dynamics and group and individual psychotherapy.

4. It allows diversity of therapeutic maneuvers and forms an excellent avenue for the teaching of psychiatry and mental health.

ECONOMIC ADVANTAGES

1. Its cost (in material and personnel) is low for the medical authorities running the scheme, as well as for the patient and his relatives.

2. It provides an excellent chance for deploying meager human and material resources in the most effective and strategic manner.

There are limitations, however. Some international visitors to this Nigerian experiment have repeatedly put forward the argument, among others, that such a scheme can operate only in nonindustrial agrarian communities like those in Africa and Asia, where the threshold of community tolerance is high, and that, with the advent of social change, difficulties may ensue.

There is an expansion program for our scheme presently in force, which should enable us to provide service for about 1000 patients and to use the scheme for the training of mental health workers, the teaching of community psychiatry, and research training for undergraduate medical students. To this end, the building of medical-student hostels and flats for doctors and nurses on the peripheries of the villages is being planned. It is also intended that the present village clinics be expanded to provide a limited number of in-patient beds, essentially for treating acutely ill patients with physical complications such as we often encounter in African countries.

In conclusion, I should like to emphasize that this experiment is a modest one that has proved useful to our community and in which the community has a great deal of confidence. There is, therefore, no doubt that the greater the confidence of the community members in the *nature* and *form* of treatment they can obtain and in the *people* who will treat them, the more spontaneous is their willingness to come forward for treatment and to encourage other people to do the same. In the same way, the greater the responsibility that is given to the community in the care and management of its mentally ill, the better and more sympathetic its response and the greater its understanding.

Although our community psychiatric practice and research in Nigeria obviously raise many questions and unfortunately provide few answers, they have contributed significantly to our understanding of many of the problems of mental ill health in the emerging nations of Africa.

Notes

1. T. A. Lambo, "Malignant Anxiety," *Journal of Medical Science* (1960).
2. S. Cloete, *The African Giant* (London: 1960).
3. Lambo, "Characteristic Features of the Psychology of the Nigerian," *West African Medical Journal*, IX (1960), No. 3, 95-104.
4. S. R. Burstein, "Public Health and Prevention of Disease in Primitive Communities," *The Advancement of Science*, IX (1952), No. 33, 75-81.
5. Lambo, "Neuro-Psychiatric Observations in the Western Region of Nigeria," *British Medical Journal*, 2 (December, 1956), 1385.
6. Alexander Leighton, Lambo, *et al.*, *Psychiatric Disorder among the Yoruba* (Ithaca: 1963).
7. Lambo, "A Form of Social Psychiatry in Africa," *World Mental Health*, 13 (November, 1961), No. 4.

Ari Kiev

Implications for the Future

IN ADDITION to the intrinsic merits of the enclosed papers and the light they shed on certain common elements of psychological treatments, their significance lies in their contribution to a number of theoretical and practical issues pertaining to the larger question of culture and psychiatry. These papers range over such broad issues as personality formation, socio-cultural stress systems, psychological illness, and its management. The most important considerations appear, however, to be those pointing to the cultural matrix and cultural aspects of psychotherapy. Awareness of these cultural elements is of special significance today both for consideration of contemporary psychotherapies and for the larger question of introducing Western psychiatry into other parts of the world.

§ The Impact of Culture on Personality: Psychopathology

The papers in this anthology, in dealing with the pathogenesis, the symptomatology, and the treatment of psychiatric illness in a variety of settings, have underscored the wide ranging impact of culture on human behavior. We have seen how, from birth onward the infant's biological functions are molded to culturally prescribed limits and patterned after accepted models, accounting ultimately for shared attributes among people from the same culture. For example, autonomy, initiative, and aggression are suppressed early in the life of Turkish villagers, which leads in adulthood to their projection onto the unseen *jinns* in the culturally sanctioned areas of sorcery and magic. In the same way, cultural sanctions encourage the development of certain behavior patterns that would be considered unusual in Western society—the possession behavior of Orisa cult initiates or Eskimo shamans, for example.

Cultural factors also influence the patterning of sick roles, which may at times serve to satisfy needs no longer being met through conventional channels. By falling sick in a traditionally Mexican way, the Mexican-American is relieved from responsibility for forgetting his origins. Being ill with *susto* may restore, through reaffirmation of traditional Mexican patterns and family solidarity, the anxious and conflict-ridden to the good graces of the community. Similarly the now obsolete Apache hunting and raiding traditions find their main expression among the Navaho today in such patterns of deviance and psychopathology as "crazy violence." Although this behavior is associated with alcoholic intoxication, it expresses previously valued elements of willfulness, honesty, and courage. Here the instinctual drives that were idealized and sanctioned in the past now create conflicts and are expressed in self-destructive ways, in contrast to the restitutive functions such ethnic factors play in Mexican-American folk illnesses.

The significance of cultural factors is highlighted further by the perpetuation of traditional folkways in the face of rapid social change. Although the Yemenite *mori*, for example, has little importance and few functions in Israel, he continues to be preferred over modern experts as a source of psychological help for the Yemenite immigrants. Psychological and social problems created by rapid industrialization and urbanization in Sierra Leone have in similar fashion been met by the influx of diviners, native doctors, and Islamic holy men, as well as by the development of voluntary organizations modeled after the native secret societies. Because of the clashing demands of the traditional secret societies and the changing role identifications of the urban Africans, these new voluntary groups have established new norms to meet old and new needs in new but familiar ways. Similarly, the Ihamba cult in Northern Rhodesia has spread precisely where hunting is in decline and has allowed the Ndembu to maintain in fantasy the values, symbols, and trappings of a highly ritualized activity that is rapidly losing its economic importance. For those experiencing guilt and anxiety because of their participation in the new industrial trade and cash economy, the Ihamba cult serves as a culturally meaningful method of reducing anxiety.

Worth noting too is the emphasis in these various papers on the larger social significance of illness in the cultures examined, which contrasts strongly with its reduced social significance in the more advanced Western societies. Because illness often suggests that something is wrong in the community, the sickness of a single individual often arouses collective fear and community action. In the Western world, by contrast, medicine has become increasingly secularized, and as Ackerknecht has observed "has lost its 'sacred' character, its social control function, its subjective influence on society, its meaning in moral terms."[1] The effect of such secularization can be seen in the hospital experiences of patients who, as Simmons and Wolff have noted, "are classified according to their illnesses, fitted into a tightly organized and scheduled system of hospital practices, and pressed into lines of conformity that are new and disturbing. Then in their emergencies they are cut off measurably from the tried and trusted contacts and supports of family and community. Indeed in the patient's darkest hours, physically, mentally and emotionally he is likely to feel, and perhaps also to be left, rather much alone, especially if these periods come at night."[2]

DISRUPTION OF CULTURE

While there has been general agreement that the incidence of psychosis does not vary greatly from one country to another, the actual number of cases of psychosis coming to the attention of public-health authorities has increased in most countries in recent years, apparently due, according to some authorities, to the breakdown of the extended family, migration to urban areas, and the strains of rapid industrialization.

In line with suggestions that the Westernization of underdeveloped areas is the only situation in which social factors are clearly reflected in an increased incidence of mental illness, several papers in this volume focus specifically on problems related to acculturation, urbanization, and industrialization. From a consideration of these phenomena it becomes clear that social change can have significantly disruptive effects. Change often brings a partial halt to the secure pursuit of familiar life goals and a consequent reduction in the significance of old values and symbols. Change also implies some confusion about new situations, associated with problems of adaptation or adoption of new methods, as well as potential difficulty in the acceptance of new values. To the extent that these demands are difficult ones to meet, change will be stressful for the group and for the individual. The degree of stress depends to some extent on the degree of difference between the old and new situation.

For adequate psychological functioning and for purposes of maintaining the integrity of a society, individuals develop certain expectations about the certainties in their world—in terms both of natural and of interpersonal events. Associated with these expectations are certain sentiments and values that influence them with varying degrees of emotional significance. Those expectations and values that lead to uncertainty or confusion or to unfavorable outcomes generate unpleasant emotions like anxiety, panic, and despair, while expectations and values leading to security generate feelings of hope and faith.

In a situation of rapid social change, these values, sentiments and accustomed ways of doing things are thrown into a state of upheaval, which produces emotional upheaval as well, for as Frank has noted: "In order to function successfully and enjoy life, a person must possess an integrated set of assumptions that correspond to conditions as they actually are. For it is only to the extent that a person can successfully predict the results of his acts that he can behave in such a way as to maximize chances for success and minimize those for failure."[3]

In a situation of social change, old traditional customs and values often become obsolete, while at the same time individuals are required to adjust to new values and folkways. For some, this change represents a challenge—for others, an overwhelming disruptive emotional experience. When efforts to cope with new threats and challenges lead to failure, individuals naturally turn to those sources of comfort that were successful in combatting unpleasant emotional states in the prechange period.

Along these lines it is of special interest to note the variety of data presented in these papers attesting to the relationship between social change and mental illness. Various forms of social change, including migration, industrialization, and urbanization have been recognized as partial causes of increased incidence of mental illness. In a recent review of the literature dealing with these same issues, Murphy noted that the nature of the relationship between sociological events and rates of mental illness still remains uncertain.[4] He found that there were almost as many studies suggesting that social change leads to an increase in mental disorders as there were studies suggesting it leads to a decrease. Only in instances of contact between Western and non-Western cultures did there seem to be clear-cut evidence of an increased rate among those undergoing change, compared to members of the same group not experiencing similar change—a fact underlining the significance of culture contact and conflict in the development of mental illness. In such situations, the breakdown of old ways and traditions seems to be greatest, and opportunity for utilizing old ways of adapting least. Insofar as change sometimes leads to an improvement rather than a worsening of mental health, it seems likely that change itself is less significant for mental health than a number of associated factors.

One critical aspect of social change is the individual's expectations and perceptions of society and his assessment of his own role in it. A valuable line of inquiry focusing on the interplay of these factors has been carefully elucidated in the studies of Wolff and Hinkle, which have been focused on an intensive review of medical and life-history data of individuals from a number of groups undergoing marked social change.[5] More frequent episodes of illness appear to be largely the result of physiological and psychological changes associated with attempts to adapt to extremely difficult life situations, rather than simply the results of fatigue, injury, poor diet, or other factors. Wolff and Hinkle found that the bulk of both psychiatric and physical illness episodes occurs at times when individuals perceive their life situations as unsatisfying, threatening, too demanding, and productive of conflict—which prevents them from making satisfactory adjustments. They concluded that the critical factor in the development of illness was not actual social or environmental stress but the individual's perceptions of stress.

These studies furthermore emphasize, although not explicitly, the significance of life-history data in the accurate assessment of the stress potential of sociological and historical events. Careful consideration of the individuals studied reveals that stressful events more often than not have highly personal meanings related no less to earlier life experiences than to the immediate and realistic "catastrophic" events.

During the Cornell study of refugees who had fled Hungary following the October, 1956, revolution, this writer had an opportunity to interview about seventy individuals. Their participation in the revolution and subsequent emigration did not appear to stem from political or ideological considerations but were more in keeping with earlier established patterns of life adjustment. One man, for example, viewed the revolution and his defection as an opportunity to solve domestic difficulties that paralleled those in his own disturbed childhood, despite the fact that he had achieved considerable academic and political recognition under the Communist regime.

§ Therapeutic Aspects of Cultural Factors

Along with consideration of the deleterious psychological effects attendant upon the disruption of social systems, some of the papers have considered the critical stabilizing and therapeutic roles played by various folk medical systems, which provide in traditional or modified form channels for anxiety reduction and treatment for individuals in need. These studies' special significance is to underline the integral role of medical systems in the social system—the fact that most cultures contain their own mental health resources.

Dr. La Barre's examination of confession throughout the Western Hemisphere highlights the effects of cultural variations on one technique and underlines the fact that apparent differences count less than do the presence of certain common elements. The knowledge gained from such "natural experiments" has been further expanded and tested in a number of practical programs seeking to utilize such resources. A case in point is Dr. Lambo's program in Abeokuta, where patients are billeted in surrounding villages and visit the hospital for treatment only during the day. In this setting, provisions for highly valued animal sacrifices and native rituals and the co-operation of native medicine men allow maintenance of continuity between the modern treatment of illness and the more traditional notions of etiology and treatment.[6]

In similar fashion, the use of native doctors as assistants to public health service doctors contributed to the rapid adoption of Western medicine by American Indians, while today, the marginality of the acculturated bilingual Navaho is used for bridging gaps in communications and techniques between Navaho and American society in the Cornell-Navaho Field Health Research Project.

The fact that treatment is culturally based and directed at the alleviation of symptoms is not, however, by any means always beneficial. Bush surgery and toxic drugs may in fact do actual harm. The use of amulets or suggestive, abreactive, and dissociative experiences, although it may cause no direct harm, may do indirect harm by delaying the use of prompt and effective modern treatment. At the recent Pan African Psychiatric Conference in Abeokuta, Margetts emphasized that, "One must differentiate spiritual, suggestive, dancing and abreactive healing such as the zar of North Africa and Ethiopia, the ayana of North Kenya, the pepo of the Arabs and coast Swahili of Kenya, from the treatment of the primitive medicine man as the dokita of Nigeria or the mganga of the Swahili speaking tribes in the East. While there might be some rationale in accepting, with caution, the purely psychological type of healer, there are many pitfalls if modern emerging countries encourage him, and real dangers if they promote the native medicine man who uses material substances or cutting procedures."[7]

As for the introduction of Western medicine into new areas, it appears that, in some instances, customs require that modern treatments be given in customary forms for a given culture—such as decoctions, pills, or powders rather than injections, for example. In some instances, it is essential to strip modern techniques to their bare essentials and find new rationalizations for them in order that they may fit the specific needs of the culture to which they are to be introduced.

Related to this point is experience that suggests that the egalitarianism and inquisitiveness of Western doctors, qualities encouraged in the West, are often disappointing to those who view the doctor as an omniscient person of higher station, one on whom patients can be completely dependent.

From these considerations, it seems not unreasonable to ponder in planning for the future the value of various subcultural institutions that might profitably be articulated into treatment programs. Most cultures, according to Wallace, sanction a number of activities that provide for the release of tension and permit individuals to "act out" in normally prohibited ways.[8] While such activities (the arts, games, feasts, ceremonies, and so forth) may be rationalized in various ways, they often provide for the satisfaction of needs not ordinarily met in the routine course of events. In the same way, myths, beliefs, ideologies, and other projective systems can also bind such potentially disruptive emotions as fear, anxiety, hate, envy, and doubt—thereby maintaining a certain degree of functional stability in a culture and effectively serving certain preventive psychiatric purposes.

While such techniques, which Wallace has labeled "cathartic strategies," serve certain quasi-therapeutic needs in stable societies, certain "control" or suppressive strategies and belief systems serve a similar purpose in less secure or unstable groups by introducing a sense of order and organization into the society through a process of "superego reinforcement." According to Wallace, techniques for accomplishing this goal generally depend upon "hysterical conversion." "Sermons depicting the terrors of hellfire, mass rallies, compulsory confession and penance, 'thought reform' induced by a combination of threat, confession and indoctrination, continuous moral exhortation and encouragement, instruction conveyed symbolically in rites de passage—devices such as these are more effective in inducing marked 'improvement' in behavior in demoralized populations than is mere threat of punishment for delinquency."[9]

§ Culture and Psychotherapy

Moving from consideration of the broad use of cultural institutions to more specific examination of psychological treatments reveals the presence of certain general patterns not ordinarily emphasized in examinations of the therapeutic elements of psychological treatments. While views about etiological factors and the requisite therapeutic efforts are necessarily influenced by the culture, it appears likely that most healers would agree about which individuals are in need of help. Symptoms of uncontrollable anxiety, depression, and agitation would be recognized almost everywhere as evidence of disorder, as would such gross breaks of contact with reality as delirium or acute schizophrenia. In addition, it appears likely that most healers in most societies are concerned first with the control of violence both to the community and to the self, next with the reduction of fear and anxiety, and last with the reintegration of the withdrawn (schizophrenics and depressives) into the community.

Shepherd has drawn attention to the great range of conceptions that can be found throughout the Western world, where, anthropologically speaking, countries have reached relatively the same stage of evolution and technological complexity. Indeed, as he has noted, "universal agreement on the broad principles of therapy, however, extends to very few conditions, all of them with a clearly defined physical basis." He notes that an explanation merely in terms of "national preference" does not do justice to questions of why the Dutch have concentrated on administrative measures designed to treat patients out of hospital; the Swiss and Germans have devoted so much attention to the intensive psychotherapy of schizophrenics; insulin therapy has waned more rapidly in England than in Austria; sleep treatment has been carried out so energetically in some French hospitals; and ECT has such low status while there is a ukase on prefrontal lobotomy in the Soviet Union.[10]

In all the examined societies, treatment procedures are governed by particular rules and follow prescribed patterns comprising the relationships among the healer, the patient, and the group. Judging from the similarity of certain mechanisms operating in these situations, it appears likely that the various culturally determined concepts and customs that give the theories and treatments their local stamp are less significant intrinsically than because they articulate the treatment with other cultural institutions.

In the cultural context, the mysteries of illness and healing procedures are made understandable and rationalized and thus become less frightening. The accuracy of diagnosis and the efficacy of the treatment count less here than does the simple fact that anxiety, fear, and doubt, all of which may contribute to an illness by complicating symptoms and reactions, are dispelled. In their place are substituted the prospect of help, a sense of hope that may contribute directly to the patient's improvement.

Such basic features of psychological treatment may be more important elements of treatment than the features that differentiate them. The healer in all instances can bring a tremendous amount of personal influence and arouse a multitude of emotions in the patient, as well as in the group, during a healing situation. This use of influence to arouse emotion may have therapeutic value. In addition, the healer's ability in most instances to use the beliefs and ideas of the group as a fulcrum for influencing treatment increases the chances for successful reintegration of the patient into the community.

A consideration of these cultural aspects of psychological treatment is especially significant for the investigation of contemporary psychotherapy. The high value placed on democracy and science in America is reflected, according to Frank, in the theory and practice of psychotherapy. The democratic ideal is made up of such values as personal betterment and freedom from the tyranny of traditional values. It accounts in part for the public's acceptance of such values of psychiatry as self-betterment, freedom from inhibition, and a certain degree of independence of thought and action. At the same time, the scientific ideal reinforces the democratic ideal by rejecting dogmatism, and upholding objectivity and intellectual comprehension, which, as Frank has suggested, may not be entirely advantageous for psychotherapy. Such an orientation results in an over-evaluation of the cognitive aspects of psychotherapy, an undue stress on the niceties of interpretation and an avoidance of therapeutically valuable emotion-arousing techniques like group rituals, dramatic activities, and direct influence of the physician.[11] In keeping with the Protestant ethic, great emphasis is placed on patient participation or "work" in therapy, the extent of progress being the responsibility of the patient, while egalitarian values are operative in the psychotherapist's avoidance of the traditional authoritarianism and direct influence of the physician. Such factors suggest that examination of the subtle interplay of values with psychotherapeutic theory and practice is of the utmost importance for increasing both knowledge of the operation of psychotherapy and the effectiveness of psychiatric treatment programs.

§ Implications for the Future

The papers in this volume, in emphasizing that psychological treatments involve much more than the application of knowledge and procedures derived from theoretical and accumulated clinical experience, suggest the importance of examining such nonrational elements as beliefs, rituals, and symbols, which influence the practice of psychiatry both in Western settings and in underdeveloped areas.

In keeping with the breadth of subject covered by these papers, areas suggested for further investigation are similarly wide-ranging. They extend from the need for large-scale epidemiological enquiries into the incidence and prevalence of both major and minor psychiatric illness in various cultures to the need for more microscopic examination of the role of cultural stress systems in the development of psychopathological patterns of mood, thought, and behavior. Extensive and careful observations of the part played by social and cultural values and forces in psychotherapeutic transactions are also needed. Here the role of both the patient's and the therapist's values must be delineated in terms of receptivity or resistance to psychological inquiry, as well as in terms of patterns of communication during therapy. At the same time, attention must also be focused on the contribution of sociocultural factors not only to the pathogenesis and development but also to the perpetuation of psychiatric disorders, which in turn can only help to further clarify phenomena observed during therapy.

More too must be learned about the importance of cultural factors in introducing changes into underdeveloped areas, for the customary symbols and folkways of community life cannot be disrupted in the name of "progress" without deleterious psychological consequences. While promising inroads have already been made along these lines—by a number of studies that have pointed to the effects of hospital *milieu* and social structure on symptomatic behavioral parameters—as well as hospital statistical data—the nature of the specific relationships between the therapeutic *milieu* and improved psychological functioning nevertheless remains to be elucidated, as do the differential responses of patients from varying cultural backgrounds. In view of the growing enthusiasm among the various disciplines for collaborative inquiries into such questions, there is some cause for optimism.[12]

Notes

1. Erwin H. Ackerknecht, "Primitive Medicine's Social Function," Paul Rivers, ed., *Miscellania* (Mexico: 1958).

2. Leo W. Simmons and Harold G. Wolff, *Social Science and Medicine* (New York: Russell Sage Foundation, 1954), p. 177.

3. Jerome D. Frank, *Persuasion and Healing, A Comparative Study of Psychotherapy* (Baltimore: The Johns Hopkins Press, 1961).

4. H. B. M. Murphy, "Social Change and Mental Health," E. Gruenberg, ed., *Causes of Mental Disorders: A Review of Epidemiological Knowledge* (New York: Milbank Memorial Fund, 1961).

5. Lawrence E. Hinkle, Jr., *et al.*, "Studies in Human Ecology," *American Journal of Psychiatry*, 114 (1957), 212-20; and Hinkle, *et al.*, "Hungarian Refugees: Life Experiences and Features Influencing Participation in the Revolution and Subsequent Flight," *American Journal of Psychiatry*, 116 (1959), 16-9.

6. The experiences of China and India, where traditional and modern medical

practices have been integrated to a considerable extent, are of interest in demonstrating how two different systems can function side by side. When the Communist government came to power in China, it encouraged the study, investigation, and use of Chen Chin therapy (acupuncture and cauterization) for rheumatism, malaria, hypertension, tuberculosis, and Parkinsonism. This orientation is reinforced by Pavlov's concept of restoring a disturbed balance between cortical excitation and inhibition by stimulating the peripheral nervous system through the skin. See D. W. James, "Chinese Medicine," *The Lancet*, 1 (1955), 1068-9.

Similarly, in India ancient Ayurvedic medicine, which is believed to rest on embryological, physiological, pathological, and therapeutic conceptions and which serves about 80% of the population, is sometimes practiced by Western-trained physicians. See Morris E. Opler, "The Cultural Definition of Illness in Village India," *Human Organization*, 22 (Spring, 1963), No. 1, 32-5.

7. Edward L. Margetts, *Psychiatry and Mental Health in Africa—Prospects for the Future.* Paper presented at the First Pan-African Psychiatric Conference, Abeokuta, Nigeria, 1961.

8. Anthony F. C. Wallace, *Culture and Personality* (New York: Random House, Inc., 1962).

9. *Ibid.*, p. 193.

10. Michael Shepherd, "Comparative Psychiatric Treatment in Different Countries," D. Richter, J. M. Tanner, Lord Taylor, and O. L. Zangwill, eds., *Aspects of Psychiatric Research* (London: Oxford University Press, 1962), pp. 110-24.

11. Frank, *op. cit.*

12. William Caudill, *The Psychiatric Hospital as a Small Society* (Cambridge, Mass.: Harvard University Press, 1958); M. Greenblatt, R. York, and E. L. Brown, *From Custodial to Therapeutic Patient Care in Mental Hospitals* (New York: Russell Sage Foundation, 1955); Maxwell Jones, *Social Psychiatry* (London: Tavistock Publications, Ltd., 1952); Shepherd, *A Study of the Major Psychoses in an English County* (Maudsley Monograph Series [London: Chapman & Hall, Ltd., 1957]); and A. Stanton and M. Schwartz, *The Mental Hospital* (New York: Basic Books, Inc., 1954).

Index

Index